W.B. Saunders Company   1985

Philadelphia   London   Toronto   Mexico City   Rio de Janeiro   Sydney   Tokyo

SECOND EDITION

IMMUNOLOGY
Basic Processes

Joseph A. Bellanti, M.D.

Professor of Pediatrics and Microbiology
Director, International Center for
    Interdisciplinary Studies of Immunology
Georgetown University School of Medicine
Washington, D.C.

W. B. Saunders Company: West Washington Square
                            Philadelphia, PA   19105

                            1 St. Anne's Road
                            Eastbourne, East Sussex BN21 3UN, England

                            1 Goldthorne Avenue
                            Toronto, Ontario M8Z 5T9, Canada

                            Apartado 26370—Cedro 512
                            Mexico 4, D.F., Mexico

                            Rua Coronel Cabrita, 8
                            Sao Cristovao Caixa Postal 21176
                            Rio de Janeiro, Brazil

                            9 Waltham Street
                            Artarmon, N.S.W. 2064, Australia

                            Ichibancho, Central Bldg., 22-1 Ichibancho
                            Chiyoda-Ku, Tokyo 102, Japan

Library of Congress Cataloging in Publication Data

Bellanti, Joseph A., 1934–

Immunology: Basic Processes

Rev. ed. of: Immunology, basic processes. 1979.

1. Immunology.   I. Bellanti, Joseph A., 1934–
   Immunology, basic processes.   II. Title. [DNLM: 1. Immunity. QW 504 B3115]

QR181.B388 1985   616.07′9   84–3121

ISBN 0–7216–1244–X

Listed here is the latest translated edition of this book together
with the language of the translation and the publisher.

Portuguese (*1st Edition*)—Editora Interamericana Ltda., Rio de Janeiro, Brazil

Cover illustration by Margaret Siner and Jane Hurd

Immunology: Basic Processes   ISBN   0-7216-1244-X

Last digit is the print number: 9   8   7   6   5   4   3   2   1

This edition is dedicated with affection to my parents, my wife Jacqueline, and my children Dawn, Lisa, Jeannine, Loretta, Maria, Joseph (who was born during the First Edition), and little Tony (who was born during the Second Edition) and to my grandchildren Jeannine, Shannan, Mark, and Kristen (who were born during the preparation of the Third Edition).

Contributors

Joseph A. Bellanti, M.D.
Professor of Pediatrics and Microbiology, and Director, International Center for Interdisciplinary Studies of Immunology, Georgetown University School of Medicine, Washington, D.C.
Introduction to Immunology; General Immunobiology; Immunogenetics; Antigen-Antibody Interactions; Cell-Mediated Immune Reactions; A Unifying Model for Immunologic Processes

George M. Bernier, M.D.
Joseph M. Huber Professor and Chairman of Medicine, Dartmouth Medical School; Chairman of Medicine, Dartmouth-Hitchcock Medical Center, Hanover, New Hampshire.
Antibody and Immunoglobulins: Structure and Function

Lynn H. Caporale, Ph.D.
Assistant Professor of Biochemistry, Georgetown University Medical Center, Washington, D.C.
The Complement System

Herbert B. Herscowitz, Ph.D.
Professor of Microbiology, Georgetown University Schools of Medicine and Dentistry, Washington, D.C.
Immunophysiology: Cell Function and Cellular Interactions in Antibody Formation

Anne L. Jackson, Ph.D.
Becton-Dickinson Monoclonal Center, Mountain View, California.
Antigens and Immunogenicity

Josef V. Kadlec, S.J., M.D.
Assistant Professor of Pediatrics and Microbiology, Georgetown University Medical School; Member, International Center for Interdisciplinary Studies of Immunology, Georgetown University Hospital, Washington, D.C.
Introduction to Immunology; General Immunobiology

Paul Katz, M.D.
Associate Professor of Medicine, and Director, Division of Rheumatology, Immunology, and Allergy, Georgetown University School of Medicine; Attending Physician, Georgetown University Hospital, Washington, D.C.
Immunomodulation: Immunopotentiation, Tolerance, and Immunosuppression

Steven L. Kunkel, Ph.D.
Assistant Professor, Department of Pathology, University of Michigan Medical School, Ann Arbor, Michigan.
The Complement System

Ross E. Rocklin, M.D.
Professor of Medicine, Tufts University School of Medicine; Chief, Allergy Division, New England Medical Center, Boston, Massachusetts.
Cell-Mediated Immune Reactions

Kenneth W. Sell, M.D., Ph.D.
Clinical Professor of Pediatrics, Georgetown University School of Medicine, Washington, D.C.; Scientific Director, National Institute of Allergy and Infectious Diseases, National Institutes of Health, Bethesda, Maryland.
Immunogenetics

Carl-Wilhelm Vogel, M.D.
Assistant Professor of Biochemistry and Medicine; Member, International Center for Interdisciplinary Studies of Immunology, and Vincent T. Lombardi Cancer Center, Georgetown University Schools of Medicine and Dentistry, Washington, D.C.
The Complement System

Peter A. Ward, M.D.
Professor and Chairman, Department of Pathology, University of Michigan Medical School, Ann Arbor, Michigan.
The Complement System

James N. Woody, Capt., MC., U.S.N., M.D., Ph.D.
Professor of Pediatrics and Microbiology, Georgetown University School of Medicine, Washington, D.C.; Director, Transplantation Research Program Center, Naval Medical Research Institute, Bethesda, Maryland.
Immunogenetics

Chester M. Zmijewski, Ph.D.
Associate Professor, Department of Pathology and Laboratory Medicine; Associate Director, Department of Pathology and Laboratory Medicine; Director, Immunology, University of Pennsylvania, Philadelphia, Pennsylvania.
Antigen-Antibody Interactions

Preface

The Second Edition of *Immunology: Basic Processes* comprises the first of three sections of a larger book entitled *Immunology III,* which, in addition to the fundamental principles, discusses mechanisms and clinical applications. *Immunology: Basic Processes* is directed to undergraduate, predoctoral, nursing, and medical technology students as well as to any readers wishing a contemporary overview of the elementary concepts of immunology.

All chapters have been completely updated and revised. New sections have been added to Chapters 3 (Immunogenetics), 6 (Complement Activity), 7 (Immunophysiology: Cell Function and Cellular Interactions), and 10 (Immunomodulation: Immunopotentiation, Tolerance, and Immunosuppression). These changes reflect our increasing awareness of the genetic diversity of antibody and immunoglobulins as well as the use of monoclonal antibodies to identify new antigenic and cell surface receptors.

Many persons have contributed to the preparation of the Second Edition, and I wish to express my indebtedness to them. First, I would like to thank Dr. Philip L. Calcagno, who has been most generous and gracious in his support and encouragement of this endeavor. I would like to express my sincere appreciation to Miss Jane Hurd and Miss Margaret Siner for the continued development of imaginative figures that illustrate the concepts of the chapters of this book so vividly. Others who have read sections of the manuscript or who have made helpful suggestions include the following: Mrs. Barbara Zeligs, Dr. Lata Nerurkar, Dr. Anne Morris Hooke, Dr. Daniel Sordelli, Dr. Cristina Cerquetti, Dr. Robert M. Chanock, Dr. Robert H. Purcell, Dr. John Gerin, Dr. Anthony Fauci, Dr. Lawrence D. Frenkel, Dr. John Dwyer, and Dr. David M. Asher.

Particular appreciation is owing to a special friend who stayed at my side throughout the revision of the book and who made this oftentimes tedious task a joy with his uplifting spirit and steadfast and gentle determination as the book progressed through its many drafts, illustrations, and galley and page proofs. Father Josef Kadlec, priest, physician, ethicist, microbiologist, immunologist, and friend: Thank you for persevering with me in this endeavor.

My appreciation is also extended to my other colleagues at Georgetown and to my clinical and research fellows and house staff, who have contributed to my intellectual life and to the life of the Immunology Center. I owe a special debt of gratitude to students of all ages for whom the book is written. Learning represents a joy of discovery shared by the student and the teacher, and it is in this spirit that the book is written. It is a product of conversations that I have had with every student I have met. It is the questions they ask in the lecture hall, in the laboratory, in the clinic, and at the bedside that have provided me with the incentive to write. Although many individuals have contributed information to this text, I alone assume responsibility for any errors found within these pages.

I wish also to thank Diane Hargrave Goldstein for her diligent typing of the entire manuscript.

Finally, I wish to express my thanks and appreciation to Mr. Albert Meier, to Ms. Constance Burton, and to Mr. Frank Polizzano and other colleagues at W. B. Saunders Company for their patience, support, suggestions, and inspiration during the lengthy preparation of this revision.

JOSEPH A. BELLANTI

Contents

Chapter 1

Introduction to Immunology

Joseph A. Bellanti, M.D., and Josef V. Kadlec, S.J., M.D.

HISTORICAL BACKGROUND

The concepts of immunology are ancient and pragmatic and are derived primarily from the study of resistance to infection. It was known for centuries before the discovery of the germ theory of infectious disease that recovery from illness was accompanied by the ability to resist reinfection. Thus, the elements of classical immunology preceded bacteriology and contributed to it. In more recent years, contributions to immunology have come from both the basic sciences, e.g., biochemistry, anatomy, developmental biology, genetics, pharmacology, and pathology, as well as from the study of clinical entities, e.g., allergy, infectious diseases, organ transplantation, rheumatology, immune deficiency diseases, and oncology. These fields, in turn, have been enhanced by the application of immunologic principles. Shown in Figure 1–1 is a schematic representation of some major milestones important in the development of immunology.

Preceding modern medicine, Chinese physicians in the eleventh century observed that the inhalation of smallpox crusts prevented the subsequent occurrence of the disease. Later, the technique of variolation, the intradermal application of powdered scabs, was used in the Middle East, where its primary intent was esthetic—"preserving the beauty of their daughters." This primitive immunization reached England in the eighteenth century through Pylarini and Timoni and was later popularized by Lady Mary Wortley Montagu (Fig. 1–2). Wide variations in vaccination procedures, however, occasionally led to death, which prevented the full acceptance of this form of therapy.

The future of modern immunobiology was assured when Edward Jenner (Fig. 1–3), as a medical student, made the surprisingly sophisticated discovery that inoculation with cowpox crusts protected humans from smallpox. This important finding resulted from Jenner's observation that milkmaids who had contracted cowpox were resistant to infection with smallpox.

The enhancement and further development of preventive immunization were made possible by Louis Pasteur (Fig. 1–4), who coined the term "vaccine" (from *vacca*: L., cow) in honor of Jenner's contribution. Pasteur's researches led to the development of the germ theory of disease, from which he developed techniques for the *in vitro* cultivation of microorganisms. This work produced material that could now be used for vaccines: living, heat-killed, and attenuated (living but with reduced virulence). During these investigations, Pasteur observed that old cultures (attenuated) of fowl cholera organisms when inoculated into fowl produced no disease. Surprisingly, these fowl were resistant to subsequent infection with the organism and were

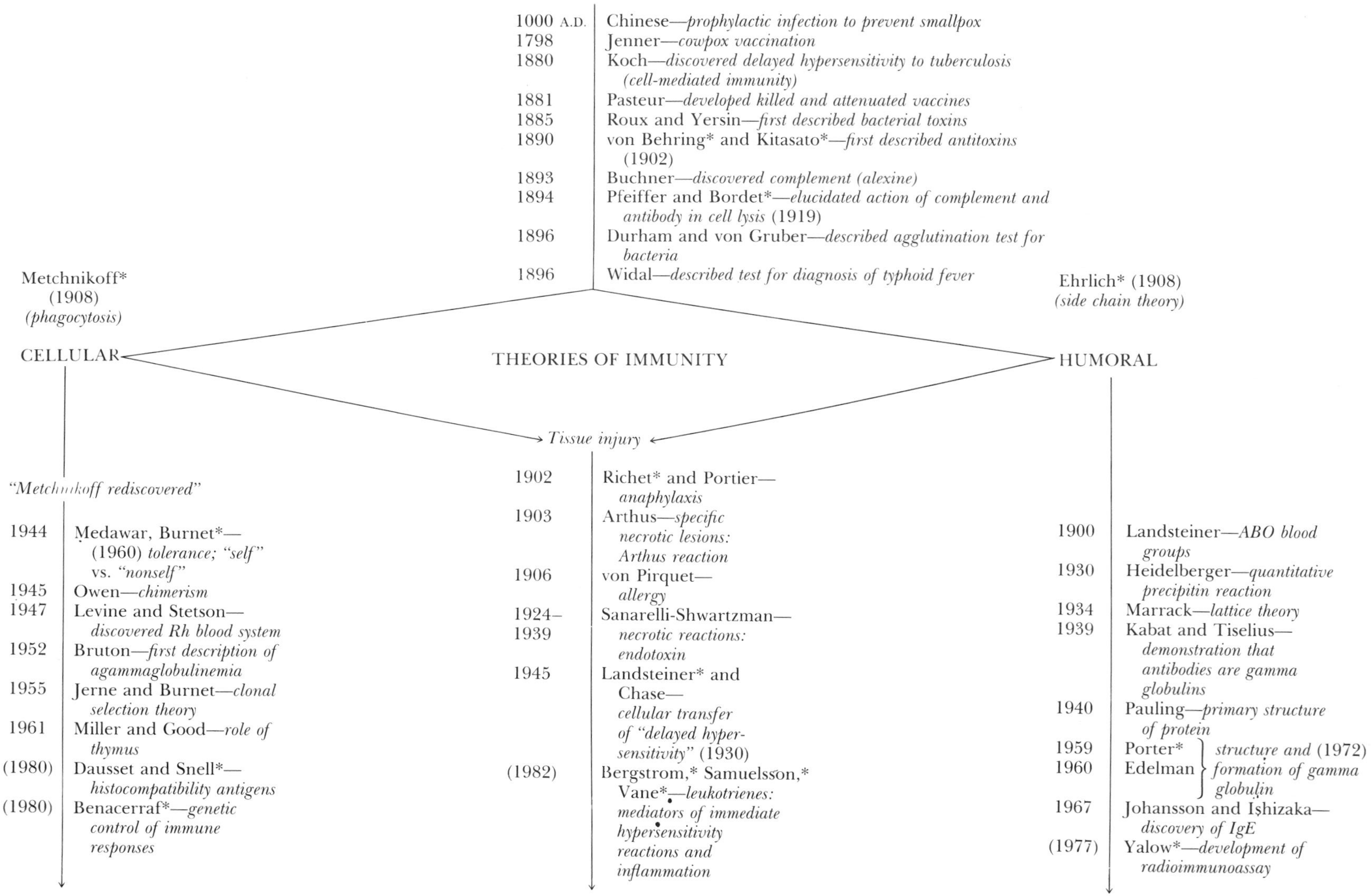

THEORIES OF IMMUNITY

Ehrlich* (1908) (side chain theory)

Metchnikoff* (1908) (phagocytosis)

Tissue injury →

HUMORAL

1000 A.D.	Chinese—prophylactic infection to prevent smallpox
1798	Jenner—cowpox vaccination
1880	Koch—discovered delayed hypersensitivity to tuberculosis (cell-mediated immunity)
1881	Pasteur—developed killed and attenuated vaccines
1885	Roux and Yersin—first described bacterial toxins
1890	von Behring* and Kitasato*—first described antitoxins (1902)
1893	Buchner—discovered complement (alexine)
1894	Pfeiffer and Bordet*—elucidated action of complement and antibody in cell lysis (1919)
1896	Durham and von Gruber—described agglutination test for bacteria
1896	Widal—described test for diagnosis of typhoid fever

1900	Landsteiner—ABO blood groups
1930	Heidelberger—quantitative precipitin reaction
1934	Marrack—lattice theory
1939	Kabat and Tiselius—demonstration that antibodies are gamma globulins
1940	Pauling—primary structure of protein
1959	Porter*— } structure and (1972) formation of gamma globulin
1960	Edelman*—
1967	Johansson and Ishizaka—discovery of IgE
(1977)	Yalow*—development of radioimmunoassay

1902	Richet* and Portier—anaphylaxis
1903	Arthus—specific necrotic lesions: Arthus reaction
1906	von Pirquet—allergy
1924–1939	Sanarelli-Shwartzman—necrotic reactions: endotoxin
1945	Landsteiner* and Chase—cellular transfer of "delayed hypersensitivity" (1930)
(1982)	Bergstrom,* Samuelsson,* Vane*—leukotrienes: mediators of immediate hypersensitivity reactions and inflammation

CELLULAR

"Metchnikoff rediscovered"

1944	Medawar, Burnet*—(1960) tolerance; "self" vs. "nonself"
1945	Owen—chimerism
1947	Levine and Stetson—discovered Rh blood system
1952	Bruton—first description of agammaglobulinemia
1955	Jerne and Burnet—clonal selection theory
1961	Miller and Good—role of thymus
(1980)	Dausset and Snell*—histocompatibility antigens
(1980)	Benacerraf*—genetic control of immune responses

Nobel Prize winners in immunology are indicated by an asterisk,* and the date of award is shown in parentheses.

Figure 1–1. Major milestones in immunology.

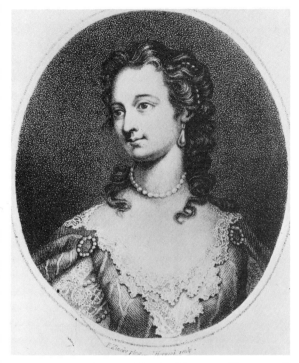

Figure 1–2. Lady Mary Wortley Montagu. (Courtesy of National Library of Medicine.)

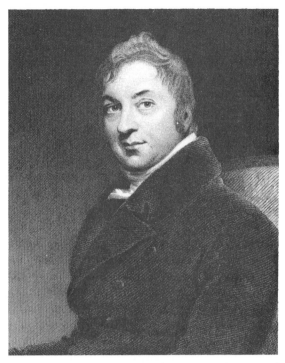

Figure 1–3. Edward Jenner (1749–1823). (Courtesy of National Library of Medicine.)

solidly immune. This use of living, attenuated, or heat-killed cultures is still our therapy of choice in the prophylaxis of many infectious diseases (Fig. 1–5), a process referred to as *active immunization.*

Later, Robert Koch (Fig. 1–6) discovered the tubercle bacillus during his studies of the bacterial etiology of infectious diseases. While attempting to develop a vaccine for tuberculosis, he observed the phenomenon known today as delayed hypersensitivity or cell-mediated immunity (Chapter 9).

Following the isolation of the diphtheria bacillus, Roux and Yersin demonstrated the existence of a potent soluble exotoxin elaborated by this organism (Fig. 1–7). This toxin was used by von Behring (Fig. 1–8) and Kitasato to inoculate animals that produced in their serum a toxin-neutralizing substance called *antitoxin.* This neutralizing capability

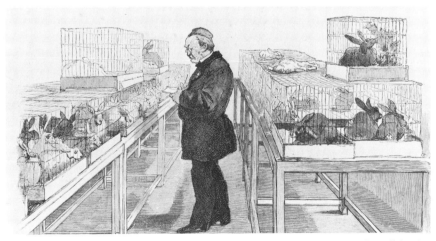

Figure 1–4. Louis Pasteur (1822–1895). (Courtesy of National Library of Medicine.)

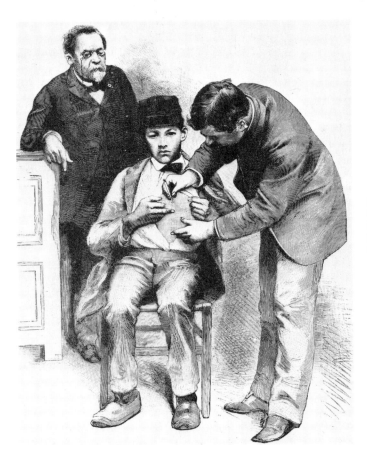

Figure 1–5. Louis Pasteur, to left, watches as an assistant inoculates a boy for "hydrophobia" (rabies). (Wood engraving in "L'Illustration" from Harper's Weekly *29*:836, 1885; courtesy of National Library of Medicine.)

could be transferred by the serum to uninoculated animals, a process called *passive immunization.* Their work formed a model for the modern techniques of preventing disease through passive immunization (immunotherapy). Pfeiffer and Bordet's work differentiated a substance in serum, distinct from antibody, called *complement* that also participates in the destruction of bacteria. The observations of Durham and von Gruber that serum could clump or agglutinate bacteria formed the basis for tests for the diagnosis of infectious specific agglutination reactions, such as the test described by Widal for the diagnosis of typhoid fever (Widal test).

Up to the turn of the century, the French and German schools dominated these areas of immunologic research. At that time there emerged two divergent vantage points from which immunology was observed and later developed: (1) the *humoral,* whose emphasis was the study of chemical products (i.e., antibodies) elaborated by cells, and (2) the *cellular,* whose emphasis was the biologic effects of intact cells involved in the host's response to foreignness (see Fig. 1–1). Paul Ehrlich

(Fig. 1–9) proposed the humoral theory of antibody formation, and Elie Metchnikoff (Fig. 1–10) almost simultaneously developed the cellular theory of immunity. Both were correct, since in the individual both cellular and humoral factors are intimately interwoven and interdependent.

Ehrlich's side-chain theory proposed the pre-existence of receptors on the living cell surface that reacted with toxins; the excess receptors eventually could be released into the circulation as antibody (Fig. 1–11). It is ironic that one of the major areas of immunologic research today is the study of receptors on immunocompetent cells (Chapter 7). Subsequently, the major emphasis in immunology was directed at the identification, characterization, and biologic function of humoral factors (see Fig. 1–1).

Metchnikoff's theories of cellular immunity held that the body's scavenger cells, the phagocytes, were the prime detectors of foreign material as well as its primary defense system. His concepts went unrecognized for several decades but today represent an area of intensive immunologic research. Both cel-

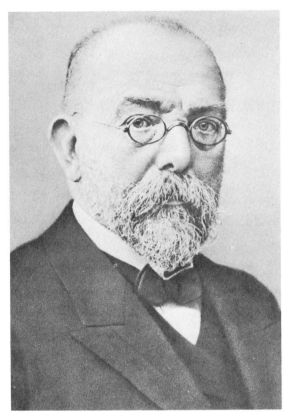

Figure 1–6. Robert Koch (1843–1910). (Courtesy of National Library of Medicine.)

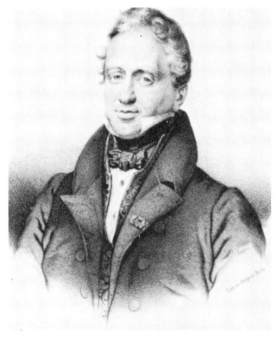

Figure 1–7. Pierre Paul Emile Roux (1853–1933). (Courtesy of National Library of Medicine.)

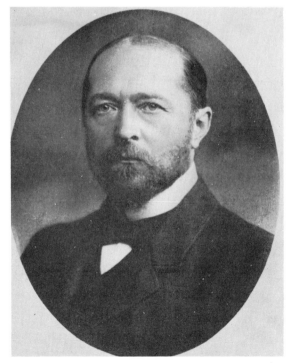

Figure 1–8. Emil Adolf von Behring (1854–1917). (Courtesy of National Library of Medicine.)

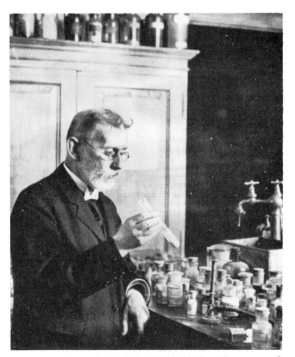

Figure 1–9. Paul Ehrlich (1854–1915). (Courtesy of National Library of Medicine.)

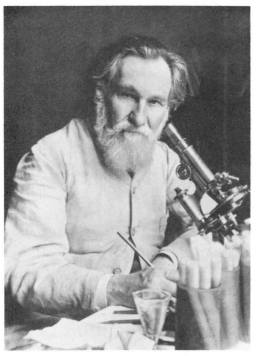

Figure 1–10. Elie Metchnikoff (1845–1916). (Courtesy of National Library of Medicine.)

lular and humoral factors are involved in understanding the principles underlying the immunologic processes that result in protection or tissue injury.

Today, there still remain two schools of immunologic investigation. The humoral school reached its peak with the discovery and characterization of the protein molecules that contain antibody activity, the *immunoglobulins* (Chapter 5). This work has culminated in the elucidation of the total amino acid sequence of almost all antibody molecules. At the same time, the cellular area is now being actively investigated from the standpoint of protection against infectious agents and graft rejection as well as immunity to tumors in man. The cellular-humoral dichotomy is also illustrated by the clinical observations of increased susceptibility to infection seen in individuals with congenital defects of the immunologic system. Some lack the humoral protective function but retain the cellular; others are deficient in cellular but have normal humoral activity; still others are defective in both humoral and cellular functions. Clearly, both areas are of pro-

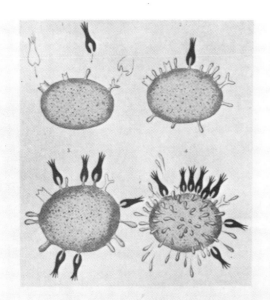

Figure 1–11. Diagrammatic representation of the side-chain theory, showing the presence of pre-existing receptors on the cell surface *(A)*, which when produced in excess *(B)* could be released as antibody. (From Croonian Lecture, "On Immunity with Special Reference to Cell Life," Proc. R. Soc. Lond. (Biol.), *66*:424, 1906; courtesy of National Library of Medicine.)

Illustration continues on opposite page

DIAGRAMMATIC REPRESENTATION OF THE SIDE-CHAIN THEORY
(PLATES I AND II)

Fig. 1   "The groups [the haptophore group of the side-chain of the cell and that of the food-stuff or the toxin] must be adapted to one another, *e.g.*, as male and female screw (PASTEUR), or as lock and key (E. FISCHER)."

Fig. 2   ". . . the first stage in the toxic action must be regarded as being the union of the toxin by means of its haptophore group to a special side-chain of the cell protoplasm."

Fig. 3   "The side-chain involved, so long as the union lasts, cannot exercise its normal, physiological, nutritive function . . ."

Fig. 4   "We are therefore now concerned with a defect which, according to the principles so ably worked out by . . . Weigert, is . . . [overcorrected] by regeneration."

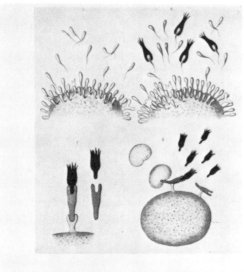

DIAGRAMMATIC REPRESENTATION OF THE SIDE-CHAIN THEORY
(cont.)

Fig. 5 ". . . the antitoxins represent nothing more than the side-chains, reproduced in excess during regeneration and therefore pushed off from the protoplasm—thus coming to exist in a free state."

Fig. 6 [The free side-chains (circulating antitoxins) unite with the toxins and thus protect the cell.]

Fig. 7 ". . . two haptophore groups must be ascribed to the 'immune-body' [haemolytic amboceptor], one having a strong affinity for a corresponding haptophore group of the red blood corpuscles, . . . and another . . . which . . . becomes united with the 'complement' . . ."

Fig. 8 "If a cell . . . has, with the assistance of an appropriate side-chain, fixed to itself a giant [protein] molecule . . . there is provided [only] one of the conditions essential for the cell nourishment. Such . . . molecules . . . are not available until . . . they have been split into smaller fragments. This will be . . . attained if . . . the 'tentacle' . . . possesses . . . a second haptophore group adapted to take to itself ferment-like material . . ."

Figure 1–11. *Continued.*

found importance to man. Although one or the other aspect will be stressed at times throughout this book, cellular and humoral factors of immunity are interrelated and interdependent.

Immunity and Hypersensitivity

The term *immune* is derived from the Latin *immunis* (free from taxes or free from burden). In classical usage, immunity referred to the relative resistance of the host to rein-

fection by a given microbe. It is now evident that immune responses are not always beneficial, nor are they associated solely with resistance to infection. On the contrary, they can even confer unpleasant and harmful effects on the host. The noxious effect has been called *hypersensitivity* or *allergy*. Listed in Figure 1–1 are some of the pioneers who contributed to this field of tissue injury. The immunologic system is equipped not only to perform a *defense* function against infectious agents but also to concern itself with the more diverse biologic functions of *homeostasis* and *surveillance* (Table 1–1).

At the turn of the century, von Pirquet put forward a hypothesis to explain the multifaceted aspects of the immune response. He coined the term "allergy" to mean "altered reactivity" of the host; one change was recognized as immunity, and the other as hypersensitivity. Von Pirquet made no distinction between beneficial and harmful responses and suggested that they were all manifestations of a common biologic process of sensitization, which he encompassed by the term "allergy". He restricted the use of the term "immunity" to mean protection from infectious agents and the term "allergy" for a more generalized reactivity of the host to foreign substances. Over the years, allergy and immunity have become reversed in their meanings; immunity has come to mean that which von Pirquet defined originally as allergy, and allergy has come to mean hypersensitivity. Nevertheless, von Pirquet's concepts of the broad scope of the immune response are now accepted in immunology.

IMMUNOLOGY IN THE MODERN SENSE

A contemporary definition of immunity would include "all those physiologic mecha-

Table 1–1. **Functions of the Immune System**

Function	Nature of Immunologic Stimulus	Example	Aberrations Hyper-	Hypo-
Defense	Exogenous	Microorganisms	Allergy	Immunologic deficiency disorders
Homeostasis	Endogenous or exogenous	Removal of effete and damaged cells	Autoimmune disease	—
Surveillance	Endogenous or exogenous	Removal of cell mutants	—	Malignant disease

nisms that endow the animal with the capacity to recognize materials as foreign to itself and to neutralize, eliminate, or metabolize them with or without injury to its own tissues." The responses of immunity may be classified into two categories: (1) *nonspecific* immunologic responses and (2) *specific* immunologic responses. Specific immune responses depend upon exposure to a foreign configuration and the subsequent recognition of and reaction to it. Nonspecific responses, on the other hand, occur following initial and subsequent exposure to a foreign configuration, and while selective in differentiating "self" from "nonself," they are not dependent upon specific recognition.

In the modern view, immunologic responses serve three functions—defense, homeostasis, and surveillance (see Table 1–1). The first is involved in resistance to infection by microorganisms, the second in removal of worn-out (effete) "self" components, and the third in perception and destruction of mutant cells.

The first function, defense against invasion by microorganisms, has occupied the thinking of immunologists for more than 100 years. If the cellular elements of defense are deployed successfully, the host will emerge victorious in the struggle with microorganisms. However, when these elements are *hyperactive,* certain undesirable features, such as allergy or hypersensitivity, may be seen. Conversely, when these elements are *hypoactive,* there may be an increased susceptibility to repeated infections, as seen in the immunologic deficiency disorders.

The second function, homeostasis, fulfills the universal requirement of all multicellular organisms to preserve uniformity of a given cell type. It concerns itself with normal degradative or catabolic functions of the body charged with the removal of damaged cellular elements, such as circulating erythrocytes or leukocytes. These may be damaged during the course of a normal life span or may arise as a consequence of injury. Aberrations of homeostasis are exemplified by the autoimmune diseases, in which these mechanisms are unduly enhanced.

The third function of the immune system is the most recently recognized and concerns itself with surveillance. This function monitors the recognition of abnormal cell types, which constantly arise within the body. These mutants may occur spontaneously or may be induced by certain viruses and chemicals. The immune system is charged with the recognition and disposal of newly acquired configurations, most of which occur on cell surfaces. Failure of this mechanism has recently been assigned a causal role in the development of malignant disease. Since it is becoming increasingly apparent that all three functions are under genetic control (Chapter 3), an understanding of the pathogenesis of many immunologically mediated diseases must take into account these genetic principles.

Modifying Factors

There are a number of factors that modify immune mechanisms: genetic, age, metabolic, environmental, anatomic, physiologic, and microbial (Table 1–2). The host immune mechanisms may be viewed *in toto* as a composite protective umbrella consisting of various components that shield the host from the injurious effects of noxious environmental agents (Fig. 1–12). Defects may be seen in any one facet, e.g., phagocyte dysfunction, or in all facets, e.g., malnutrition.

Genetic Factors. The whole of the immune response is under genetic control (Chapter

Table 1–2. **Elements Involved in Immunologic Processes**

Modifying Factors	Type of Response	Type of Encounter	Examples
Genetic Age Metabolic Environmental and nutritional Anatomic Physiologic Microbial	Nonspecific immunity	All	Phagocytosis, inflammatory response, cellular immunity, fever, acute phase phenomena (CRP, sedimentation rate)
	Specific immunity	Initial and subsequent	Humoral, cell-mediated immunity (delayed hypersensitivity)

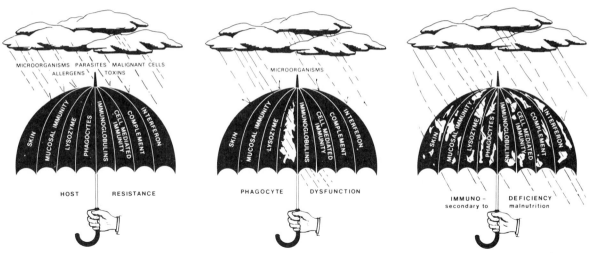

Figure 1–12. Host protective factors and examples of primary and secondary immunodeficiency. A concert of nonspecific barriers and antigen-specific immune responses protect man from extraneous and internal injurious agents *(left panel)*. Primary, often inherited, deficit of a protective mechanism, for example, phagocyte defect, results in repeated infections *(center panel)*. Malnutrition robs the host of many host defenses *(right panel)*. Some bulwarks of immunity are impaired more often and to a greater extent than others. (From Chandra, R. K.: Malnutrition and immunocompetence: An overview. *In* Bellanti, J. A. (ed.): Acute Diarrhea: Its Nutritional Consequences in Children. New York, Raven Press, 1983. Reproduced with permission of the publisher.)

3). For example, certain strains of guinea pigs are capable of responding to a given antigen (responders), whereas others are not (nonresponders). In addition, there are genetic differences in susceptibility to infection that may have similar bases. Strains of rabbits have been bred, one susceptible, the other resistant, to infection with *Mycobacterium tuberculosis*. In man, moreover, there are racial differences in susceptibility to tuberculosis. One of the exciting recent developments in immunology has been the identification of a genetic complex (i.e., the major histocompatibility complex [MHC]) that controls both immune responsiveness and the expression of histocompatibility antigens on cells (Chapter 3). The identification of these genetic markers is finding clinical application in the diagnosis and treatment of many diseases whose pathogenesis has been unclear in the past, e.g., ankylosing spondylitis and lymphomas.

Age Factors. Chronologic age influences immunity, and direct evidence is accumulating that a hypofunctional state of the immune system occurs in the very young and the very old. For example, these two age groups are uniquely susceptible to the ravages of infection. Generalized sepsis due to *Escherichia coli* is not an uncommon event in the newborn period. Presumably, this is the result of a number of factors, including an incompletely developed specific immune system and deficiencies of nonspecific immunity, such as a thin integument and a poor inflammatory response. Similarly, fatal pneumonia due to *Streptococcus (Diplococcus) pneumoniae* and influenza is a common event during old age. Underlying cardiac, pulmonary, and metabolic derangements (e.g., diabetes mellitus) as well as a primary hypofunction of the immune system predispose this group to infection with these pathogens. This provides the rationale for immunization of this group with pneumococcal and influenza vaccines. Also, the decrease in many of the immunologic functions, such as immunoglobulin concentrations and cell-mediated immunity, in the elderly may be associated with the known higher incidence of autoimmune phenomena and malignancy in this age group.

Metabolic Factors. In addition to the well-recognized susceptibility of the patient with uncompensated diabetes mellitus to bacterial infection, certain hormones have been shown to affect the host immune response. In both hypoadrenal and hypothyroid states there is an increased susceptibility to infection. Moreover, patients treated with steroids are unduly susceptible to bacterial diseases (e.g., staphylococcal infection) as well as to certain viral diseases (e.g., varicella). Steroids appear to affect many modalities of the immune response, having an inhibitory effect on phagocytosis and inflammation as well as on humoral and cellular immunity (Chapter 10).

Environmental and Nutritional Factors. The increased rate of infectious diseases due to poor living conditions is well known. An increased rate of infection may be related to a greater exposure to pathogens as well as to diminished resistance caused by malnutrition. In studies conducted in children in the developing countries, nutritional deprivation at an early age has been shown to be associated with developmental failure of the immune response, predominantly the cell-mediated immune response which presents as recurrent infections, particularly respiratory and gastrointestinal. Recently, a new acquired immune deficiency syndrome (AIDS) has been described in homosexual males and other groups, which has been associated with recurrent opportunistic infections and malignancy. Although at present the precise cause of the syndrome as well as its therapy is unknown, the most plausible etiology is a transmissible agent (e.g., a variant of human T-cell leukemia virus family, HTLV-III) that may be destroying the immune system, particularly its cell-mediated component. The occurrence of the syndrome also points to the contribution of other factors, e.g., lifestyle, environment, intravenous drug use, and transfusions. The solution of these complex problems will require the broader consideration of many factors, e.g., social, economic, and political as well as medical.

Anatomic Factors. The first line of defense against invasion by microbes is usually provided by the *skin* and the *mucous membranes.* These tissues act in nonspecific immunity by providing a physical barrier to invasion. The intact skin appears to be a more effective barrier than the mucous membranes. The increased susceptibility to infections following burns or secondary to eczema is a well-known clinical finding. The skin and the mucous membranes may allow penetration by certain pathogens, e.g., the tubercle bacillus, which can pass across the intact gastrointestinal mucosa after ingestion, leading to local infection and regional lymph node enlargement.

Microbial Factors. Following colonization of the body surfaces, both internal and external, a "normal" flora develops. Not only is this flora essential for the production of metabolites, e.g., vitamin K, but it also contributes to the production of "natural" antibodies to these organisms. The flora also acts to suppress the overgrowth and the subsequent infection by pathogenic and possibly virulent organisms. The well-recognized overgrowth of virulent staphylococci in patients treated with so-called broad-spectrum antibiotics illustrates the effect of a disturbed ecologic microbial balance in man.

Physiologic Factors. The gastric juice is an unfavorable milieu for many pathogenic strains of bacteria, which are destroyed in the stomach following ingestion. Some bacteria, such as the typhoid bacilli, are not affected, survive digestion, and produce disease. Ciliary action in the respiratory tract is another important physiologic mechanism of resistance. Normal urine flow clears bacteria from the urinary tract, preventing infection. It is well known that the obstructed urinary tract or respiratory tract (e.g., cystic fibrosis) is more susceptible to infection, probably owing to the absence of this clearing action.

Certain skin secretions of normal individuals have been shown to be bactericidal. This is believed to be due in part to the acidity of the skin produced by *lactic acid.* After puberty the skin appears more resistant to infection with certain fungi (dermatophytes). This may result from an increase in saturated fatty acids in the skin. In postpubertal skin, there are also increased amounts of unsaturated fatty acids known to be bactericidal.

Lysozyme is an enzyme that has been shown to have bactericidal activity. The enzyme is found in many types of cells and body fluids and functions by virtue of mucolytic properties that cleave acetylamino-sugars, the backbone of both gram-positive and gram-negative bacteria. Certain basic polypeptides (with large amounts of lysine) have been shown to kill anthrax. There are other chemical substances in the body that kill, injure, or inhibit bacteria and viruses.

The blood contains a number of protective substances that act in a nonspecific manner. Bactericidal substances in blood have been demonstrated that do not appear to be specific antibody, since they are present without prior exposure to a foreign configuration. These have been called *natural antibodies.* Their precise origin is not known, and, indeed, the concept of preformed antibodies has been a subject of controversy. One explanation is that these antibodies are stimulated following exposure to closely related materials. It is known, for example, that isohemagglutinins—the antibody to blood groups—(Chapter 3) may develop as a result of exposure to enteric bacilli containing blood group—like substances in their structure.

Another set of protective functions are derived from the complement system, a cascading group of serum proteins with biologic functions (Chapter 6). Deficiency of a number of the complement components may be associated with a variety of clinical disorders, including recurrent infection, edema, or autoimmune diseases.

Still another set of protective functions are provided by tissue mucoproteins with viricidal activity, which prevent attachment of certain viruses to host cells. A family of proteins, the *interferons,* originally thought to inhibit viral replication by protection of host cells, are now known to have much broader cellular effects and are receiving increasing attention in the autoimmune diseases and malignancy.

Nonspecific Immune Responses: Inflammation and Phagocytosis

The first encounter of the host with a foreign configuration leads to a stereotyped response that consists of mobilization of phagocytic elements into areas where the foreign configuration has been introduced (Table 1–2). This may occur as an isolated event or as part of the inflammatory response.

Inflammation. Following any one of a variety of tissue injuries, a spectrum of cellular and systemic events occur in which the host attempts to restore and maintain homeostasis under the adverse environmental influences. This reaction is referred to as inflammation. Accompanying the inflammatory response are a number of systemic events that involve fever as well as a series of hematologic phenomena. The febrile response is believed to reflect enhanced metabolic activity following injury. One mechanism is believed to be the release of endogenous pyrogen from host leukocytes. An increased leukocyte count occurs during bacterial infections or tissue injury. Tissue necrosis, for example, with myocardial infarction, is associated with a "left shift," i.e., a predominance of polymorphonuclear leukocytes with many young forms, e.g., bands. In general, bacterial products cause more tissue injury than do viruses and induce the greatest febrile response.

Increased blood fibrinogen, activation of the Hageman factor, and increased fibrinolytic activity and erythrocyte rouleaux formation are each associated with one of the most useful indices of the acute-phase response—the erythrocyte sedimentation rate (ESR). This parameter is affected by any factor causing erythrocyte rouleaux formation, such as increased gamma globulin, e.g., multiple myeloma. A rapid sedimentation rate is most commonly associated, however, with a raised fibrinogen level.

Other changes in serum globulins occur during illness, such as an increase in the alpha and beta globulins. One of these, the C-reactive protein (CRP), is elevated in the early phases of many illnesses. It was originally discovered by virtue of its interaction with the C, or carbohydrate, substance of *Streptococcus (Diplococcus) pneumoniae,* but it is now recognized that CRP is released from many types of tissues following injury.

Phagocytosis. Once mobilized, the phagocytic cells mount an attack on their target by a process called phagocytosis (cell-eating), a multiphasic act requiring the following steps: recognition of the material to be ingested, movement toward the object (chemotaxis), attachment, ingestion, and subsequent intracellular digestion by a number of antimicrobial mechanisms (Chapter 2). A series of complex biochemical reactions occur involving utilization of certain humoral factors (e.g., opsonins) as well as complement, a maze of interacting serum proteins which, when triggered, lead to the generation of a number of products active in each of these functions (Chapter 6). Knowledge of these steps has assumed great clinical importance with the recent discovery that there occur in the human inborn errors of leukocyte function. This family of neutrophil dysfunction syndromes may involve deficiencies in complement, antibody, or intracellular enzymes concerned with antimicrobial activity.

Specific Immune Responses

Definitions. The specific immune responses are concerned with the recognition and ultimate disposal of foreignness in a highly discriminatory fashion. The final outcome of the encounter between host and a foreign configuration is dependent upon the properties of the substance (size, structure, chemical nature, amount) and also upon properties of the host (age, genetic constitution) (Fig. 1–13). The foreign material may interact with the host in a number of ways. It may become localized or completely removed nonspecifically by phagocytes, e.g., inert carbon particles, without any further response. It may also lead to a specific immune response in which the material is referred to as an *immunogen* or *antigen* (Chapter 4). On the other hand, after interaction with the host the material may induce a state of unresponsiveness, in which case it is referred to as a *tolerogen*. The resulting condition, *immunologic tolerance*, will be considered in Chapter 10.

General Characteristics of the Specific Immune Response. The *specific immune response* is the reaction of the host to a foreign substance and encompasses a series of cellular interactions expressed by the elaboration of specific cell products. There are three general characteristics of the specific immune response that distinguish it from the nonspecific responses: (1) *specificity*, (2) *heterogeneity*, and (3) *memory*.

Specificity is the highly discriminatory selectivity by which the products of the immune response will react solely with the configuration identical or similar to that which initiated the response. Landsteiner first demonstrated specificity and showed that antibody could distinguish closely related substances; it is this property of the specific immune response that distinguishes one antigen from another. Operationally, the immune response can distinguish and differentiate antigens originating from different species *(species specificity)*, from different individuals *(individual specificity)*, or from different organs *(organ specificity)*.

The second characteristic of the specific immune response is heterogeneity, in which a vast array of cell types and cell products are induced to interact with a diversity of response commensurate with the variety of cell types. The heterogeneity of cell types gives rise to the elaboration of an equally heterogeneous population of cell products, e.g., antibody. This heterogeneity of antibody contributes a fine degree of homeostatic control with which the host can respond in a highly variable and specific manner to foreign structures.

The third hallmark of the specific immune response is memory. Memory is the property that results in an accelerated and augmented specific response through proliferation and differentiation of sensitized cells upon subsequent exposure to an immunogen. This leads to an enhanced elaboration of cell products.

Nonspecific responses, on the other hand, represent the initial encounter with foreignness, and upon subsequent encounter merely repeat the same general response to the substance. Unlike the specific responses, the nonspecific responses include a limited number of pre-existent cell types. The specific responses are characterized by the induction and interaction of a variety of new cell types specific for the inducing antigen. The nonspecific immune responses do not include the property of memory.

Specific Immune Responses: Humoral and Cell-Mediated

There are two types of effector mechanisms that mediate specific immune responses (Fig. 1–14): (1) those mediated by a cell product of the lymphoid tissues referred to as antibody *(humoral immunity)* and (2) those mediated by specifically sensitized lymphocytes themselves *(cell-mediated immunity)*.

Following an immunogenic stimulus a series of cellular events occur prior to the expression of the *specific immune response*. For ease of discussion, we may divide these events into two general areas: (1) the *afferent limb*, in which there takes place the processing of the immunogen by macrophages and cellular interactions between lymphocytes and macrophages culminating in the activation of lymphocytes, and (2) the *efferent limb*, in which the specifically activated lymphocytes proliferate and differentiate in the expression of specific humoral and cell-mediated immunity. These events are described in detail in Chapter 7.

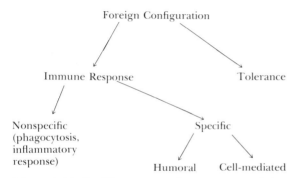

Figure 1–13. Possible outcome of an encounter of the host with a foreign configuration.

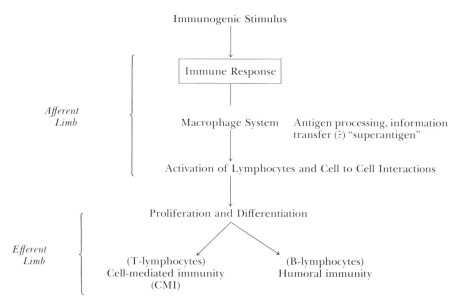

Figure 1–14. Effector mechanisms that mediate specific immunologic responses.

Humoral Immunity. Humoral immunity is mediated by a group of lymphocytes that differentiate in bone marrow and are referred to as bone marrow–derived or B-lymphocytes. Antibody is a product of B-cell elements (B-lymphocytes and plasma cells) and is either cell-bound or secreted as an extracellular product. It has the capability of reacting with the configuration responsible for its production (immunogen or antigen) (Chapter 4). In the human, antibody is associated with five major classes of proteins (immunoglobulins) that can be differentiated from one another on the basis of size, biologic function, or biochemical properties (Chapter 5). The presence of antibody is determined by measuring some functional parameter of the interaction between antigen and antibody (Chapter 8). For example, some antibodies can neutralize the effect of a toxin (antitoxin), others can punch holes in cell membranes (cytolytic antibodies), and still others are measured *in vivo* by eliciting a hypersensitive reaction (anaphylactic antibody) such as the IgE. It is believed that the humoral effector mechanism is derived embryologically in the chicken from the bursa of Fabricius. In the human, the location of this tissue is not known with certainty, but it is nevertheless referred to on occasion as the gut-associated lymphoid tissue (GALT).

Other Humoral Factors: Biologic Amplification Systems. Immunologic reactions may also involve other humoral factors that can augment or amplify the response without the direct participation of cells. The best known example is the complement system, in which a variety of factors, both cell-bound and soluble, come into play and set the stage for protective mechanisms and, in some cases, detrimental events. Most complement factors act by triggering the inflammatory response. Under certain conditions this leads to the removal of infective agents; however, under other conditions the result is tissue damage. The complement system will be described in detail in a later section (Chapter 6).

The kallikrein system is yet another component of the amplification system and represents a well-defined system of proteins in plasma, activated by a reaction of antigen with antibody. Presumably through the activation of the Hageman factor and the permeability factor of Miles, the enzyme kallikrein interacts with its substrate, an alpha-2-macroglobulin, to produce different vasoactive peptides, e.g., the bradykinins. Another humoral factor, slow-reacting substance (SRS-A), is a humoral factor liberated by the interaction of antigen with sensitized cells and has recently been identified as one of the arachidonic acid metabolites, i.e., leukotriene. All these agents increase capillary permeability.

Certain proteins of the coagulation sequence also may act to amplify the immune response during the interaction of antigen with antibody. Increase in the rapidity of clotting in plasma following such interaction has been attributed to activation of the Hageman factor, although an earlier step in the coagulation sequence may be directly activated by an antigen-antibody complex. Finally, there is some evidence that the fibrinolytic system may be activated in plasma by the antigen-antibody interaction, but the precise mechanism for the conversion of plasminogen to plasmin is unknown.

Cell-Mediated Immunity. Cell-mediated immunity is the second major type of effector mechanism underlying specific immune responses (see Fig. 1–13). This is mediated by a group of lymphocytes that differentiate under the influence of the thymus and are therefore referred to as T-lymphocytes. This effector arm of specific immunity is carried out directly by specifically sensitized lymphocytes or by specific cell products that are formed upon interaction of immunogen with specifically sensitized lymphocytes. These specific cell products, the lymphokines, include migration inhibitory factor (MIF), cytotoxin, interferon, and several others and are believed to be the effector molecules of cellular immunity (Chapter 9).

CONCEPT OF IMMUNOLOGIC BALANCE

In order to understand immunologically mediated disease, the immunologic system may be viewed as a dynamic multicompartmental network of elements with ever-changing morphologic components and functions (Chapter 11). It should be kept in mind that much of the work in experimental immunology has been performed with nonreplicating antigens. Normally, many immunologic stimuli are self-replicating, such as bacteria, viruses, and organ transplants. Thus, data obtained in the laboratory may not be directly applicable to natural phenomena occurring in humans. A second point is that not all configurations confronting the host are immunogenic, i.e., lead to a specific immune response. Some substances are taken up by phagocytic cells and may be completely degraded before they can lead to a specific immune response.

As with all physiologic mechanisms, the immunologic response may be viewed as an adaptive system in which the body attempts to maintain homeostasis between the internal body environment and the external environment.

Following confrontation of the host with a foreign configuration (stimulus) there is a period of disequilibrium. Immunologic balance is restored by the appropriate immunologic response. A pertubation occurs if the stimulus and the response are inappropriate for each other. Any derangement in homeostasis results in the production of undesirable sequelae referred to as immunologic imbalance. The clinical appearance of immunologic imbalance is manifested as immunologically mediated disease.

Overwhelming sepsis is an example of a situation in which the amount of replicating antigen exceeds the capacity of lymphoreticular tissue response. Immunologic unresponsiveness or paralysis may also occur when the host is confronted with antigen in a form not easily catabolized, e.g., the pneumococcal polysaccharide. The net result is referred to as high-zone paralysis (Chapter 10). This may be the mechanism by which the host maintains nonreactivity to its own bodily constituents, i.e., "self-tolerance."

The converse is also seen and occurs when too little antigen leads to an immunologic imbalance. This is known as low-dose tolerance. The clinical counterpart of low-dose interaction is perhaps best exemplified by the interaction of certain microorganisms with the host. Certain fungi, e.g., dermatophytes, can establish a type of infection in which insufficient replication occurs to stimulate the immunologic apparatus. Consequently, these organisms live in peaceful coexistence with the host, usually at body surfaces, and persist in this relationship for many years. Disordered homeostasis due to the magnitude or type of antigen is at present a subject of intense interest in relation to organ transplantation and maternal-fetal interactions.

The second major cause of immunologic imbalance is related to aberrancy of cells of the immunologic system, e.g., immune deficiency disorders or products of the immune response. There may be a failure to produce sufficient numbers of effector cells or cell products, or they may be functionally defective in type. Failure may be genetic (e.g., congenital agammaglobulinemia) and may be controlled by certain loci in the major histocompatibility complex (MHC), e.g., immune response (Ir) locus, which specifies the synthesis of certain cell surface antigens that control cellular interactions. Failure also may be acquired, e.g., acquired immune deficiency syndrome (AIDS). The recent discovery of subpopulations of T-cells that regulate the immune response, e.g., T-helper and T-suppressor cells, and imbalance in ratios in certain disease states further exemplify the importance of an understanding of the host's immunologic system in balance. The net result is immunologic imbalance, recurrent infections, and a predisposition to malignant tumors and autoimmune disease. These aberrations also occur as a consequence of acquired cases of immunosuppression, e.g., chemical immunosuppressive agents.

Aberrations may involve the production of cell products. There may be overproduction of a product normally present in trace amounts. An example of this is the allergic individual who produces too much IgE immunoglobulin and manifests immediate-type hypersensitivity. Qualitative aberrations may also occur with natural infection; for example, following streptococcal tonsillitis, antigen-antibody complexes may be produced that damage the kidney (acute glomerulonephritis). Lastly, these aberrations may be produced iatrogenically as a complication of vaccines. Certain vaccines may produce hypersensitivity rather than protective immunity.

Suggestions for Further Reading

History of Immunology

Bulloch, W.: The History of Bacteriology. London, Oxford University Press, 1938.

Burnet, F. M.: Cellular Immunology. Cambridge, Melbourne University Press, 1969.

Edsall, G.: What is immunology? J. Immunol., *67*:167, 1951.

Ehrlich, P.: On immunity with special reference to cell life. Proc. Soc. Lond. (Biol). *66*:424, 1906.

Grabar, P.: The historical background of immunology. *In* Stites, D. P., Stobo, J. D., Fudenberg, H. H., et al. (eds.): Basic and Clinical Immunology. 4th ed. Los Altos, Lange Medical Publications, 1982.

Marx, J. L.: Strong new candidate for AIDS agent. Science *224*:475, 1984.

Metchnikoff, E.: Immunity in Infective Diseases. London, Cambridge University Press, 1905.

Immunology in the Modern Sense

Bellanti, J. A., and Dayton, D. H.: The Phagocytic Cell in Host Resistance. New York, Raven Press, 1975.

Chandra, R. K.: Malnutrition and immunocompetence: An overview. *In* Bellanti, J. A. (ed.): Acute Diarrhea: Its Nutritional Consequences in Children. New York, Raven Press, 1983.

Davis, B. D., Dulbecco, R., Eisen, H. N., et al.: Immunology. *In* Davis, B. D., et al. (eds.): Microbiology. New York, Harper & Row, 1973.

Gell, P. G. H., Coombs, R. R. A., and Lachman, P. T.: Clinical Aspects of Immunology. Oxford, Blackwell Scientific Publications, 1975.

Humphrey, J. H., and White, R. G.: Immunology for Students of Medicine. Philadelphia, F. A. Davis, 1970.

Kabat, E. A.: Structural Concepts in Immunology and Immunochemistry. New York, Holt, Rinehart and Winston, 1975.

Roitt, I. M.: Essential Immunology. Oxford, Blackwell Scientific Publications, 1974.

Rose, N. R., Milgrom, F., and van Oss, C. J.: Fundamentals of Immunology. New York, Macmillan Publishing Company, 1973.

Sell, S.: Immunology, Immunopathology and Immunity. Hagerstown, Md., Harper & Row, 1975.

Samuelsson, B.: Leukotrienes: Mediators of immediate hypersensitivity reactions and inflammation. Science, *220*:568, 1983.

Stites, D. P., Stobo, J. D., Fudenberg, H. H., et al. (eds.): Basic and Clinical Immunology. 4th ed. Los Altos, Lange Medical Publications, 1982.

Chapter 2

General Immunobiology

Joseph A. Bellanti, M.D., and Josef V. Kadlec, S.J., M.D.

ANATOMIC ORGANIZATION OF THE IMMUNE SYSTEM

Cell Types and Effector Mechanisms Involved in Nonspecific Immune Mechanisms

In order to carry out the functions of immunity, a ubiquitous immunologic cell system has appeared within the vertebrates: the *lymphoreticular system*. This collection of cellular elements is distributed strategically throughout the tissues as well as lining lymphatic and vascular channels. Its cells are housed within the *blood, tissues, thymus, lymph nodes,* and *spleen* (internal secretory system), and in those body tracts exposed to the external environment—the *respiratory, gastrointestinal,* and *genitourinary* systems (external secretory system) (Fig. 2–1).

The tissues contain a variety of cell types, each performing a separate function either directly or through the elaboration of a cell product(s). The system may be activated by a variety of stimuli that have the common characteristic of being recognized as foreign by the host. The stimuli may be presented to the host either exogenously (e.g., microorganisms) or endogenously (e.g., effete cells or transformed neoplastic cells).

Following activation, a spectrum of cellular and humoral events occurs that constitutes the nonspecific and specific immune responses (Chapter 1). The nonspecific immune responses consist of phagocytosis and the inflammatory response; if the stimulus leads to the production of specific cell products (e.g., antibody, lymphokines) by specialized groups of lymphocytes, the foreign configurations are referred to as immunogens or antigens (Chapter 4). A number of effec-tor mechanisms involving several cell types, cell products, and soluble serum factors may be called into play by the host following the encounter and recognition of a foreign configuration (Table 2–1). The cellular constituents include *mononuclear phagocytes, granulocytes, platelets,* and *lymphocytes.* The origins of these cells are pluripotential hematopoietic stem cells located within the bone marrow, fetal liver, and yolk sac of the fetus. The cell types, differentiation, and tissue localization of these cells are shown in Table 2–2. For ease of discussion, these cells will be grouped into a functional classification according to the following categories: *phagocytic cells, mediator cells,* and *lymphocytes.*

PHAGOCYTIC CELLS

The process of phagocytosis is part of the nonspecific immune response (Chapter 1) and represents the host's initial encounter with foreignness. Endocytosis is a more general term and includes both *phagocytosis* (ingestion of particles) and *pinocytosis* (uptake of nonparticulates, e.g., fluid droplets). Both represent the process of engulfment and uptake of particles or fluid from the environment, and those groups of specialized cells that carry out these functions are commonly referred to as phagocytic cells. In some cases, subsequent digestion of these materials into smaller fragments facilitates their elimination (Fig. 2–2). In the human, phagocytosis is carried out primarily by *mononuclear phagocytes, neutrophils,* and, to a lesser extent, *eosinophils.*

Mononuclear Phagocytes. The mononuclear phagocyte system (MPS) consists of a generalized group of cells that are widely distributed throughout the body where they can effectively eliminate foreign materials and debris from the blood, lymph, and tis-

ORGANIZATION OF THE IMMUNE SYSTEM
(lymphoreticular tissues)

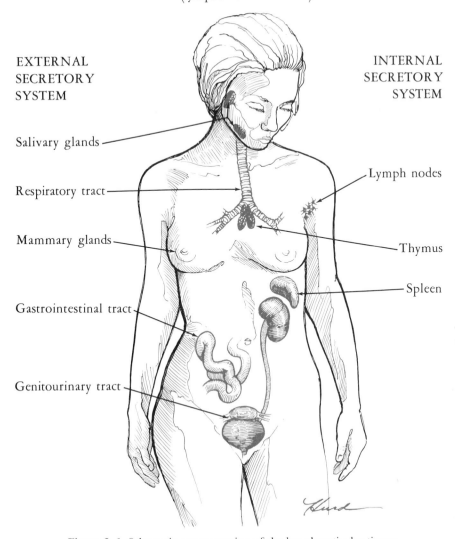

Figure 2–1. Schematic representation of the lymphoreticular tissues.

Table 2–1. Cell Types and Effector Mechanisms Triggered by or Involved in Immune Reactions

| Cell Type | Humoral Factors | |
	Agents Responsible for Mobilization of Cells	Cell Product
Nonspecific		
Mononuclear phago-cytes	Chemotactic factors, macrophage activat-ing factor (MAF)	Processed immunogen
Granulocytes		
Neutrophils	Chemotactic factors (complement-associ-ated and bacterial factors) lymphocyte-derived	Kallikreins (producing kinins). SRS-A, basic peptides
Eosinophils	Specific chemotactic factors (e.g., ECF-A), and other chemotactic factors as for neutrophils	Histaminase, aryl sulfatase, phospholipase D, eosinophil-derived inhibitor (EDI)
Basophils	?	Vasoactive amines
Platelets	Factors producing platelet aggregates (thrombin, collagen)	Vasoactive amines
Specific		
B-lymphocytes	Antigen	Antibody
T-lymphocytes	Antigen	Lymphokines, e.g., MIF, interferon, cyto-toxin, "transfer factor," and others

Table 2–2. Differentiation and Localization of Cells Involved in Immune Processes*

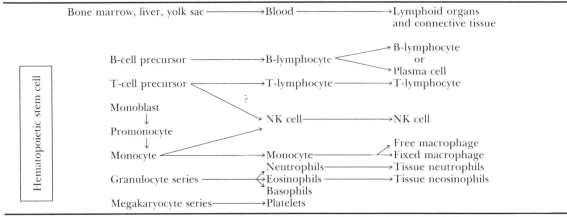

Bone marrow, liver, yolk sac ——————→Blood ——————————→Lymphoid organs
and connective tissue

Hematopoietic stem cell			
	B-cell precursor ——————→	B-lymphocyte	B-lymphocyte or Plasma cell
	T-cell precursor ←	T-lymphocyte ——————	T-lymphocyte
	Monoblast ↓ Promonocyte ↓ Monocyte ←	NK cell ——————	NK cell
		Monocyte ————	Free macrophage Fixed macrophage
	Granulocyte series ————	Neutrophils ———— Eosinophils ———— Basophils	Tissue neutrophils Tissue neosinophils
	Megakaryocyte series————	Platelets	

*(Adapted from van Furth, R.: Mononuclear Phagocytes in Immunity, Infection and Pathology. Oxford, Blackwell Scientific Publications, 1975.)

sues. The term MPS has been suggested to replace the less precise term reticuloendothelial system (RES), which was coined by Aschoff to define those morphologic elements of the immune system that are phagocytic as determined by clearance of particles (Fig. 2–3). The mononuclear phagocytes include both monocytes of the circulating blood (Fig. 2–4) and macrophages found in various tissues of the body.

The mononuclear phagocytes are produced from a stem cell in the bone marrow. Here they undergo proliferation and are delivered to the blood after a period of maturation through a *monoblast → promonocyte → monocyte* phase. Following a brief time in the blood (approximately one to two days), the monocytes migrate to the main site of their action in the tissues where they differentiate further into macrophages. Here they can divide, thus differing from granulocytes. The blood monocyte serves as an intermediate cell in the monocyte-macrophage transition.

The transition of monocyte to macrophage is also accompanied by morphologic, biochemical, and functional changes. During

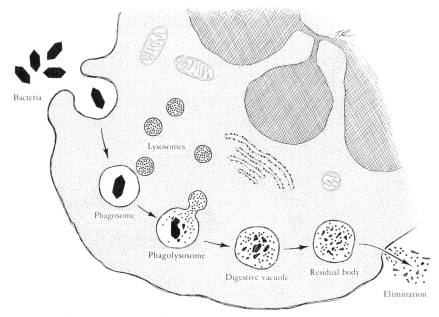

Figure 2–2. Schematic representation of phagocytosis showing ingestion process and intracellular digestion.

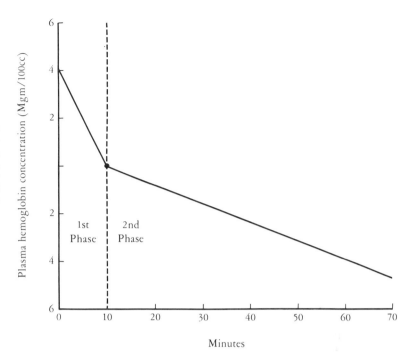

Figure 2–3. Plasma hemoglobin clearance in a group of 40 apparently healthy human subjects. (After Gabrieli, E. R., and Snell, F. M.: Reflection of reticuloendothelial function in studies of blood clearance kinetics. J. Reticuloendothel. Soc., 2:141, 1965.)

differentiation, the cell enlarges in size and in the number and complexity of intracellular organelles (e.g., Golgi apparatus, mitochondria, lysosomes, and lipid droplets). In addition, during maturation, the cell increases in the content of lysosomal enzymes, such as acid phosphatase, beta-glucuronidase, cathepsin, lysozyme, and aryl sulfatase, as well as related mitochondrial enzymes, e.g., cytochrome oxidase. The energy sources for the cells of the MPS are dependent upon the degree of cellular maturity, the level of endocytic activity, and the environment. With the notable exception of the alveolar macrophage, which derives its energy primarily from aerobic metabolism, all other cells of the MPS derive their energy for particle uptake through the glycolytic pathway.

The macrophages are highly specialized to carry out their function in the ingestion and destruction of all particulate matter by the process of endocytosis. These cells remove and destroy certain bacteria, damaged or effete cells, neoplastic cells, colloidal materials, and macromolecules. The phagocytic process is sometimes facilitated by antibody, since particles coated with antibody are ingested more efficiently; complement, a series of sequentially reacting serum proteins, may also be involved as an amplifier of phagocytosis (Chapters 5 and 6). The term *opsonin* is used to describe this phagocytic-enhancing principle of both antibody and complement.

The circulating monocytes are attracted to an area of injury (chemotaxis) by a number of factors, some of which are derived from the complement system or secreted by the T-lymphocytes (Table 2–1). Here they may further differentiate into macrophages and may be activated in a variety of ways—either following endocytosis or through humoral substances, including antibody, complement, or products of lymphocytes (lymphokines) (Chapter 9). Once activated, the cells assume heightened metabolic activity (activated macrophages) and display enhancement of function, e.g., microbicidal activity. Some workers believe that, in addition to a role in defense and surveillance, the macrophage system is important in the initial recognition and processing of antigen, steps that may be necessary for the induction of specific immunologic responses (Chapter 7).

Neutrophils or Polymorphonuclear Leukocytes. In the human the circulating granulocytes comprise three varieties of morphologically identifiable cells that are involved in a number of immunologic reactions in tissue; these include the neutrophil, the eosinophil, and the basophil (Table 2–1). Of these three, only the neutrophil and, to a lesser extent, the eosinophil are primarily phagocytic.

Neutrophils or polymorphonuclear (PMN) leukocytes (Fig. 2–5) normally account for 60 to 70 per cent of the total leukocyte count in

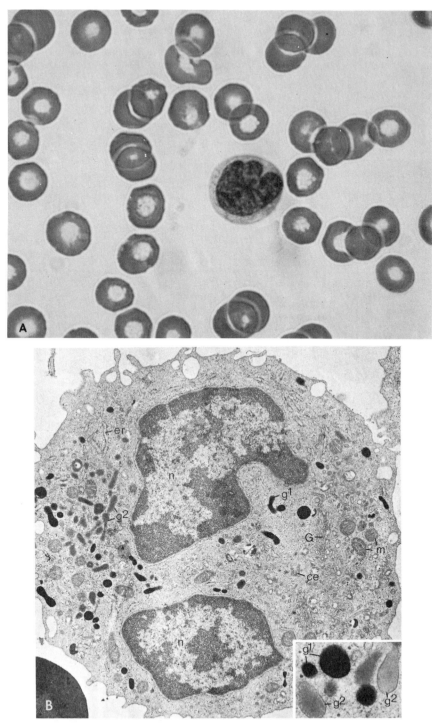

Figure 2–4. Monocyte from peripheral blood. *A,* Light micrograph, Wright-Giemsa stain, × 1400. Note the lobulated nucleus. (Courtesy of Dr. Theodore I. Malinin.) *B,* Electron micrograph, × 16,200 examined for peroxidase. Note the presence of two types of granules (g¹), peroxidase-positive and (g²) peroxidase-negative; the endoplasmic reticulum (er); Golgi complex (G); the mitochondria (m); the centriole (ce); and the nucleus (n). (From Bainton, D. F.: *In* Dingle, J. T. (ed.): Lysosomes in Biology and Pathology. Vol. 5. New York, North-Holland, 1976.)

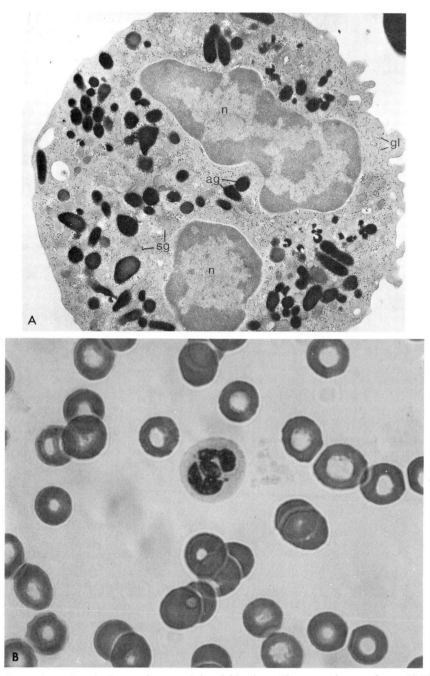

Figure 2–5. Polymorphonuclear leukocyte from peripheral blood. *A,* Electron micrograph, × 13,500, showing a lobulated nucleus (n) and cytoplasmic granules reacted for peroxidase. Note the presence of two types of granules: the peroxidase-positive azurophilic (ag) and the peroxidase-negative specific granules (sg); and the glycogen particles (gl) that are dispersed throughout the cytoplasm. (From Bainton, D. F.: *In* Dingle, J. T. (ed.): Lysosomes in Biology and Pathology. Vol. 5. New York, North-Holland, 1976.) *B,* Light micrograph, Wright-Giemsa stain, × 1400, showing fully segmented nucleus. (Courtesy of Dr. Theodore I. Malinin.)

the peripheral blood of the adult human. Unlike the macrophage, the neutrophil is an end cell of myeloid differentiation and does not divide. The neutrophils arise in the bone marrow from a common ancestral stem cell and, after a series of divisions, undergo a maturation through various stages—myeloblast → promyelocyte → metamyelocyte → band cell → mature PMN. Unlike the situation with the monocyte-macrophage series, however, there appears to be a large storage compartment in the bone marrow that can be called upon as needed to replenish cells in the circulation. After a short period in the blood (about 12 hours), the PMN's enter the tissues, where they complete their life span of a few days. Normally, there is no return of these cells from the tissues back to the blood. Some of the cells in the vascular pool do not circulate freely, presumably because they are temporarily sequestered in small blood vessels or adhere to the walls of larger vessels (marginal pool).

With maturation of the cells, there is a sequential appearance of two distinct classes of granules: the primary (azurophilic) and the secondary or specific granules (Fig. 2–5). The primary granules are electron-dense structures approximately 0.4 micron (μ) in diameter that appear early in maturation and have many features in common with lysosomes of other tissues. They contain myeloperoxidase, arginine-rich basic (cationic) proteins, sulfated mucopolysaccharides, acid phosphatase, and several other acid hydrolases. The secondary or specific granules are not truly lysosomes; they are smaller (about 0.3 μ in diameter) and are less dense than the primary granules. They are rich in alkaline phosphatase, lysozyme, and aminopeptidase. In the intermediate stage of neutrophil maturation, both populations of granules are seen. As maturation proceeds, however, the secondary granules increase in number and appear to predominate. Both types of granules are important in the breakdown of ingested material and in the killing of microorganisms. Granulocyte production and release appear to be under the control of cellular and humoral factors.

The Eosinophils. The eosinophilic granulocytes make up 1 to 3 per cent of the circulating blood leukocytes and are distinguished by large cytoplasmic granules that stain intensely red with eosin (Fig. 2–6). They share many features with the neutrophil, arise from a common progenitor cell, and display a similar morphogenesis. In contrast to the neutrophil, however, the eosinophils mature in the bone marrow in three to six days before release into the circulation, following which they circulate with a half-life of approximately 30 minutes. The eosinophils have a half-life of 12 days in tissues, where they fulfill their major function. Like the neutrophil, the eosinophils do not return from tissues to the circulation but are eliminated through the mucosal surfaces of the respiratory and gastrointestinal tracts. With maturation of these cells, there occurs a transition from primary (azurophilic) granules to large cytoplasmic granules, which have a crystalloid substructure (Fig. 2–6). The granules of the eosinophil do not contain lysozyme and phagocytin as found in PMN's. They are rich in acid phosphatase and peroxidase activity. In addition, the eosinophil granule contains in its crystalline core a unique protein, the eosinophilic basic protein (EBP), of approximately 11,000 daltons, found to be toxic to certain parasites (e.g., *Schistosoma*), as well as to normal host cells (e.g., tracheal epithelium). Although the cells have the capacity to phagocytose a variety of particles, including microorganisms and soluble antigen-antibody complexes, the process appears to be less efficient than with neutrophils. In spite of its well-known association with allergic and parasitic diseases, the specific role of the eosinophil is not known with certainty. Major roles postulated include the ingestion of immune complexes and their involvement in limiting inflammatory reactions, presumably by antagonizing the effects of certain mediators. For example, aryl sulfatase B from eosinophils has been shown to inactivate SRS-A released by mediator cells. Furthermore, the eosinophil has been implicated directly as a putative cell of tissue injury, possibly through the release of its toxic components, e.g., EBP. The eosinophils have been found to participate in antibody-mediated cytotoxicity reactions of importance in the clearance of certain parasitic organisms, e.g., *Schistosoma*. The regulation of eosinophils involves a complex set of mechanisms, including products of T-lymphocytes, complement components, mast cell products (e.g., ECF-A) as well as a variety of arachidonic acid metabolites (e.g., HETE's). As a general rule, eosinophilia is more common in atopic diseases in which increased levels of IgE are found than in other immunologically mediated disorders.

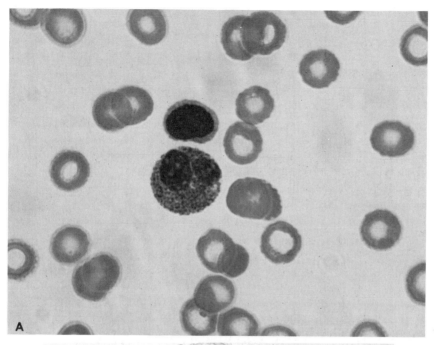

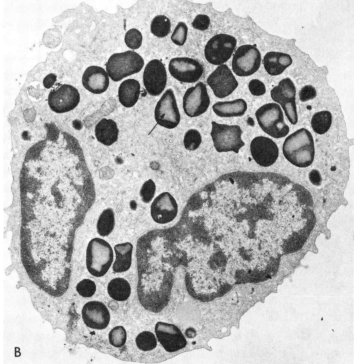

Figure 2–6. *A,* Eosinophilic leukocyte and a small lymphocyte from peripheral blood. Light micrograph, Wright-Giemsa stain, × 1400. (Courtesy of Dr. Theodore I. Malinin.) Note the bilobed nucleus and the prominent granules of the eosinophil. *B,* Electron micrograph of a human eosinophil from normal bone marrow, × 33,000, reacted for peroxidase. Note the presence of large granules that have a predominance of peroxidase staining filling the granule contents except for the area occupied by the crystalline core *(arrow).* (From Bainton, D. F.: *In* Dingle, J. T. (ed.): Lysosomes in Biology and Pathology. Vol. 5. New York, North-Holland, 1976.)

MEDIATOR CELLS

Certain cells of the body also participate in immunologic reactions through the release of chemical substances (mediators) that have a variety of biologic activities, including increased vascular permeability, contraction of smooth muscle, and enhancement of the inflammatory response. These cells are referred to as mediator cells and constitute a heterogeneous collection of morphologic types, including *mast cells, basophils, platelets, enterochromaffin* cells, and certain of the phagocytic cells, e.g., neutrophils.

Basophilic granulocytes (Fig. 2–7), which make up only 0.5 per cent of the blood leukocytes, and the platelets, the non-nucleated hemostatic elements of the blood, are the two major mediator cells in the circulation. They have been shown to contain a variety of vasoactive amines, such as histamine and serotonin. The basophils are distinguished by their large purple or blue-black granules that ultrastructurally are electron-dense and homogeneous and that, when mature, show a characteristic banded pattern. These granules contain acid mucopolysaccharides (e.g., heparin), which are responsible for the tinctorial phenomenon of metachromasia. Little is known of their production, distribution, or life span. Although they resemble the mast cells morphologically, they differ in several respects.

The basophil and mast cell are important sources of mediators, e.g., histamine, which are involved in immediate hypersensitivity. The elaboration of these agents is thought to be triggered by contact of these cells with antigen-antibody complexes through complement-dependent or complement-independent mechanisms. The release of these mediators can occur by direct impact of an environmental agent (e.g., compound 48/80) or indirectly through the interaction of antigen with membrane-bound IgE. The release appears to be mediated by cyclic 3',5'-adenosine monophosphate (cyclic AMP) (Chapter 7). Substances that increase cyclic AMP lead to a decrease in the release of mediators; substances that decrease intracellular levels of cyclic AMP lead to an increased release. These vasoactive amines appear to be involved in tissue injury. Following interaction of antigen with antibody in tissues such as the renal glomerulus, for example, there is a release of these substances that results in permeability changes that lead to accelerated deposition of circulating soluble antigen-antibody complexes. The release of histamine and serotonin therefore appears to be involved in an immunologic cascade, in which there may be amplification of injury mediated by antigen-antibody complexes. Findings of this nature may have important clinical implications. In animals undergoing experimental forms of immunologic injury (serum sickness), treatment with antihistamines or serotonin antagonists leads to a protection of the animals from immune complex-induced type nephritis.

Chemotaxis, Phagocytosis, and Metabolic Changes and Antimicrobial Systems of Phagocytic Cells

The primary role of the phagocytic cells in the body economy is the localization and removal of foreign substances, such as microorganisms. Several integrated functions may be required to achieve these goals. First, the cells must reach the site of the foreign configuration (chemotaxis). They must then ingest the foreign substance (phagocytosis). Finally, after a series of metabolic steps, they must destroy the foreign substance or inhibit the replication of the microorganism (microbial killing).

CHEMOTAXIS

There are three phenomena involved in cell movements: *motility, locomotion,* and *chemotaxis*. Motility refers to a cell that moves; locomotion refers to movement from one place to another; and chemotaxis refers to unidirectional locomotion toward an increasing gradient of attractant (chemoattractant). A phagocytic cell adherent to glass, for example, can be a highly motile cell but may not be exhibiting locomotion or chemotaxis. A cell that is undergoing random locomotion may not be exhibiting chemotaxis. There are a variety of *in vivo* and *in vitro* techniques for measurement of locomotion and chemotaxis.

The polymorphonuclear leukocyte responds to at least three different chemotactic

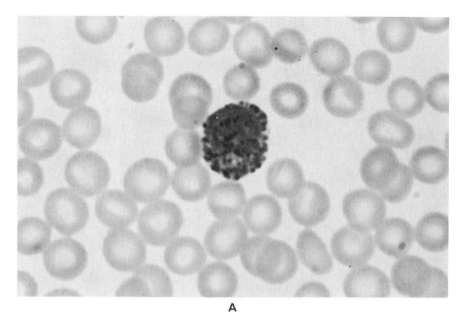

A

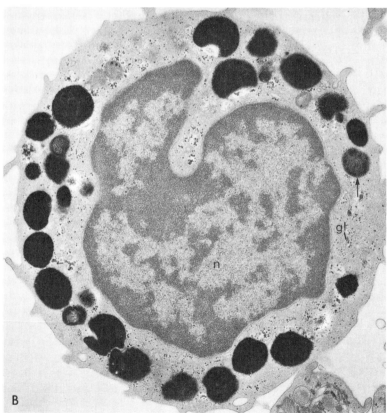

B

Figure 2–7. Basophilic leukocyte from peripheral blood. *A*, Light micrograph, Wright-Giemsa stain, × 1400, showing large granules in the cytoplasm. *B*, Electron micrograph, × 14,800, reacted for peroxidase. Note the unusually large nucleus (n), scattered glycogen particles (gl), and peroxidase-positive granules, some of which may appear speckled (*arrow*). (From Bainton, D. F.: *In* Dingle, J. T. (ed.): Lysosomes in Biology and Pathology. Vol. 5. New York, North-Holland, 1976.)

stimuli derived from the complement system, as well as bacterial and lymphocyte-derived factors (Table 2–1). The neutrophils also are directly or indirectly involved in the production of a substance known as slow-reactive substance (SRS-A), now identified as leukotrienes C_4, D_4, and E_4, humoral factors capable of causing the contraction of smooth muscle. Other factors produced by the granulocyte include the kinins, small polypeptides that are vasoactive. These substances are important pharmacologic mediators of immediate hypersensitivity reactions.

A number of substances chemotactic for monocytes and macrophages have also been described (Table 2–1). These include products of the complement system as well as of the lymphocyte series, e.g., macrophage-activating factor (MAF). Moreover, a substance that is inhibitory for chemotaxis of monocytes has been described in extracts of tumor tissues.

There are a number of substances that are chemotactic for eosinophils that are similar to those for neutrophils. These include antigen-antibody complexes; complement-derived chemotactic factors; products of the lymphocyte series, e.g., lymphokines; and an eosinophilic chemotactic factor of anaphylaxis (ECF-A), a substance released from tissue mast cells and peripheral basophils that may be very important in the pathogenesis of immediate-type hypersensitivity reactions. ECF-A has also been shown to be released from PMN leukocytes.

PHAGOCYTOSIS

The next step in the sequence is phagocytosis, the process by which a particle is ingested by a cell. This process can be divided into two steps: the *attachment phase* and the *ingestion phase*.

During the attachment phase, firm contact is established with the particle. This can occur between the particle and phagocyte directly through unenhanced processes, in which case it is largely dependent upon surface properties of the particle to be phagocytosed, e.g., hydrophobicity and surface tension. In other cases, attachment involves the participation of two types of receptors on the plasma membrane of the phagocyte: (1) a receptor for the Fc fragment of an immunoglobulin molecule; and (2) a receptor for the C3b, a

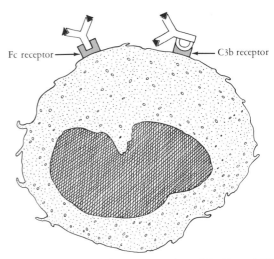

Fc receptor ⟶   ⟵ C3b receptor

Figure 2–8. Schematic representation of the Fc and C3b receptors.

component of complement. These are shown schematically in Figure 2–8.

Many bacteria that are unencapsulated are rapidly taken up by phagocytes and destroyed. Encapsulated strains such as the pneumococcus, however, are taken up poorly and hence not destroyed. This resistance to engulfment is related to the protective capsule of the bacterium and ensures its survival within the host. When certain serum proteins, e.g., complement or antibodies (opsonins), are present, the attachment of the coated bacterium is facilitated by the surface receptors and the phagocytic uptake is enhanced.

The ingestion process is the next step of phagocytosis and represents the engulfment of the particle. The phagocyte invaginates its plasma membrane and the particle is then taken up into the cytoplasm and enclosed within a vacuole (phagosome), the wall of which is made up of inverted plasma membrane (see Fig. 2–2). In addition, actin- and myosin-like proteins that appear to participate in the ingestion process through the formation of microfilaments have been isolated.

MORPHOLOGIC EVENTS ASSOCIATED WITH PHAGOCYTOSIS

Following the formation of the phagosome, the membrane enclosing the particle gradually pinches off from the surface membrane and is internalized within the cell, forming the phagocytic vacuole (see Fig. 2–2). The

Table 2–3. **Enzymes and Other Substances Found Within Neutrophils***

Acid phosphatase	Hyaluronidase
Acid ribonuclease	Lysozyme
Acid deoxyribonuclease	Collagenase
Cathepsins B, C, D, E	Aryl sulfatases A and B
Phosphoprotein phosphatase	Phospholipases
Organophosphate-resistant esterase	Acid lipase
β-Glucuronidase	Lactoferrin
β-Galactosidase	Phagocytin and other related bactericidal proteins
β-N-acetylglucosaminase	Endogenous pyrogen
α-L-fucosidase	Plasminogen activator (?urokinase)
α-1,4-glucosidase	Hemolysin(s)
α-mannosidase	Mucopolysaccharides and glycoproteins
α-N-acetylglucosamidase	Basic proteins: (a) Mast cell-active (b) Permeability-
α-N-acetylgalactosaminidase	inducing independent mast cells
Myeloperoxidase	

*(Adapted from Cochrane, C. G.: Immunologic tissue injury mediated by neutrophilic leukocytes. Adv. Immunol., 9:97, 1968.)

lysosomal granules within the leukocytes come into apposition with this phagosome, and the membranes of the two structures fuse into a phagolysosome. The granules rupture, discharging their enzymatic contents into the vacuole, and come into contact with the ingested particle. This process has been termed degranulation and represents the morphologic counterpart of the transfer of enzymes from the lysosomal granule to the phagosome. The leukocyte granules (primary) are analogous to the lysosomes of other cells and contain several hydrolytic enzymes and other bactericidal substances (Table 2–3). First, these ranges of acidity are achieved by the cell during the "respiratory burst" associated with phagocytosis as described below. Second, most of the enzymes found within the primary granules have pH optimum within this acid range. These facts suggest that the fall in pH during phagocytosis might trigger the digestive process by liberating hydrolytic enzymes that function best at a low pH.

METABOLIC EVENTS ASSOCIATED WITH PHAGOCYTOSIS

Following the formation of the phagocytic vacuole, a series of biochemical reactions is initiated in phagocytic cells. The metabolic pathways that are primarily involved include the glycolytic pathway and the hexose monophosphate (HMP) shunt (Fig. 2–9). In addition, alveolar macrophages utilize the tricarboxylic acid pathway, which provides

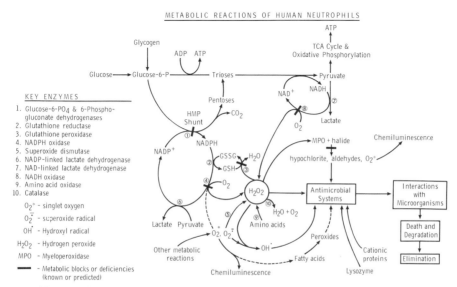

Figure 2–9. Metabolic pathways of leukocytes. (Courtesy of Dr. Lata Nerukar.)

their main energy source. Collectively, the stimulation of these pathways is termed the respiratory burst and consists of the following: (1) an increase in glycolysis; (2) a marked increase in HMP shunt activity; and (3) an elevation in oxygen consumption and H_2O_2 and lactic acid production. The increase in lactic acid production is in part responsible for the fall in pH within the phagosome, as previously described. Accompanying the respiratory burst is an enhanced RNA and phospholipid turnover, events important in protein synthesis and membrane formation. These changes are most prominent in neutrophils but also are seen to a lesser extent in the mononuclear phagocytes.

The biologic significance of the preferential utilization of these pathways by certain phagocytic cells, e.g., PMN's, may be to facilitate their function in tissues in which oxygen may be limited. In contrast, the utilization of the TCA cycle by other phagocytic cells, e.g., alveolar macrophages, may be an adaptation to their aerobic environment.

The precise initiating events that result in the metabolic changes following particle uptake are not known, but appear to involve perturbations of the plasma membrane. Several surface-active agents such as deoxycholate, digitonin, and concanavalin-A can also induce a respiratory burst similar to that seen following particle uptake. The extraordinary feature of this phenomenon is that the initiation of the respiratory burst is detectable within seconds after particle uptake and actually precedes the morphologic events, suggesting that the biochemical changes may be required for subsequent events to occur. In addition, the activation of the macrophages can be produced by several other agents, e.g., adjuvants, microorganisms, lymphokines, and bacterial products. The features of the enhanced metabolism of this "activated macrophage" are the same as those described with particle uptake.

One of the proposed key enzymes involved in the metabolism of phagocytic cells is NADPH oxidase (Fig. 2–9). This enzyme may serve a twofold function: (1) It provides a source of NADP, which may be the limiting factor regulating HMP shunt activity; or (2) it may be involved in the formation of H_2O_2, which is an essential component in the microbicidal reactions. In addition, NADP also participates in many other metabolic functions, such as glutathione production, RNA and lipid metabolism, and membrane for-

mation, events essential for phagocytic cell function. Other enzyme systems are involved in the conversion of NADPH to NADP, including glutathione peroxidase, which oxidizes reduced glutathione (GSH) to its oxidized form (GSSG) in the presence of H_2O_2. The GSSG is further reduced to GSH and in turn converts NADPH to NADP (Fig. 2–9).

With the respiratory burst there occurs an enhanced production of H_2O_2 or superoxide anion (O_2^-). The superoxide anion undergoes dismutation in the presence of an enzyme, superoxide dismutase, with further production of H_2O_2 (Fig. 2–9). The production of H_2O_2 is more prominent in PMN's than in tissue or alveolar macrophages and appears to be extremely important in microbicidal function of PMN's. Defects in H_2O_2 production associated with failure in the induction of the respiratory burst have been observed in the leukocytes of children with a variety of neutrophil dysfunction disorders, e.g., chronic granulomatous disease (CGD). A useful diagnostic test of phagocytic function has been developed based upon these biochemical considerations. The reduction of nitroblue tetrazolium (NBT) to a blue formazan derivative provides a useful functional test of leukocyte HMP activity and is abnormally low in CGD.

ANTIMICROBIAL MECHANISMS OF PHAGOCYTIC CELLS

In order to successfully destroy and eliminate microorganisms, e.g., bacteria, following their ingestion, the next step in the process is the killing and destruction of the microorganism by the phagocytic cell. The observation that anaerobic conditions only partially impair bactericidal activity led to the discovery that both oxygen-dependent and oxygen-independent antimicrobial mechanisms exist within phagocytic cells. Klebanoff has proposed a classification of these antimicrobial systems on the basis of their oxygen requirements. The oxygen-dependent mechanisms can be further subdivided on the basis of their utilization of myeloperoxidase. This classification of antimicrobial systems of phagocytic cells is shown in Table 2–4.

A system consisting of H_2O_2, halide, and MPO has been shown to have powerful microbicidal activity contributing to the microbicidal action of phagocytic cells, primarily the PMN's (Fig. 2–9). The role of this system in mononuclear phagocytes is less clear. The

Table 2–4. Antimicrobial Systems of Phagocytic Cells*

I. O_2-dependent	II. O_2-independent
a. Myeloperoxidase (MPO)-mediated	a. acid
b. MPO-independent	b. lysozyme
1. H_2O_2	c. lactoferrin
2. superoxide anion (O_2^-)	d. granular cationic proteins
3. hydroxyl radical (OH^-)	
4. singlet oxygen (O_2*)	
5. ascorbate-peroxide-metal ion	
6. amino acid oxidation	

*(After Klebanoff, S. J.: *In* Bellanti, J. A., and Dayton, D. H. (eds.): The Phagocytic Cell in Host Resistance. New York, Raven Press, 1975.)

proposed mechanism of action of the MPO-H_2O_2-halide complex is thought to involve the formation of aldehydes and hypochlorite or halogenation of bacterial proteins, the net effect of which leads to the death of the microorganism. The significance of this reaction is apparent in several clinical disorders of neutrophil function in which a failure of production of H_2O_2 leads to defective bacterial killing and the clinical spectrum of recurrent infection, e.g., CGD, which suggests that there are mechanisms other than the MPO-H_2O_2-halide system operative in antimicrobial activity. These other systems have been referred to as back-up systems. In the case of low concentrations of H_2O_2, the action of MPO can be replaced by catalase. Such alternate pathways may be important in macrophages, in which the role of MPO is less clear. It is of interest that in children with CGD the characteristic spectrum of bacteria causing infection includes those that are catalase-positive and peroxide-negative, e.g., *Staphylococcus aureus*. In contrast, organisms that are catalase-negative and peroxide-positive, e.g., *Haemophilus influenzae,* do not cause serious infection in these children. It has been postulated that these latter organisms can provide an alternative source of H_2O_2, which in effect can partially correct the cellular defects.

Among the MPO-independent systems, H_2O_2 itself exhibits antimicrobial activity, and since it is produced during the phagocytic event it may in part contribute to the overall killing capacity of the phagocytic cell (Table 2–4). The superoxide radical (O_2^-) that is generated during phagocytosis is formed by the univalent reduction of molecular oxygen and is an extremely toxic and reactive moiety important in bactericidal activity. Subsequent dismutation of O_2^- by superoxide dismutase (SOD) leads to the formation of H_2O_2.

$$O_2 \xrightarrow{e} O_2^-$$

$$O_2^- + O_2^- + 2H^+ \xrightarrow{SOD} O_2 + H_2O_2$$

The superoxide radical, in addition to its own bactericidal activity, may through dismutation produce H_2O_2, which is microbicidal. This indicates that O_2^- acts as an intermediate to H_2O_2 production and indirectly contributes to the MPO-mediated system. Singlet oxygen (O_2*) is an electronically excited state of molecular oxygen that emits light (chemiluminescence) when it reverts to the triplet ground state (O_2). This biochemical finding has also been used in the functional assessment of phagocytic cells. The source of this singlet oxygen (O_2*) may be an MPO-mediated reaction involving the formation of hypochlorite. Singlet oxygen might also react with certain unsaturated chemical groups, e.g., ethylene groups, forming dioxytanes across double bonds that are unstable, and may be toxic to microorganisms

$$\rangle C=C \langle \xrightarrow{O_2^*} \rangle \overset{\overset{\displaystyle O-O}{\displaystyle |\quad|}}{C-C} \langle$$

and thus responsible for the killing by MPO-mediated systems. Other proposed antimicrobial mechanisms include an ascorbate-peroxide system, which may function in synergism with lysozyme and may even be more potent in the presence of metallic ions such as cobalt and copper. The oxidation of amino acids may also add to the generation of H_2O_2.

The mononuclear phagocytes lack significant myeloperoxidase activity and must therefore resort to other microbicidal mechanisms. Although little is known of the microbicidal mechanisms of mononuclear phagocytes at present, they do exhibit the metabolic burst and H_2O_2 and O_2^- generation displayed by PMN's, but to a lesser extent.

The oxygen-independent mechanisms also seem to contribute to the killing capacity of the phagocytic cells, since anaerobiosis does not totally impair their microbicidal activity (Table 2–4). Although there is evidence that lysozyme may be involved directly in the killing of bacteria, the action of this enzyme may also be to function in a digestive manner after the killing of the bacteria. Lactoferrin, an iron-binding protein, leukin, and phago-cytin, found in the specific granules of the PMN but not in mononuclear phagocytes, also have been shown to have bacteriostatic properties. The granular cationic proteins also exhibit antimicrobial activity, presumably after binding to the microorganisms, a function that is also lacking in macrophages. Finally, the formation of lactic acid as a result of the respiratory burst reduces the intracellular pH and thus provides conditions favorable for the action of digestive enzymes rather than functioning directly as a microbicidal agent.

Cell Types and Effector Mechanisms Involved in Specific Responses

LYMPHOCYTES AND PLASMA CELLS

The lymphoid cells of the immune system differ from the preceding group of cells by their ability to react specifically with antigen and to elaborate specific cell products. The lymphoid cells include plasma cells and lymphocytes (Figs. 2–10 and 2–11). These cells, once sensitized, become "committed" and are referred to as immunocytes. By definition, an immunocyte is a cell of the lymphoid series that can react with antigen with the production of specific cell products called antibody or a cell-mediated event such as delayed hypersensitivity, e.g., tuberculin reaction (Chapter 9).

The traditional classification of lymphocytes as small, medium, and large was based on the concept that morphologically similar cells had the same functions, life cycles, and metabolic behavior. In recent years, however, it has become apparent that even lymphocytes that appear morphologically identical constitute several cell populations that are extremely heterogeneous in function.

The lymphoid cell line traces its origin to a pluripotential stem cell that in the fetus is found within the yolk sac, bone marrow, and liver and in the adult in the bone marrow. These cells produce two classes of committed stem cells: (1) a committed hematopoietic stem cell that can give rise to the erythroid elements, granulocytes, or megakaryocytes; and (2) a committed lymphoid stem cell pre-

cursor that can give rise to cells of the lymphoid series (Table 2–2). The commitment to any of these pathways is dependent upon the microenvironments in which these stem cells develop.

DEVELOPMENT OF THE LYMPHOID TISSUE

Available evidence indicates that the lymphoid system consists of two compartments: (1) a *central* compartment involved in the differentiation of the lymphoid stem cells into lymphocytes capable of reacting with antigen (antigen-reactive cell); and (2) a *peripheral* compartment in which these cells can subsequently react with antigen (Fig. 2–12). The central lymphoid system consists of three components: (1) the *bone marrow*, (2) the *thymus*, and (3) a component whose identity is known with certainty only in birds (the bursa of Fabricius) and that in mammals is designated as the *bursal equivalent tissue*. The peripheral lymphoid system consists of lymph nodes, spleen, and gut-associated lymphoid tissue. In contrast to the differentiation of lymphocytes in the peripheral compartment, which is antigen-dependent, the maturation of lymphoid elements in the central compartment can occur in the absence of antigen (Fig. 2–12).

In higher vertebrates two types of lymphocytes may be found in peripheral lymphoid tissues that are dependent upon their sites of differentiation in the central lymphoid compartment. One type, which develops in the thymus, differentiates into small lymphocytes referred to as T-lymphocytes, which are involved in antigen recognition in cell-mediated immune reactions, including delayed hypersensitivity. The other population of lymphocytes is derived from stem cells, which differentiate in the bursa of Fabricius in birds and in the mammalian (bursal) equivalent and consist mainly of small lymphocytes referred to as B-lymphocytes, the plasma cells, and their progeny. In higher mammals, the location of the bursal equivalent is unknown, and several sites have been postulated, including the bone marrow. Such bursal equivalent– or bone marrow–derived lymphocytes are termed B-lymphocytes. Thus, the bone marrow component of the central lymphoid tissues may serve not only as a site of production of pluripotential lymphoid stem cells but also as a microenvironment for the differentiation of stem cells into antigen-reactive B-lymphocytes as well as a site for mature recirculating lymphocyte populations.

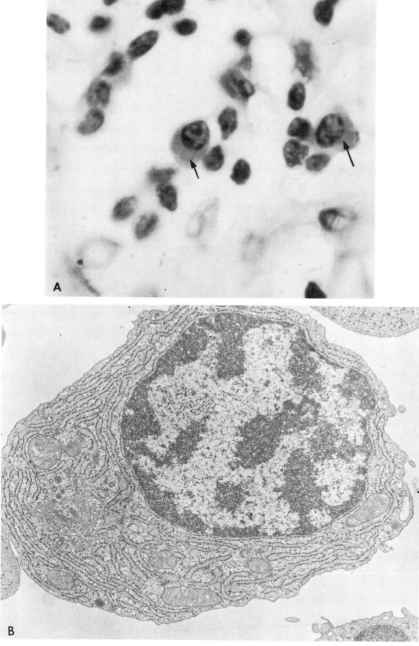

Figure 2–10. *A,* Plasma cells from section of aorta with chronic inflammation. Hematoxylin and eosin stain, × 1000. (Courtesy of Dr. Theodore I. Malinin.) *B,* Electron micrograph of plasma cells showing well-developed endoplasmic reticulum, × 11,000. (Courtesy of Dr. Dorothy F. Bainton.)

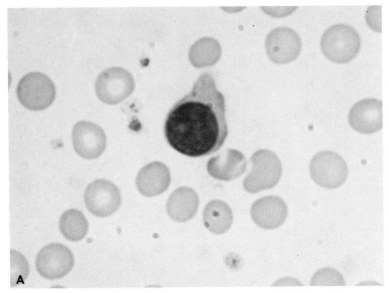

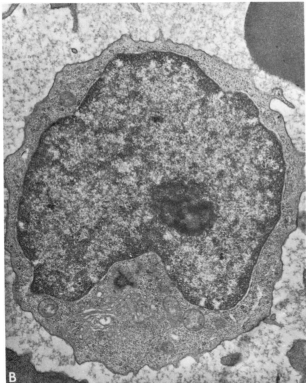

Figure 2–11. *A*, Lymphocytes from peripheral blood. Wright-Giemsa stain, × 1400. *B*, Electron micrograph of a resting lymphocyte, × 11,000. (Courtesy of Dr. Dorothy F. Bainton.)

CELLULAR ELEMENTS

Lymphocytes thus comprise two lines of immunocompetent cells, one concerned with cell-mediated immunity (T-lymphocytes) and the other with humoral immunity (B-lymphocytes) (Fig. 2–12). Ordinarily, in the absence of stimulation the B-lymphocyte does not replicate. Under an appropriate stimulus, such as antigen, it transforms into a large, metabolically more active "blast" cell, which has been termed "an active lymphocyte" or "a large pyroninophyllic" cell (Chapter 7). Plasma cells are characterized by their RNA-rich cytoplasm and eccentrically placed nuclei. Ultrastructurally, the cytoplasm contains

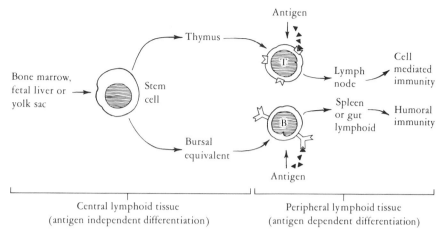

Figure 2–12. Development of the lymphoid system.

an extensive system of endoplasmic reticulum studded with ribosomes (Fig. 2–10). This structure is characteristic of cells active in protein synthesis, and the product of these cells is immunoglobulin.

T-lymphocytes are involved in such cell-mediated immune reactions as graft versus host (GVH), delayed hypersensitivity, and tumor rejection, and develop in an alternative pathway of development. These cells are incapable of differentiating into plasma cells but give rise to a cell capable of producing a variety of factors that trigger inflammatory or cell-mediated damaging reactions leading to cell-mediated events. These factors include migration inhibitory factor (MIF), a substance chemotactic for mononuclear and granulocytic cells, a cytotoxic factor capable of injuring a variety of cell types, interferon, and several other factors whose biologic roles are not yet well defined, e.g., interleukin-2 (Chapter 9). Some are released upon interaction of sensitized lymphocytes with appropriate antigens; others may remain cell-bound. In either case, they lead to the destruction of foreign target cells or to the damage and destruction of host cells. In addition to the function of releasing these various factors, the T-lymphocyte is now recognized to exist as a family of different T-cell subsets. These are identified by specific surface antigenic markers recognized by monoclonal antibodies or by functional assays of the cells. As described below, two major populations of T-cell subsets include the T-inducer ("helper cells") and the T-cytotoxic/suppressor ("suppressor cells" or "killer cells"). Recently a group of cells have been

identified as "natural killer (NK) cells," which are defined by their ability to kill tumor cells without previously being sensitized. The origin of the NK cells is unclear, but they share many of the surface membrane characteristics not only of thymocytes but also of monocytes. Thus, it is apparent that the lymphocytes possess the most diversified function of all cells of the immune system.

Following stimulation of either B- or T-lymphocytes, an alternate pathway of differentiation leads to the production of a subpopulation termed memory cells. Upon re-encounter with specific immunogens, these cells have the capacity to proliferate and differentiate into cell lines responsible for either humoral or cell-mediated immunity (Chapter 7).

The conversion of small lymphocytes to blast cells provides the basis for one of the most useful tests employed in clinical immunology, i.e., the test of immunocompetency of patients suspected of having a variety of immune deficiency disorders. In addition, other tests allow the identification of specific lymphocytes as B- or T-lymphocytes (Chapters 7 and 9). The transformation of the lymphocyte to the activated lymphocyte can be induced by a variety of stimuli including specific antigen, in either a soluble or a cell-associated form, e.g., lymphocytes from a genetically unrelated individual in a mixed lymphocyte response (MLC), or on a graft in graft rejection, or on a tumor cell in tumor rejection; or by antilymphocyte sera or by nonspecific mitogens, some of which selectively stimulate B-lymphocytes, others T-lymphocytes. These reactions take place by virtue of receptors on the surface of lymphocytes, which are described in greater detail in Chapters 3, 7, and 9.

The Structure of Organs That House Immunologic Cells: The Peripheral Lymphoid Tissue

The immune system contains some cells concerned with the initial response to foreign configurations and other cells that function in subsequent encounters. The system is equipped to perform nonspecific events, such as phagocytosis, as well as responses carried out in a specific manner by cells of the lymphoid tissues.

The lymphoreticular cells are strategically located in areas of the body best suited to deal with foreign configurations, which may confront the host *exogenously* or may arise *endogenously* (Fig. 2–1). For example, the foreign configuration may be a microorganism entering the host by such natural portals as the gastrointestinal, respiratory, or genitourinary tract. The lymphoid tissue is arranged in a unique manner in these areas. When the configuration arises *endogenously* within a host, e.g., a worn-out·erythrocyte or a tumor cell, elements are mobilized into the lymphatics or the blood stream, where they quickly come into contact with immune effector cells.

The encounter between a configuration and a cellular element involved in immunity appears to be a random event. There are two anatomic features that increase the chance occurrence of these random events. The first feature is that some elements of the system are in constant motion and are recirculating continuously (the phagocytes and lymphoid cells). The second is that certain organs, such as the lymph nodes and spleen, contain a system of conduits through which a continuous recirculation of lymph or blood occurs.

Thus, the system is well organized to carry out its functions in defense, homeostasis, and surveillance. Four types of peripheral lymphatic tissues are important in this regard: (1) the lymph nodules, (2) the lymph nodes, (3) the spleen, and (4) the thymus. Although all four seem to be engaged in lymphopoiesis, only the first three respond actively to antigenic stimulation. The thymus, in contrast, stands autonomous in this regard and appears to be a master central lymphoid organ concerned with embryogenesis and orchestration of the remainder of the peripheral lymphoid tissues.

LYMPH NODULE

Lymph nodules consist of collections of lymphoid elements scattered in the submucous tissues of the respiratory passages, the intestine, and the genitourinary tracts. They are particularly well developed in structures such as the tonsils, which stand guard at the entrance of the gastrointestinal and respiratory tracts, and also in the Peyer's patches, collections of lymph nodules in the gastrointestinal tract. Their structure is demonstrated in Figure 2–13. This type of lymphoid tissue is arranged somewhat differently from that in lymph nodes, insofar as it lacks a connective tissue capsule. These nodules are not well developed in the fetus or in germ-free animals, but develop following exposure to antigens. Their development is believed to be related in some way to exposure of the host to antigens in the environment.

Since lymph nodules contain phagocytic elements as well as lymphoid elements, they are capable of reacting in nonspecific as well as in specific immunity. In the lymphoid cells that line these tracts, there occurs synthesis of the secretory IgA immunoglobulins. This class of immunoglobulin has been shown to be important at mucosal surfaces (Chapter 5). These tracts, contiguous with the exterior, elaborate a secretory form of antibody and provide the host with a cell product well suited to function at body surfaces and to deal with pathogens in the external environment. The IgE globulins have also been shown recently to be synthesized by cells in the same locations. Both IgA and IgE globulins are cell products of the external secretory system (Fig. 2–1).

LYMPH NODES

If a foreign configuration can overcome the initial barriers provided by the skin, mucous membranes, and lymph nodules, it may be handled in three additional ways: (1) It may be attached by wandering macrophages in the connective tissue; (2) it may provoke an inflammatory response with cellular accumulations, e.g., neutrophils; or (3) it may be taken up directly into the lymph or blood. The lymph represents a collection of tissue fluids flowing in lymphatic capillaries into a series of even larger collecting vessels called

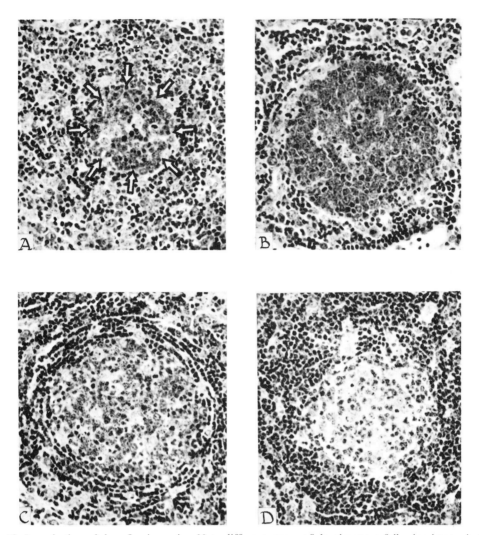

Figure 2–13. Lymphatic nodules of guinea pigs. Note different stages of development following immunization with *Listeria monocytogenes.* Hematoxylin and eosin stain, × 1100. (From Bloom, W., and Fawcett, D. W.: Textbook of Histology. 10th ed. Philadelphia, W. B. Saunders Company, 1975.)

the *lymphatics.* These vessels connect with and pass through a series of structures, the lymph nodes. During this voyage, the lymph becomes progressively enriched with lymphocytes, so that when it finally empties into the blood stream via the thoracic ducts, the fluid is significantly different from the tissue fluids of its origin. Lymphocytes are also added from postcapillary venules and become part of the *recirculating pool.*

The *recirculating pool* consists of a group of lymphocytes found in the circulating blood, lymph, and lymph nodes, which traverse a circumscribed pathway from the blood to the lymph and then back to the blood. The recirculation of lymphocytes from the blood to the lymph occurs through a unique anatomic structure of lymph nodes, the postcap-

illary venule. These venules, found in the lymph node cortex, are distinguished by their elongated endothelial cell structure. Unlike other interepithelial cell transfers, such as that of the polymorphonuclear neutrophil, the lymphocyte passes from the blood to the lymph by a remarkable process in which the endothelial cell invaginates the lymphocyte and allows it to pass directly through the cell (Fig. 2–14). The recirculating pool of small lymphocytes consists primarily of T-cells that are characterized by their long life spans and are believed to function as memory cells.

Lymph nodes are oval structures distributed throughout the body (Fig. 2–15); through them pass the motile carriers of specific genetic information, the lymphocytes. When enlarged, the lymph nodes be-

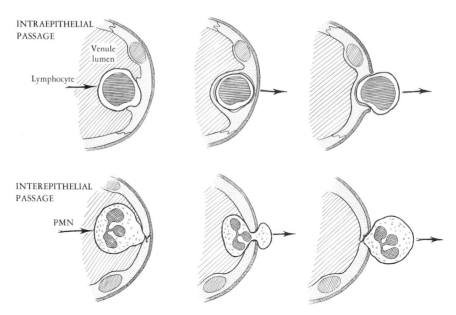

Figure 2–14. Schematic representation of intraepithelial passage of a small lymphocyte and interepithelial passage of a polymorphonuclear leukocyte.

come physically palpable, providing a useful diagnostic sign of infection or malignant disease. The structure of a lymph node is shown in Figure 2–15. It consists of two main portions, an outer portion (cortex) and an inner portion (medulla). The node is surrounded by a connective tissue capsule from which extensions protrude centrally (trabeculae). The capsule provides support and a conduit along which blood vessels run. Weblike structures (reticular fibers) extend from these connective tissue elements into the substance of the node; these contain phagocytic elements of the macrophage system. In the periphery, the node is made up of large numbers of lymphocytes organized into nodules. In the center of the nodules are collections of actively dividing cells termed *germinal centers*. Deeper cortical zones contain the postcapillary venules with their characteristic cuboidal endothelial cells through which passage of lymphocytes from blood lymph occurs (Fig. 2–16). Thus, in the lymph node, lymphocytes enter through both the vascular system and the lymphatics (Fig. 2–16). In mutant strains of mice born without thymuses (nude mice) or following the thymectomy of neonatal animals, there is a depletion of lymphoid elements in these paracortical or subcortical regions; therefore, this region has become known as a *thymic-dependent region* and contains the T-lymphocytes important in cell-

mediated immunity. In contrast, upon removal of the bursa of Fabricius (in birds) or the bursal equivalent tissues (in the mammal), there is a failure of formation of the outer cortical regions containing the germinal centers, as well as the deeper medullary region; therefore, these regions have been called the bursal equivalent regions and contain the B-lymphocytes important in antibody synthesis. Following antigen stimulation, antibody synthesis can be noted in both the medullary and the far cortical regions of the node. Although it is tempting to compartmentalize the node according to function, this is undoubtedly an oversimplification of a more complicated process, since elements of each type of tissue may be present in both regions. Nonetheless, the importance of these findings for clinical medicine is illustrated in numerous disease states such as the DiGeorge syndrome, in which T-lymphocytes are absent owing to the congenital absence of the thymus, or X-linked agammaglobulinemia, in which a deficiency of B-lymphocytes occurs as a result of a failure of development of the bursal equivalent tissue.

There are two basic functions of the lymph nodes. The first function is the filtration of foreign material performed as lymph percolates through the multichanneled structure. This removes particulate matter, and some products of phagocytic degradation become

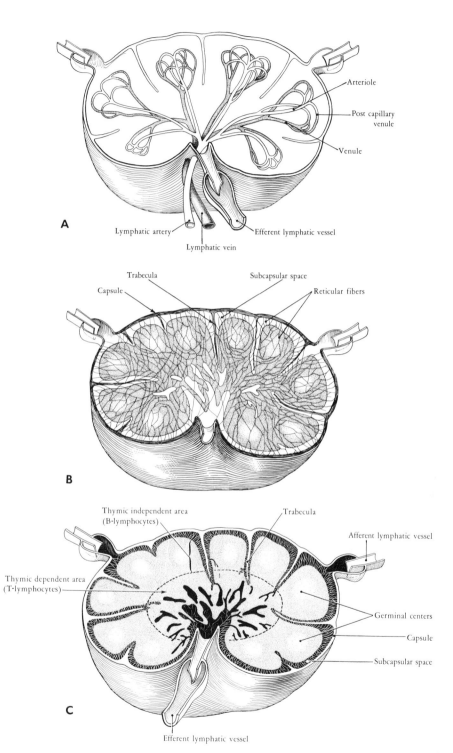

Figure 2–15. Structure of lymph node, schematic. *A*, Circulation; *B*, supporting structures (reticular fibers); and *C*, general areas of thymic-dependent (T-cell) and -independent (B-cell) areas.

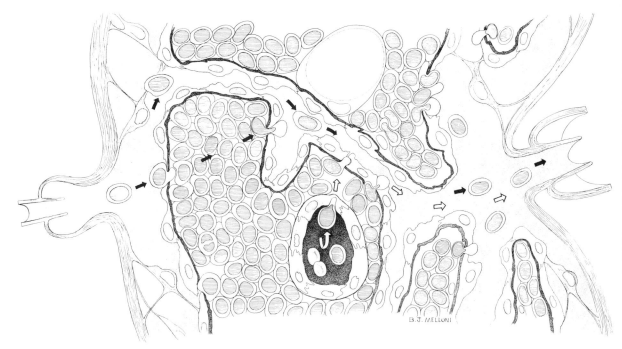

Figure 2–16. Schematic representation of circulation of lymphocytes within a lymph node. Note the dual entry of lymphocytes: from the vascular to lymphatic via postcapillary venule, and from afferent lymphatic vessels.

immunogenic. The second function is the circulation of lymphocytes, which are formed in the central lymphoid pool.

SPLEEN

If these first two barriers are inadequate, foreign constituents may gain access to the blood, either by direct invasion of small vessels (capillaries, venules) or via lymph stream channels emptying into the blood. The spleen is the sole lymphatic tissue specialized to filter blood. This organ has a number of *nonimmunologic* and *immunologic* functions. It removes effete or worn-out cells from the circulatory system (homeostatic function), converts hemoglobin to bilirubin, and releases iron into the circulation for reutilization. Like the lymph nodes, the spleen is a component of the peripheral lymphoid system, produces lymphocytes and plasma cells, and is important in the mediation of specific immunologic events. Yet the organ is important early in life, when other elements of the lymphoreticular system are incompletely developed. Removal of the spleen has been shown to be associated with overwhelming bacterial infections not only in infants and children but also in young adults.

The spleen is surrounded by a connective tissue capsule from which trabeculae extend into its interior (Fig. 2–17). The interior (pulp) is filled with two kinds of tissue: the *white* pulp and the *red* pulp. The white pulp contains lymph nodules and is the chief site of lymphocyte prodution in the spleen. The germinal follicles found in this region contain B-lymphocytes and are considered bursal equivalent tissues. Other lymphocytes surrounding the follicles and periarteriolar sheaths of the white pulp contain T-lymphocytes and are referred to as the thymic-dependent regions. Red pulp, on the other hand, surrounds the white pulp and contains large numbers of erythrocytes consonant with its filtration function. The arterial blood supply enters through the hilus and follows along trabeculae until the smaller arteries become surrounded by sheaths or collars of lymphocytes (white pulp). They then give off capillaries to the lymph nodules. The blood passes through the red pulp, containing elements of the reticuloendothelial system active in phagocytosis. These structures are shown in Figure 2–17. In addition to its phagocytic function, the spleen is capable of responding to antigenic stimulation. Following the intravenous injection of rabbits with antigen, one can demonstrate cells actively engaged in antibody synthesis in the sheaths surrounding arteries and also in lymph nodules.

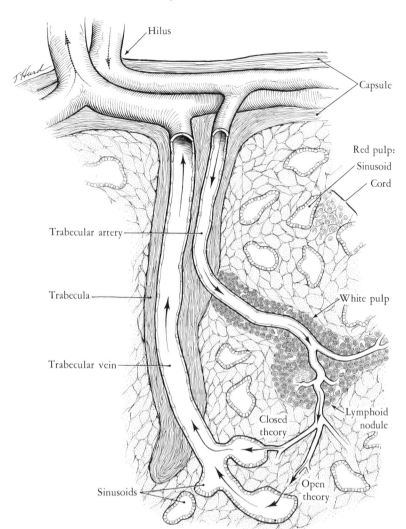

Figure 2–17. Schematic representation of structure of spleen.

THYMUS

The thymus is responsible for the development of lymphocytes involved in cell-mediated immune responses (thymus-derived or
T-lymphocytes). The gland appears to be a
master organ important in immunogenesis
in the young and in orchestrating the total
lymphoid system throughout life. This central lymphoid organ differs in a number of
respects from other lymphoid tissues. All the
lymphoid tissues described thus far are ad-
vantageously and strategically positioned for
contact with foreign configurations that may
enter or arise within the host. The thymus,
on the other hand, is protected from rather
than exposed to antigen. In addition, the rate
of mitotic activity in the thymus is greater
than in any other lymphatic tissue, yet the
number of cells leaving it is fewer than the

number accounted for by this high rate of
mitosis. The assumption made from these
findings is that a large number of lymphocytes produced within the thymus die within
its substance. Although originally considered
to be a mechanism for removal of "forbid-
den" autoreactive lymphocyte clones, this
function of the thymus probably represents
homeostatic activity involved in the production of T-lymphocytes. The role of the thymus in the development of the immunologic
system is described more fully in Chapters 3
and 9.

The thymus consists of two lobes surrounded by a thin capsule of connective tissues (Fig. 2–18). The capsule extends into
the substance of the gland, forming septa
that partially divide the lobes into lobules.
Peripheral portions of the lobule (cortex) are
heavily infiltrated with lymphocytes. More

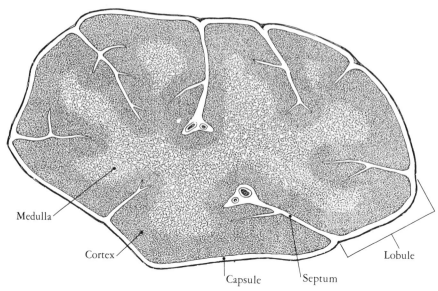

Figure 2–18. Schematic representation of thymus gland, showing division into cortex and medulla.

central portions (medulla) contain fewer lymphocytes but more epithelial elements. Within the substance of the thymus are cystic structures containing keratin (Hassall's corpuscles). The thymus is believed to perform two main functions: the production of lymphocytes within the cortex and the production of a humoral substance(s) by epithelial elements of the gland. These humoral substances (or hormones) may induce differentiation of lymphocytes directly within the thymus or may control their differentiation in the periphery. Although the thymus gland has a cortex and a medulla, neither contains germinal centers or plasma cells in the normal situation. These may appear when the gland is abnormal, e.g., in thymoma or in certain autoimmune diseases.

Unlike other lymphoid organs, the thymus is composed of two tissue types: lymphoid and epithelial. The lymphoid cells are of mesenchymal origin, and the epithelial cells

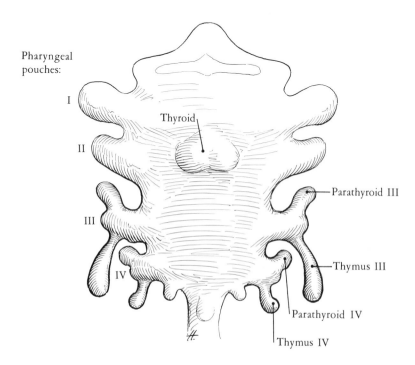

Figure 2–19. Embryology of the thymus gland from III to IV pharyngeal pouches. Note close proximity of site of differentiation of thyroid gland (II–III) and parathyroid glands (III–IV).

are of endodermal origin. The thymus initially develops as a continuous epithelium of cells from the third and fourth pharyngeal pouches Then the mesenchyme-derived lymphoid cells seed this epithelial thymus and convert this structure into a lymphoepithelial organ. The process of differentiation in the human begins as a ventral outpocketing from these pouches about the sixth week of fetal life (Fig. 2–19). It is noteworthy that the parathyroids begin their development about the same time from the same pouches. A

caudal migration of epithelium occurs with further differentiation. Failure of this migration is seen in one of the immunologic deficiency disorders—thymic dysplasia. By the tenth week, the thymic epithelium is differentiated into a compact epithelial structure interlaced with a fibrous reticular network. The epithelial cells are secretory cells with a well-developed Golgi apparatus, a rough endoplasmic reticulum, and a large nucleus with multiple nucleoli (Fig. 2–20). With further development, the thymus is infiltrated

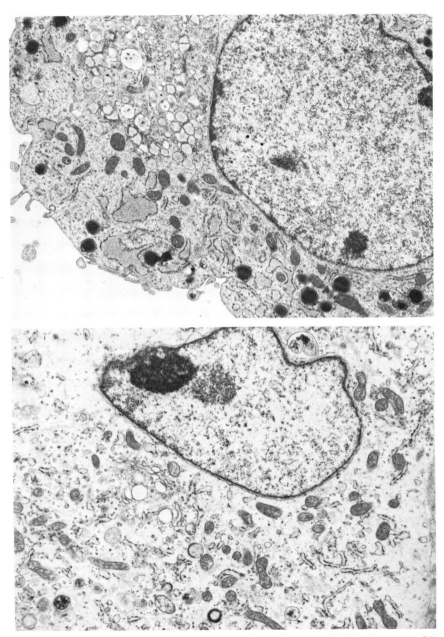

Figure 2–20. Electron micrograph of a thymus epithelial cell in culture, × 11,000. (Courtesy of Sam Waksal.)

with precursor cells migrating from the liver and yolk sac during fetal life and bone marrow during adult life. Large lymphoblastoid cells first enter the subcapsular cortex and subsequently undergo further differentiation as they migrate through the different areas of the thymus. The clinical importance of the simultaneous embryogenesis of parathyroid glands and the thymus is seen in another of the immunologic deficiency disorders of man, the DiGeorge syndrome. Infants with this disorder are born not only lacking in thymic function but also without parathyroid glands. Thus they present with hypocalcemic tetany in the newborn period and with subsequent failure of the development of cell-mediated immunity.

Thymocytes develop within the thymic microenvironment, and autoradiographic studies show that they migrate from cortical areas to medullary areas. This maturation process is characterized by changes in surface (differentiation) antigens as well as functional properties (Table 2–5). In the mouse, one of the more important surface antigens is the Thy-1 (Θ) antigen on thymocytes, which also exists on peripheral T-lymphocytes. Less differentiated thymocytes contain large amounts of Thy-1 and TL (thymus leukemia) antigens and small amounts of H-2 antigen on their surfaces. The more differentiated thymocytes contain large amounts of H-2, small amounts of Thy-1, and no TL antigen. The highly differentiated thymocytes in the medullary regions of the thymus acquire GVH reactivity and cortisone resistance. The thymus may exert its control over the differentiation and maturation of prothymocytes either by direct contact with these cells and the thymus epithelium or via the thymic humoral factors. These factors or thymic hormones are secreted by the epithelial cells of the thymus and may be the control mechanism over peripheral T-lymphocytes.

In man, similar changes in differentiation antigens occur. Following infiltration of the thymus with pluripotential stem cells that have migrated from the yolk sac, fetal liver, or spleen, these cells acquire new surface differentiation antigens and functions. Utilizing monoclonal antibody techniques, three discrete stages of thymic differentiation have been defined (Fig. 2–21). During intrathymic maturation, thymocytes progress through these stages and gradually acquire and then lose or retain various surface markers. The most mature thymocytes eventually differentiate into two separate populations that finally are released into the peripheral blood. These two populations are called (1) T-inducer (T_4) lymphocytes, which facilitate antibody production ("helper cells"); and (2) T-cytotoxic/suppressor (T_5/T_8) lymphocytes, which inhibit antibody production ("suppressor cells") or destroy target cells ("killer or cytotoxic cells"). These events will be more fully described in Chapters 7 and 9.

After birth, the role of the thymus continues to change. The changes in the size of the gland with age are shown in Figure 2–22. Relative to body size it is largest during fetal life and at birth weighs from 10 to 15 gm. The gland continues to increase in size, reaching a maximum of 30 to 40 gm at puberty. This follows the same pattern of change that occurs in all lymphoid tissue during childhood. It is of interest that this pattern of growth parallels the sequential appearance of T- and B-cell function during maturation. Following adolescence, the gland begins to involute. The parallel continues in that lymphoid tissues and immunoglobulins also diminish with increasing age. In addition, the development of autoimmune phenomena and malignant disease increases with advancing age with a loss of T-cell (e.g., suppressor) function. Thus the thymus and its associated lymphoid tissues and their

Table 2–5. Thymocyte Populations (Mouse)

	Size		
	Large	Small	Medium
Per cent of thymus	5–7	85–90	5–7
Location	Subcapsular	Deeper cortex	Medulla
Life span	Rapid turnover	Long-lived	Long-lived
Cortisone sensitivity	Yes	Yes	No
Thy 1 (θ)	+ + +	+ +	+
H-2	+	+	+ +
Per cent Fc +	< 1	10	9

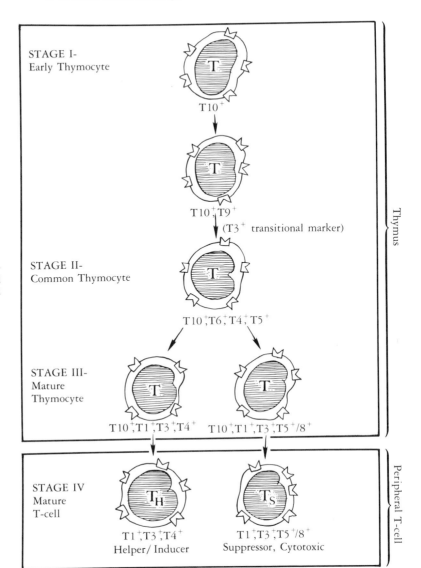

Figure 2–21. Human T-cell maturation as defined by monoclonal antibodies. (After Reinherz and Schlossman.)

products play a dynamic role from early embryogenesis throughout the life span of the individual.

The thymus thus appears to be equipped to maintain lymphopoiesis while segregated from antigen. This curious finding may be explained in part by the barrier that is made up of a continuous epithelium surrounding blood vessels in the cortex (Fig. 2–23). This epithelial membrane forms a perivascular space between the capillary endothelium and the epithelial sheath. The barrier might prevent macromolecules in the blood stream from entering the substance of the thymus gland. Although macromolecules may be prevented from entering the epithelial barrier, lymphocytes produced within the cortex are capable of passing freely through this epithe-lium into the blood system, as in other anatomic sites (e.g., postcapillary venule of the lymph nodes) (Fig. 2–23).

Thus, the thymus may be viewed as a lymphoid organ, anatomically distinct, upon which all other peripheral lymphoid organs are dependent. It is an organ actively engaged in lymphopoiesis but independent of antigenic stimulation. It appears important as a central lymphoid tissue essential for the development and maturation of peripheral lymphoid tissues. Two major functions have been attributed to the thymus: (1) that it acts by the elaboration of a hormone that expands peripheral lymphocyte populations in much the same way as erythropoietin expands erythrocyte populations, and (2) that it acts by direct seeding of peripheral lymphoid

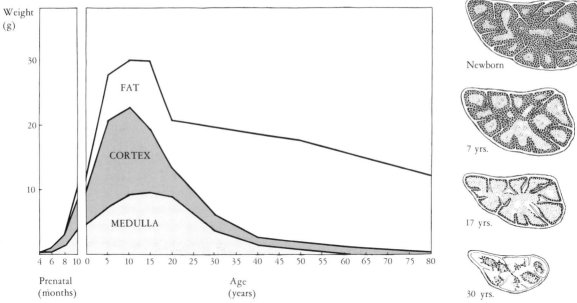

Figure 2–22. Schematic representation of changes in weight and composition of thymus gland with maturation, showing involution of the gland with age. (After Hammar, J. A.: Die normal morphologische Thymusforschung im letzten. Vierteljahrhundert. Leipzig. Barth, 1936.)

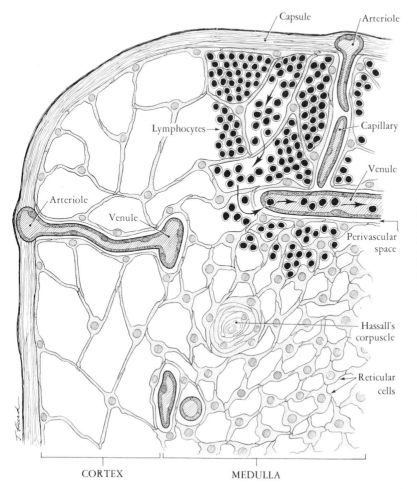

Figure 2–23. Thymus gland. Schematic representation of the perivascular epithelium surrounding blood vessels in the cortex. Note the barrier provided by this sheath and the pathways of lymphocytes formed in the cortex into the blood vessels.

tissues with lymphocytes. Recent studies have focused upon the role of the thymus as an endocrine gland, and several thymic hormones from the human and animal sources have been described. Some of these, e.g., thymosin(s), are receiving clinical trials in the reconstitution of children with a wide variety of immune deficiencies. Failure of thymic function has also been implicated in the development of neoplasms and autoimmune disease, e.g., myasthenia gravis.

DEVELOPMENT OF THE IMMUNOLOGIC SYSTEM

The development of the immunologic system may be considered as a series of adaptive cellular responses to a changing and potentially hostile environment (Table 2–6). It may be considered at several levels: *species, individual,* or *cell.*

The effect of the hostile environment ensures by selective pressures the survival of those life forms within the species that are best adapted to that environment. This adaptive process forms the basis for the *phylogeny* of the immune response. The microenvironment in which undifferentiated immunologic progenitor cells exist provides yet another type of inducing stimulus within the developing individual *(ontogeny).* The immunologically mature individual may be considered as the selected form that resulted from this type of development. Finally, when cells find themselves within the molecular milieu of antigen, a series of proliferative and differentiative events occur that are characteristic of the specific immune response. This leads to the synthesis of cell products such as antibody or mediators of cell-mediated immunity. The "memory" cells that are the result of this process may be considered the best adapted forms for the environment initiated by antigen. Moreover, the interaction of macrophages, B- and T-lymphocytes involved in immunologic processes, has genetic require-

ments (Chapter 7). Thus, the development of immune systems at all levels is the result of selective pressures exerted by a type of environment on either a species, an individual, or a cell, the net effect leading to some survival advantage of the evolving form.

Development of the Immunologic System in Evolving Species: Phylogeny of the Immune Response

PHYLOGENY OF NONSPECIFIC IMMUNITY

The most primitive manifestation of a resistance mechanism is phagocytosis. This event, which is found in the most ancient of the unicellular organisms, served a nutritive function; in higher forms, the process evolved to a *defense* function. This was clearly recorded by Metchnikoff in his writing.

Immunity is a phenomenon which has existed on this globe from time immemorial. Immunity must be of as ancient date as is disease. The most simple and primitive organisms have constantly to struggle for their existence; they give chase to living organisms in order to obtain food, and they defend themselves against other organisms in order that they may not become their prey. When the aggressor in this struggle is much smaller than its adversary, the result is that the former introduces itself into the body of the latter and destroys it by means of infection. In this case it takes up its abode in its adversary in order to absorb the contents of its host and to produce within it one or more generations. The natural history of unicellular organisms, both vegetable and animal, often presents to us these examples of primitive infection.

From the currently identifiable life forms, there arose an increasingly complex immune system, that ranged from the primitive defense of phagocytosis to the humoral and cell-mediated responses characteristic of specific immunity (Fig. 2–24).

As cellular life differentiated into more complex forms, there developed an increas-

---

Table 2–6. **Effect of Environment on the Development of the Immune Response**

Target	Inductive Environment	Process	Selected Form
Species	Macroenvironment	Phylogeny	Existing life forms
Individual	Microenvironment (thymus, bursal tissues)	Ontogeny	Immunologically mature individual
Cell	Molecular environment (antigen)	Induction of immune response	"Memory" cells

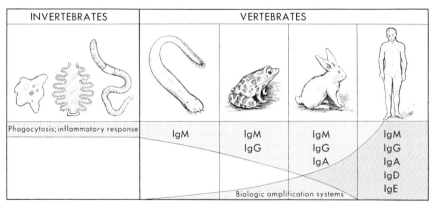

Figure 2–24. Schematic representation of phylogeny of immune response.

ing specialization of the systems concerned with recognition of foreignness. Thus, there evolved ever-increasingly complex immunologic systems. Although phagocytosis was continued as a nutritive function by endodermal cells (sponges, for example), the addition of a newly acquired mesodermal layer added a defense function. *It is the development and specialization of this mesodermal layer in higher life forms, beginning with vertebrates, in which specialization of cells destined for specific immunologic events is seen.*

In higher invertebrates a vascular system developed that allowed phagocytosis to proceed by both *fixed* and *circulating* cells (Fig. 2–24). In man, for example, there are five circulating white cells, three of which are phagocytic (monocytes, polymorphonuclear leukocytes, and eosinophils). Thus, in phylogeny, the two most important nonspecific elements, *phagocytosis* and the *inflammatory response,* were found in primitive life forms. With evolution, these defense mechanisms persisted, and were supplemented and amplified by the addition of new components—*specific immunity* and *biologic amplification systems* (e.g., coagulation system and complement). Thus, these older mechanisms were not replaced with evolution, but rather were continued and reinforced as evolving life forms added new responses.

PHYLOGENY OF SPECIFIC IMMUNITY

The first evidence of a specific immunologic system appeared in primitive vertebrates such as the hagfish (Fig. 2–24). It consisted of a disseminated lymphoid system, rather than the specialized lymphoid structures that occur in higher forms. In these early species there existed a primitive high

molecular weight antibody and cells that could manifest cell-mediated immunity. In the elasmobranchs, for example, a tissue transplant consisting of skin or scales would be promptly rejected. Similarly, the introduction of antigens into these species will elicit a high molecular weight antibody analogous to IgM immunoglobulin of higher forms (Chapter 5). During evolution, there occurred specialization of cells and supporting structures to house these tissues—the lymphoreticular tissues. The thymus is the earliest lymphoid organ to appear in phylogeny and is present in the most primitive of vertebrates. There also appeared in birds a separate anatomic structure arising from the primitive gut, the bursa of Fabricius, which is important in the development of cells that elaborate antibody in avian species. The mammalian equivalent of this organ is not known. In the human, it is useful to consider thymic-controlled tissues that elaborate cell-mediated events as *thymic-dependent* tissues and those that elaborate antibody under a separate influence as *thymic-independent* tissues. Both are important to our understanding of the maturation of immune responses and immunologic deficiency states of man.

The evolutionary order of appearance of immunoglobulin classes in many respects parallels that seen in the maturing individual (ontogeny). It also recapitulates the sequential appearance of immunoglobulin molecular forms that appear following a single antigenic exposure during the immune response (Chapter 7). These are shown in Figure 2–24. In the most primitive of vertebrates, the predominant antibody is a high molecular weight substance, analogous to the IgM globulins of the human. During phylogeny, a second class of antibody with properties similar to the IgG globulins is elaborated. The IgA immunoglobulins appear as rather late evolutionary events and are restricted to mammals. The development of a novel form of IgA immunoglobulin, the secretory IgA globulins, was also elucidated in mammals. This external antibody system has proved to be of immense importance in defense at body surfaces and appears to be a mechanism by which lower forms, such as the ungulates, receive passive antibody via colostrum. The major transfer of antibody in the human occurs primarily via the placenta; however, breast milk still continues to be a source of IgA antibody. This antibody is not absorbed by the infant's gastrointestinal tract but may be important locally within the intestine (coproantibody). Finally, still later additions seen in man are the IgD and the IgE immunoglobulins. The IgE immunoglobulins, seen also in other mammalian forms, are a unique class of antibody involved in immediate-type hypersensitivity.

With evolution there also occurred the development of an elaborate series of substances that could augment and enhance the efficiency of the ancient resistance mechanisms. These are referred to as biologic amplification systems and consist primarily of the coagulation and the complement systems (Chapter 6).

Development of the Immunologic System in the Developing Individual: Ontogeny of the Immune Response

Available evidence suggests that the maturation of the immune response in the human begins *in utero* sometime during the second to third months of gestation. The differentiation of cells destined to perform both nonspecific and specific immunologic functions seems to have a common ancestral origin. Both cell types appear to arise from a population of progenitor cells referred to as *stem cells* or *hemocytoblasts;* these are located within the hematopoietic tissues of the developing embryo (yolk sac, fetal liver, and bone marrow). Depending upon the type of microchemical environment surrounding the cells, development will occur along at least two avenues: the *hematopoietic* and the *lymphopoietic* (Fig. 2–25).

One type of microchemical environment leads to proliferation and differentiation of nonlymphoid stem cell hematopoietic precursors. The products of these cell lines are the hematopoietic elements of the peripheral blood and tissues and include the *erythrocytes, granulocytes, platelets,* and *monocytes.* The second set of progenitor cells are the stem cell lymphoid precursors that can differentiate along two pathways. The first, under the influence of the thymus, perhaps within the substance of the gland itself, includes a population of small lymphocytes that subserve the function of cell-mediated immunity (thymic-dependent or T-lymphocytes). If the lymphoid stem cells come under a second type of microchemical environment, i.e., bursal equivalent, differentiation will occur to produce a population of lymphocytes (B-lymphocytes) and plasma cells concerned with humoral immunity or antibody synthesis (Fig. 2–25).

The functional significance of this *two-compartment system* is important to clinical medicine. It provides a useful basis upon which our understanding of immunologic deficiency disorders rests. Thus, individuals displaying selective disorders of bursal equivalent tissues, the so-called aggammaglobulinemias or dysgammaglobulinemias, present with recurrent bacterial infections. Selective deficiencies of the thymic-dependent tissues, on the other hand, are also seen in man and are manifested with other types of infections, such as fungal and viral diseases. Still a third type of patient presents with combined deficiencies of both thymic-dependent and thymic-independent tissues. These individuals have profound deficiencies in both cell-mediated and antibody mediated functions and have the most serious sequelae of all the immunologic deficiency syndromes and present with a diversity of infections.

MATERNAL-FETAL RELATIONSHIPS

One of the most significant developments in phylogeny is the appearance of placentation in the species with the ability to bear live young (viviparity). This occurred in higher forms with the development of the multilayered placenta. One of the challenging problems in biology is the question of how a fetus, who inherits one half of its antigens from paternally controlled genes foreign to the mother, can be tolerated successfully during

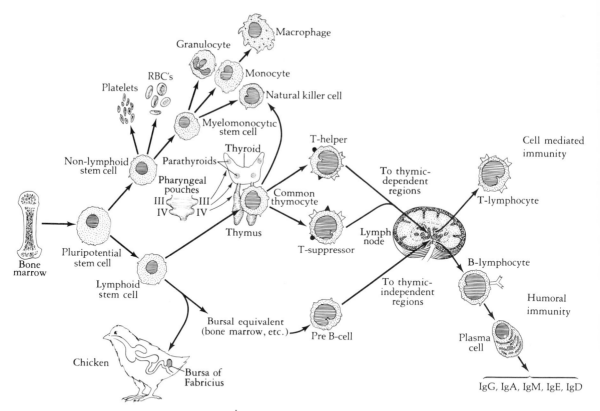

Figure 2–25. Schematic representation of ontogeny of immune response, showing differentiation of progenitor cells into hematopoietic and immunocompetent cells.

pregnancy. This has been attributed largely to the barrier function of the placenta. By acting as a mechanical barrier, the placenta usually effectively separates the formed elements of the blood of the mother from that of the fetus. There are elements, however, that do gain access to the fetus and provide protection—antibodies.

There are different pathways of transmission of maternal antibody to the fetus in different species (Table 2–7). In species with large numbers of membranes intervening between the maternal and fetal circulations, the colostral route seems to be a more important

mechanism of transfer. Conversely, as the number of layers of membrane decreases (as in man, for example), the transplacental route seems to assume greater importance. Thus, in man, the prodominant transfer of antibody occurs via the passage of the IgG immunoglobulins from the maternal circulation to that of the fetus. This is accomplished by means of an active transport mechanism of this immunoglobulin by virtue of a receptor located on the Fc fragment of the molecule (Chapter 5). In this manner, the fetus receives a library of preformed antibody from its mother, reflecting most of her ex-

Table 2–7. Relationship of Type of Placentation with Character of Maternal-Fetal Transfer of Antibody in Various Species

Animal	Number of Placental Membranes	Relative Importance of Route	
		Placental	Colostral
Horse	6	0	+ + +
Sheep, cow	5	0	+ + +
Cat, dog	5	+	+ +
Rat, mouse	4	+	+ +
Rabbit, guinea pig	3	+ + +	±
Man, monkey	3	+ + +	0

periences with infectious agents. Occasionally, fetal cells or other proteins may gain access to the maternal circulation and thus actively immunize her to the paternal allotypes (antigen) found on these substances. This process, referred to as isoimmunization, may lead to serious disease in the infant, such as hemolytic disease of the newborn, thrombocytopenia, and leukopenia.

The development of serum immunoglobulins during intrauterine life and postnatally is shown in Figure 2–26. If one analyzes the amount and type of gamma globulin found in the blood of the newborn infant at birth, one finds that the levels of immunoglobulin are equivalent to those of the mother and are made up almost exclusively of the IgG immunoglobulins. There is virtually little or no IgA and IgM globulin present in cord sera. This is because the fetus is usually protected *in utero* from antigenic stimuli. If the fetus is challenged *in utero* as a consequence of immunization or infection (e.g., congenital rubella, cytomegalic inclusion disease, toxoplasmosis), it will respond with antibody production largely of the IgM variety. The exclusion of other classes of antibody is beneficial to the fetus in many cases. For example, the exclusion of the IgM isohemagglutinins, leukoagglutinins, or the IgE antibodies of allergy prevents disease that may be produced by these antibodies. However, it also prevents the passage of other maternal antibodies that would be beneficial to the newborn, such as the IgM antibodies important in bacterial defense against gram-negative bacteria (opsonins, agglutinins, and bactericidal antibodies). This may explain, in part, the increased susceptibility of the newborn to infection with gram-negative organisms such as *Escherichia coli.*

Since the IgG immunoglobulins are passively transferred, they have a finite half-life of between 20 and 30 days, and therefore their concentration in serum falls rapidly within the first few months of life, reaching the lowest levels between the second and fourth months. This period is referred to as physiologic hypogammaglobulinemia. During the course of the first few years, the levels of gamma globulin increase because of exposure of the maturing infant to antigens in the environment. There appears to be a sequential development in gamma globulin at different rates. The IgM globulins attain adult levels by one year of age, the IgG globulins by five to six years of age, and the IgA globulins by ten years of age. This pattern of appearance of immunoglobulins recapitulates that seen in phylogeny and also appears to parallel that seen following an antigenic exposure during the primary immune response.

It is important to emphasize that the development of immunoglobulin receptors on lymphocytes during fetal life follows the same general pattern as that observed with the appearance of various immunoglobulins in the serum after birth (Table 2–8). It is notable that IgM is present on the surface of cells

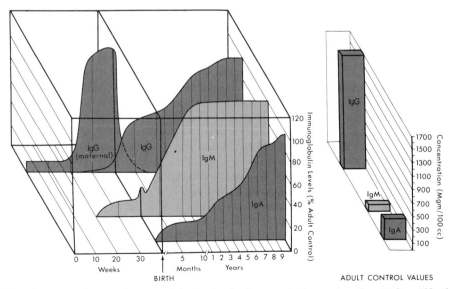

Figure 2–26. Development of serum immunoglobulins in the human during maturation. (After Alford, C. A., Jr.: Immunoglobulin determinations in the diagnosis of fetal infection. Pediatr. Clin. North Am., *18*:99, 1971.)

Table 2–8. Maturation of Human T- and B-Cells: Surface Markers and Lymphoproliferative Responses

| | | Serum Immunoglobulins | | | | | Responsiveness | | | | |
| | | | | | | | Mitogens | | | Antigens | |
	Age	IgM	IgG	IgA	IgD	IgE	PHA	Con-A	PWM	PPD	SK-SD
Fetal	10 weeks	−	−	−	−	−	+	−	−	−	−
	10.5 weeks	+	−	−	−	?	+	?	−	−	−
	12 weeks	+	+	−	−	?	+	+	−	−	−
	20 weeks	+	+	+	±	±	+	+	+	−	−
	Newborn	+	+	+	+	±	+	+	+	−	−
	Adult	+	+	+	+	+	+	+	+	+	+

as early as 10½ weeks. At birth, human immunocompetent cells have become fully responsive to mitogens (Table 2–8). (Mitogens such as phytohemagglutinin [PHA], concanavalin-A [Con-A], and pokeweed [PWM] are substances that will directly stimulate either B-or T-lymphocytes [Chapter 7].) However, the ability of cells to respond to specific antigens, such as tuberculin (PPD) or streptokinase-streptodornase (SK-SD), is limited. Only later do the lymphocytes develop the capability for cell-mediated responses against foreign antigens. Cell-mediated responses can also be measured *in vitro* by the development of lymphotoxin (LT) or macrophage inhibition factor (MIF) (Chapter 9). As can be seen in Table 2–9, at birth, cell-mediated responses are variable; LT can be produced, but MIF cannot.

From the very earliest fetal life, lymphocytes are present that can act both as responders to and stimulators of the mixed lymphocyte reaction (MLR) (Table 2–9). This suggests that the fetus can recognize transplantation antigens even before they can respond to any other foreign antigen, making all the more remarkable the inability of the fetus to react against its mother.

DEVELOPMENT OF THE IMMUNOLOGIC SYSTEM AT THE LEVEL OF THE WHOLE ORGANISM

It is now well established that the ability to respond to certain antigens is determined by the genetic constitution of the host (Chapter 3). Thus, selected strains of guinea pigs and mice fail to respond with antibody formation following immunization with normally immunogenic polypeptide antigens. The precise mechanism of this *nonresponder state* is not yet known, but is believed to be due to the suppression or deletion of genes important in immune responses.

Several studies in the mouse indicate an association between certain histocompatibility antigens and the ability to respond to immunogens (Chapter 3). Histocompatibility typing of mice allows the prediction of immune responsiveness to a wide variety of antigens other than histocompatibility antigens. The association between histocompatibility antigenic composition and immune responsiveness is under intensive study, and various data suggest that the expression of certain antigenic phenotypes may also be an expression of an individual immunologic responsiveness, e.g., association of HLA-B27 antigen with ankylosing spondylitis (Chapter 3).

In the human, the precise analog of this nonresponder state is not known. However, in certain of the immunologic deficiency states, such as the Wiskott-Aldrich syndrome, there is an inability to process certain polysaccharide antigens. It would seem reasonable that with the vast heterogeneity of the human species, variations in responsiveness from individual to individual would exist. Indeed, this appears to be the case and is manifested in clinical practice by the frequent encounter of individuals with susceptibility to infectious disease not expressed by other individuals. The susceptibility to certain autoimmune and malignant diseases is also known to occur in children with immunologic deficiency. A genetic basis may be involved in other hypersensitivity diseases of man. Only in certain individuals does acute glomerulonephritis or rheumatic fever occur following infection with Group A beta-hemolytic streptococci. This may be the human counterpart to the experimental model of serum sickness-type nephritis, which occurs after administration of repeated doses of bovine serum albumin to rabbits. Such animals could be divided into three groups: good antibody responders, moderate anti-

Table 2–9. Maturation of Human T- and B-Cells: Mixed Lymphocyte Responsiveness and Mediator Production

		MLR		Lymphokine	
	Age	Responder	Stimulator	LT	MIF
Fetal	7.5 weeks	+	+	−	−
	10 weeks	+	+	−	−
	12 weeks	+	+	−	−
	20 weeks	+	+	−	−
	Newborn	+	+	+	−
	Adult	+	+	+	+

body responders, and poor antibody responders. Limited disease was seen in the good and poor antibody responders; the most progressive and chronic forms of glomerulonephritis were seen in animals with moderate antibody production. This was presumably because of the development of antigen-antibody complexes injurious to their kidneys.

Development of the Immunologic System at the Cellular Level

Antigen itself may be considered as part of the cellular environment that induces the development of an immune responsiveness (Table 2–6). During the induction of an immune response, antigen comes in contact with an appropriate collection of lymphoid cells, following which a series of proliferative and differentiative steps are initiated (see Fig. 7–2). At the moment of presentation of antigen, at least two, and possibly three, cells are involved. The first is a macrophage, which in some cases is essential for the processing of antigen to a form that can interact with a second series of cells, those of lymphoid type. These latter cells can proliferate and differentiate to become immunocompetent cells, capable of antibody formation or cell-mediated events. Following removal of antigen, there is an involution of this population of immunocompetent cells. However, some cells remain as "memory" cells, capable of carrying out specific immunologic events during any future encounter with the same antigen. These consist of either B- or T-lymphocytes. The whole cellular burst of activity seen in the induction of an immune response may be analogous to genetically controlled differentiation seen in the development of the species or during ontogeny of the individual. The memory cells may be considered as the best adapted forms for this type of environment (Table 2–6).

These processes involve a variety of cell types. As described previously, the lymphoid cell populations that respond to antigens can basically be divided into two populations, the T- and B-lymphocytes, which can act independently as well as in cooperation to produce an immune response (Chapter 7). Specific antigen receptors exist on the surface of both T-cells and B-cells. Certain antigens can directly stimulate the B-cells so that they will subsequently produce plasma cells and antibody; other antigens require the interaction of T-cells, which provide specific and nonspecific helper substances that will allow the B-cell to mature to produce antibody. It is interesting to note that antigen, after processing by macrophages, can lead to the production of activators of helper T-cells. Further, these macrophages must be syngeneic to the T-cells in order for the help to occur. Subsequent to activation, the T-lymphocytes produce factors that can trigger the B-cells (Chapter 9). A separate population of T-lymphocytes can also act to suppress the immune response, i.e., suppressor T-lymphocytes. This appears to involve active processes in the suppression of helper T-cells.

The interaction of T-cells, in both their helper and suppressor functions, is under strict genetic control, which is mediated by genes that are located within the major histocompatibility complex. These immune response (IR) genes are related to histocompatibility identity between the various cell types involved in the immune response (Chapter 3). Immunoregulation and the multiple interactions between specific cell types are only now beginning to be understood.

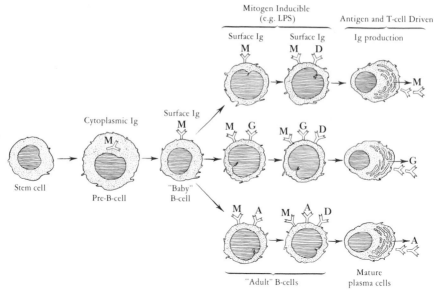

Figure 2–27. Ontogeny of B-lymphocyte system. (Adapted from Cooper, M. D., and Seligmann, M.: B and T lymphocytes in immunodeficiency and lymphoproliferative diseases. *In* Loor, F. and Roelants, G. E. (eds.): B and T Cells in Immune Recognition. West Sussex, England, John Wiley & Sons Ltd., 1977.)

The future directions of clinical immunology will, we hope, provide for the unraveling of these complex events. In the meantime, the clinician must deal with diseases that result from genetic failure to regulate immune response at each level of interaction.

Based upon evidence obtained from the human and experimental animal, Cooper and his coworkers have proposed a model of B-cell differentiation (Fig. 2–27). In this model, B-cells differentiate from a stem cell to a pre–B cell that initially expresses only cytoplasmic IgM. The next stage is represented by a cell expressing surface IgM receptors only. This "Baby B-cell" is a pivotal cell for further differentiation of cells that produce immunoglobulins. After this, two stages of differentiation exist: (1) an antigen-independent stage responsive to mitogen, and (2) an antigen-dependent T-cell driven stage that requires the presence of an IgD surface marker lost after antigenic stimulation.

To summarize, the whole of the immune response appears to be under developmental (genetic) influences. These range from the controls exerted on the evolving species (phylogeny) to those imposed on the maturing individual (ontogeny), the controls exerted within an individual and on the cell and cell products. Both immune responsiveness and unresponsiveness should be considered as genetic processes. This approach to immunology may better enable the physician to appreciate the pathogenesis of many immunologically mediated diseases, their transmissions within families, and their expected reappearances in future offspring.

Suggestions for Further Reading

Anatomic and Functional Organization of the Immune System

Bloom, W., and Fawcett, D. W. (eds.): A Textbook of Histology. 10th ed., Philadelphia, W. B. Saunders Company, 1975.

Cline, M. J. (ed): The White Cell. Cambridge, Harvard University Press, 1975.

Dingle, J. T., and Dean, R. T. (eds.): Lysosomes in Biology and Pathology. New York, American Elsevier Publishing Company, 1976.

Fauci, A. S.: The idiopathic hypereosinophilic syndrome: clinical, pathophysiologic and therapeutic considerations. Ann. Intern. Med., 97:78, 1982.

Gabrieli, E. R., and Snell, F. M.: Reflection of reticuloendothelial function in studies of blood clearance kinetics. J. Reticuloendothel. Soc., 2:141, 1965.

Van Furth, R. (ed.): Mononuclear Cells in Immunity, Infection, and Pathology. Oxford, Blackwell Scientific Publications, 1975.

Weiss, L. (ed.): Cells and Tissues of the Immune System: Structure, Functions, Interactions. Englewood Cliff, N.J., Prentice-Hall, Inc., 1972.

Chemotaxis, Phagocytosis, Metabolic Changes, and Antimicrobial Systems of Phagocytic Cells

Bellanti, J. A., and Dayton, D. H. (eds.): The Phagocytic Cell in Host Resistance. New York, Raven Press, 1975.

Cline, M. J. (ed.): The White Cell. Cambridge, Harvard University Press, 1975.

DeChalelet, L. R.: Oxidative bacterial mechanisms of polymorphonuclear leukocytes. J. Infect. Dis., *131*: 295, 1975.

Specific Immune Response

Gell, P. G. H., Coombs, R. R. A., and Lachman, P. T.: Clinical Aspects of Immunology. Oxford, Blackwell Scientific Publications, 1975.

Roitt, I. M.: Essential Immunology. Oxford, Blackwell Scientific Publications, 1974.

Stites, D. P., Stobo, J. D., Fudenberg, H. H., et al.: Basic and Clinical Immunology. 4th ed. Los Altos, Lange Medical Publications, 1982.

Suskind, R. M. (ed.): Malnutrition and the Immune Response. Kroc Foundation Series, Vol. 7. New York, Raven Press, 1977.

Phylogeny and Ontogeny

Cooper, E. L. (ed.): Contemporary Topics in Immunobiology. Vol. 4. Invertebrate Immunology. Plenum Publishing Corp., 1974.

Cooper, M. D., and Dayton, D. H. (eds.): Development of Host Defenses. New York, Raven Press, 1977.

Cooper, M. D., and Seligmann, M.: B and T lymphocytes in immunodeficiency and lymphoproliferative diseases. *In* Loor, F., and Roelants, G. E. (eds.): B and T cells in Immune Recognition. West Sussex, England, John Wiley & Sons Ltd., 1977.

Friedman, H. (ed.): Thymus factors in immunity. Ann. N.Y. Acad. Sci., *249*:1–547, 1975.

Reinherz, E. L., and Schlossman, S. F.: Regulation of the immune response-inducer and suppressor T-lymphocyte subsets in human beings. N. Engl. J. Med., *303*:1153, 1980.

Stites, D. P., Caldwell, J., Carr, M. C., et al.: Ontogeny of immunity in humans. Clin. Immunol. Immunopathol., *4*:519, 1975.

Chapter 3

Immunogenetics

James N. Woody, Capt., M.C., U.S.N., M.D., Ph.D.,
Joseph A. Bellanti, M.D., and Kenneth W. Sell, M.D., Ph.D.

INTRODUCTION

Immunogenetics include all those processes concerned in the immune response that may have a *genetic* basis. In the past, the term has been largely restricted to mean genetic markers on immunoglobulin polypeptide chains. In the light of recent developments, a more contemporary definition of immunogenetics should include *all the factors that control the immunologic responsiveness of the host to foreignness, as well as the transmission of antigenic specificities from generation to generation.*

Immune mechanisms may be viewed from an evolutionary standpoint as a series of genetic adaptations by the evolving species to changing environmental influences exerted upon it (Chapter 2). This has been referred to as *phylogeny* of the immune response. Similarly, the maturation of the immune mechanisms within the developing individual may be considered, and this has been termed *ontogeny* of the immune response. In a narrower sense, the genetic controls can be regarded at a cellular level as the proliferation and differentiation of a variety of cell types in response to antigen (Chapter 7). The action of genes can also be studied at the molecular level in terms of the unlimited variability of immunoglobulin structures that are directly encoded within DNA (Chapter 5). The heritability of antigens themselves, such as the blood group and histocompatibility antigens, is also transmitted within the chromosomes of the germ cells. Finally, of considerable importance are the recent discoveries indicating that the genes that control the expression of certain cellular antigens are nearly identical to those that control immune responsiveness.

The field of immunogenetics can be divided into two broad areas of study. The first major area concerns the genetic regulation and control of the immune system itself. Genes coding for immunoglobulins, the major histocompatibility (MHC) antigens, and the T-cell receptor(s), as well as genes coding for other mediators, interact in regulating and fostering an effective immune response. The second area with the broadest application is the use of antibodies and sensitized immune cells, the products of the immune system, as probes to detect and characterize various antigens that may show genetic variation, i.e., polymorphism. Over the past decade the analytic power of these immunologic probes has increased immensely as they have been used to study the more polymorphic genetic systems, such as the HLA or H-2 histocompatibility systems, blood groups, immunoglobulins, and complement proteins as well as cell surface glycoprotein antigens. The routine availability of exquisitely specific monoclonal antibodies (Chapter 5) and the capacity to prepare T-lymphocyte clones with an equivalent degree of specificity have fostered studies in research disciplines within and outside of immunology. Further, many of these reagents have rapidly found utility as clinical diagnostic reagents, e.g., for the detection of cell surface glycoproteins such as OKT4, which allow the identification of human T-lymphocytes as helper/inducer cells (Chapter 7). Equally important are the monoclonal antibodies capable of recognizing genetic variants of bacteria and viruses, e.g., differentiation between herpes simplex Type I and Type II. The use of sensitized cells as probes is currently limited to the detection of Class II histocompatibility (HLA) antigens with a mixed lymphocyte culture format; however, this will probably expand to include a variety of antigens.

CLINICAL IMPORTANCE OF IMMUNOGENETICS

A knowledge of the tools available, as well as their application, is essential for a thorough understanding of many clinical problems. The major blood group antigens are characterized by antibodies that detect polymorphic determinants; likewise, the human histocompatibility antigens, HLA, are defined by antibodies that detect small changes in these cell surface glycoproteins, which are coded for by the allelic genes at each of the HLA loci. The discovery of the association between HLA types and certain disease states was made possible by the use of antibody detection systems. Similar technologies are being used for diagnosis, treatment, and follow-up of clinical entities in nearly every phase of medicine, ranging from infectious diseases to oncology.

Studies on the development and functioning of the immune system have application to many clinical conditions. The maturation or ontogeny of the immune cells in a given individual is an example of genetic control of cellular proliferation and differentiation. Interruptions or alterations of these developmental sequences lead to immunodeficiency disorders, autoimmune disorders, and perhaps malignancies, as the cells escape the influence of their normal control mechanism(s). The age and maturational level at which the immune cells are of sufficient maturity to react to complex vaccine antigens, such as the polysaccharide vaccine determinants, are a function of the genetic control of this maturational process.

Genetic variability within individuals may determine their ability to respond to a vaccine or a natural infection. Studies in these areas are assuming great importance, especially as recombinant DNA and synthetic vaccines, consisting of small peptides, are being considered as third-generation vaccines. Interestingly, the histocompatibility-linked immune response genes were discovered in the evaluation of antibody responses to small peptide determinants, and animals were divided into high- and low-responder strains, based on their ability to produce antibodies to synthetic peptides (Chapter 4). The widespread use of small synthetic peptides as vaccines might segregate individuals into high and low responders, based on their genetic backgrounds. This can, of course, be overcome with proper vaccine construction; however, an understanding of the immunogenetic processes involved in generating an effective response is essential.

Genetic variation that yields exaggerated immune responses may lead to harmful consequences, such as anti-platelet antibodies in idiopathic thrombocytopenic purpura (ITP), or autoimmune islet cell destruction during the onset of diabetes in susceptible individuals. These hyperresponsive states, some of which are associated with certain HLA phenotypes, as will be described later, point out a need for a clear understanding of immunogenetics.

A knowledge of family genetic susceptibility to allergic rhinitis may aid the pediatrician in arriving at a correct diagnosis of milk allergy in an infant who presents with gastrointestinal colic (Fig. 3–1).

Effective organ and bone marrow transplantation requires a knowledge of the genetic control of histocompatibility antigens and how these antigens are transmitted within families. Many of the current transplant problems, including transplant rejec-

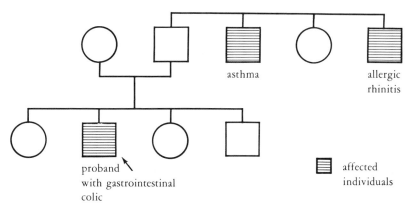

Figure 3–1. Pedigree of an infant who presented with gastrointestinal colic, showing other allergic disorders within the kindred.

asthma

allergic rhinitis

proband with gastrointestinal colic

affected individuals

tion and graft-versus-host disease, derive from an insufficient understanding of the immune system, its ontogeny, and its immunoregulatory networks. Several novel therapies, such as multiple blood transfusion prior to kidney transplantation, seem to enhance graft survival; however, such treatment regimens have poorly understood effects on the immune system, some of which may relate to genetically controlled immune responses. The impact of such drugs as cyclosporine A on graft survival appears promising; however, its impact on the entire immune network has yet to be defined. Studies on the association of HLA antigens and certain diseases suggest that "susceptibility genes" lie nearby. These leads, now strengthened and advanced by the innovative use of c-DNA (complementary DNA) probes to detect unique HLA gene sequences and restriction enzyme fragment length polymorphisms in susceptible individuals, pave the way for identifying immunoregulatory "disease susceptibility genes" at the DNA level, and open the door to understanding important pathophysiologic mechanisms of disease.

GENETICS OF IMMUNE REGULATION

The immune system is a complex network of cells that interact by direct contact and through soluble mediators. The goal of the network is to provide effective immunity for the organism and to prevent harmful internal events. A large number of genes (collectively called immune response or IR genes) exist that code for the regulatory components of the network. It was originally thought that the genes controlling the immune response were located within the genetic segment coding for histocompatibility antigens. Although the histocompatibility-linked IR genes certainly play an important role, they compose only a part of the system. Certain IR genes may code for cellular receptors for antigen as seen with the immunoglobulin molecules, which act as receptors on the surface of B-cells. The genes coding for receptors on T-cells, recently identified, are similar to immunoglobulin genes and compose a third large set of polymorphic genes. Other genes may control mediator secretion or cellular receptors. In this way, a multigenic system controls not only the ability to respond to antigens but also the level and duration of the response.

Disorders of this immunoregulatory network, whether genetic or environmental, can lead to serious consequences ranging from an inability to respond to antigenic exposure (hyporesponsive), as seen in patients with acquired immunodeficiency syndrome (AIDS), to autoimmune disorders such as systemic lupus erythematosus (hyperresponsive). Interestingly, the entire network must be effectively blocked before a foreign kidney, heart, or liver can be successfully engrafted. This iatrogenic intervention must be extremely skillful in order to avoid serious consequences. The future may see the development of innovative schemes to gently perturb this network. Examples might include the short-term blocking of T-cell surface receptors for antigen or interleukin-2, or other mediators using antibodies or receptor-binding drugs.

This chapter will focus on the major histocompatibility systems in mice (H-2) and in man (HLA) as well as on the blood group antigens and will describe their clinical relevance. Immunoglobulin genetics is described in Chapter 5; a discussion of the genetics of the T-cell receptor polymorphisms is, at best, preliminary.

THE MAJOR HISTOCOMPATIBILITY COMPLEX

The major histocompatibility complex (MHC) is a chromosomal region consisting of a series of genes that code for the cell surface expression of strong transplantation antigens. These transplantation antigens are, in general, glycoproteins that are present on the surface of most nucleated cells. The MHC in mammals is also the region where the histocompatibility-linked immune response (IR) genes are located; hence, this chromosomal segment not only controls the synthesis of the transplantation antigens and graft rejection, but also influences immune responses to infectious challenge and susceptibility to the development of immunologically mediated diseases. The two MHC systems that have been most extensively characterized are the H-2 system in the mouse and the HLA (human leukocyte antigen) system in man.

The MHC's of all mammals studied are remarkably similar; in fact, amino acid sequence homology of transplantation antigens between mouse, man, and other species is high, suggesting an evolutionary pressure for conservation of these genetic regions. The genes of the MHC in all animals thus far studied code for two general types of transplantation antigens, Class I and Class II. The complement components (Chapter 6), some of which are coded for by genes in the MHC region, have sometimes been referred to as Class III antigens.

Class I Antigens

The Class I antigen consists of a large transmembrane glycoprotein of about 350 amino acids (44K molecular weight) noncovalently associated with beta-2 microglobulin, a 100–amino acid, 12K molecular weight protein. The beta-2 microglobulin protein is coded for by genes on a separate chromosome from those coding for the Class I heavy chains. The arrangement of these molecules on the cell surface is shown schematically in Figure 3–2.

In humans, three structural genes on chromosome 6 code for the Class I type antigens. The HLA-A, HLA-B, and HLA-C genes code for the 44K heavy-chain portion of the molecule. Each of the HLA-A, -B, or -C genes has multiple alleles (i.e., alternate forms of the gene at each locus). For this reason, the HLA genes have been termed polymorphic, and each of the alleles of a particular locus has been numerically designated; for example, HLA-A1, HLA-A2, HLA-A3, and so forth represent alleles of the HLA-A gene. For a tentative assignment, the prefix "w" (workshop) has been assigned (e.g., HLA-

Bw47) to indicate that it is under consideration for acceptance as a formal allele.

In mice there are three genes on chromosome 17 within the mouse H-2 histocompatibility region that code for Class I antigens. These genes have been named K, D, and L; two other genes adjacent to the region, Qa and TLa, also code for Class I–like antigens (Fig. 3–3). The mouse and human Class I antigens are structurally similar, with 60 to 70 per cent of the amino acid sequence showing identity. This similarity has now been confirmed with the DNA sequencing technology.

The allelic Class I products are found on most nucleated cells, exceptions being sperm and trophoblastic cells, and are generally detected by their reactivity with human or mouse alloantisera. Lymphocytes are commonly used for the detection or typing because they are easily obtainable. Since the Class I antigens are similar in the mouse and human systems, the function of the Class I antigens will be described under the murine H-2 genes.

Class II Antigens

The Class II antigens consist of two noncovalently associated glycoproteins (alpha and beta chains) of about 34 and 29K molecular weights, respectively (Fig. 3–2). In humans, at least three genes have been identified that code for Class II antigens, although several more candidates currently exist. The

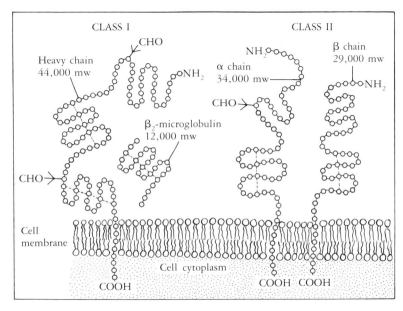

Figure 3–2. Schematic representation of Class I and Class II histocompatibility antigens within the cell membrane. Class I type glycoprotein antigens are coded for by HLA-A, B, and C genes in humans, and by H-2 K, D, L, Qa, and TLa genes in mice. Class II antigens are coded for by HLA-DR, DC, and SB genes in humans, and by IA and IE genes in mice.

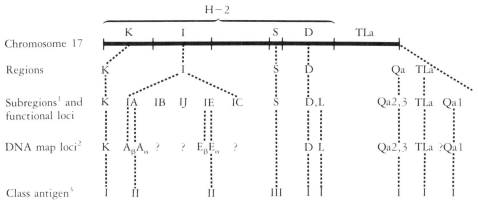

Figure 3–3. Schematic of the mouse H-2 region. (1) Subregions and functional loci were mapped by analysis with recombinant mice and by using functional immune assays such as antibody production, cellular proliferation, or delayed-type hypersensitivity reactions. (2) DNA-mapped loci were determined using DNA sequence analysis to map the position of the genes coding for their respective glycoproteins. (3) It is generally thought that the function of the Class I molecules is to serve as target antigens for immune recognition and killing. The function of the Class II antigen is to serve as restricting molecules for cellular recognition and regulatory events.

three have been designated DR, DC(DS), and SB. In mice, the genes coding for Class II antigens were mapped to a segment in the H-2 MHC called the immune (I) region (Fig. 3–3). Loci that code for the Class II antigens are prefaced by the letter I to designate this region; I-A and I-E represent the structural genes verified by DNA sequence analysis, while IB, IJ, and IC are putative genes, their location having been proposed based on functional assays. These cell surface Class II glycoprotein molecules in mice are collectively termed Ia (immune-associated) antigens, a term often used to refer to either mouse or human Class II antigens. As with the Class I antigens, a high degree of structural similarity exists between mouse and human Class II antigens. In fact, c-DNA probes made to human Class II genes have been used to identify mouse Class II genes. Since the Class II antigens are made up of two chains, alpha and beta, two genes are necessary to code for a single Class II antigen. Gene probes are currently being used to determine the precise location and relationship of the genes. Recent studies suggest that several types of alpha chains may combine with various beta chains to make cell surface "hybrid" molecules.

Using standard tests, some of the Class II antigens can be serologically detected; others are recognized only by T-lymphocytes, which proliferate in response to the foreign Class II determinants. The latter type antigens have been termed lymphocyte-defined or LD antigens, to designate the need for cellular recognition in detection, although in many cases antibodies have been found that bind to the same or similar determinants recognized by the typing cells.

The Class III antigens, or complement components, are discussed in Chapter 6.

MHC of Mice (H-2)

The MHC of mice has been extensively studied and has provided crucial information for our understanding of the human MHC. There are several reasons why the murine MHC has received a great deal of attention.

Some of the early studies on skin graft transplantation survival in mice, for which Sir Peter Medewar was awarded a Nobel Prize, launched the current era of immunogenetics. Transplantation of organs or tissues between nonidentical mouse strains invariably led to rejection of the graft, which was shown to be dependent on the number of genetic differences between animals. It was subsequently learned that certain cell surface antigens, termed histocompatibility antigens, were important in graft rejection. Of the many genetic loci coding for histocompatibility antigens, the H-2 locus was found to be the strongest, although several weaker antigens exist. For several reasons the murine system represented an ideal model for studying the role of these genes, their gene products, and the associated interactions.

1. Inbred strains of mice have been developed and maintained for many years; hence, they are uniform and genetically stable.

2. Because of their rapid breeding cycle,

large numbers of genetically identical animals can be obtained. In studying genetically controlled events, such as graft rejection, it is essential to perform the experiments with a significant number (five to ten animals per experimental group) of genetically identical animals; otherwise, the results would not be statistically valid and it would be impossible to assign functions to specific loci.

3. Inasmuch as the breeding time for mice is very short, one can perform crosses and mapping studies to determine the precise locations of genetic traits.

4. A number of co-isogeneic or congeneic strains have been developed that are genetically identical to a parent strain except for a small section of chromosome. Of particular interest are those with the same parental "background" genes except for the MHC, or H-2 region, and those with small changes within the H-2 region itself. When tested, these strains allow investigators to precisely assign immunologic functions to various loci and provide insight into immune interactions, as demonstrated in Table 3–1. Once defined in the murine system, human counterparts can be sought.

The H-2 region in the mouse is located on chromosome 17 and covers a length of DNA equivalent to 0.5 recombinant units. A schematic representation is shown in Figure 3–3, in which the K, D and L, Qa and TL genes code for Class I antigens, and the I region genes code for Class II antigens.

TERMINOLOGY

Inbred strains of mice are bred to be genetically uniform, their Class I and Class II antigen alleles having been studied and defined using serologic tests such as cytotoxicity and red cell agglutination. The H-2 genes are very polymorphic, with perhaps 50 alleles at each of the H-2K or H-2D loci. These alleles are numbered based on serologic detection. Each inbred strain of mice inherits the MHC genes as a group having a complex but limited group of alleles. It has become standard practice to designate the allelic specificities of the entire H-2 complex by a single, small-script letter; therefore, the CBA strain of mice are designated H-2^k type, which represents a unique sequence of 20 to 30 serologically defined Class I and Class II alleles (antigens). Other strains of mice have a different set of alleles and are designated by different letters, such as the Balb/c strain, which has been designated H-2^d, while the C57 Black 6 is H-2^b. Several of the strains may share a particular set of alleles; hence, the H-2^k strains of mice include not only CBA but also C$_3$H and AKR. In general, skin grafts may be successfully transplanted between strains of the same H-2 type, although slow rejection may occur owing to weaker histocompatibility antigens not associated with the H-2 complex. Of special interest are the congeneic strains, in which the background genes may derive from an H-2^b or other strains, while the H-2 genes come from an H-2^k or alternate strain. Special strains have been prepared with "isolation" of each of the subregion genes, allowing investigators to assign a specific function for that subregion locus. Such a mapping study, using the H-2 congeneic strains, is demonstrated in Table 3–1.

FUNCTION OF CLASS I ANTIGENS: MICE

What appears to be the major function of the H-2K, D, and L Class I antigens on the

Table 3–1. Mapping of the Murine Genetic Region that Controls Macrophage-T Interactions for Helper Cell Induction Using Congeneic Strains of Mice

Antigen	Macrophage Source	H-2 of Macrophage						T Cell Source	H-2 of T-cells						Antibody Response*
		K	IA	IB	IC	Ss	D		K	IA	IB	IC	Ss	D	
KLH	None			—				CBA	k	k	k	k	k	k	73
+	CBA	k	k	k	k	k	k	"							305
+	B10.A	k	k	k	d	d	d	"				"			293
+	B10.A (4R)	k	k	b	b	b	b	"				"			263
+	A.TL	s	k	k	k	k	d	"				"			327
+	AQR	q	k	k	d	d	d	"				"			303
+	B10.D2	d	d	d	d	d	d	"				"			63
+	B10	b	b	b	b	b	b	"				"			70

*Antibody response is measured as antibody-forming cells per culture.

In this experiment, macrophages must cooperate with T-cells to produce T-helper cells, which, in turn, promote an antibody response when mixed with B-cells. Since the B10.A (4R) and AQR macrophages were able to cooperate with the CBA-T cells, the genes controlling or "restricting" this interaction are mapped to the IA region. (From Erb, P., and Feldmann, M. J.: Exp. Med., *142*:460, 1975. Reproduced with permission.)

cell surface was clarified by the work of Zinkernagel and Doherty, who initially showed that these products are necessary for immune T-cell recognition of specific target antigens. They used as their main model the cellular killing of virus-infected targets, demonstrating that vaccinia-specific cytotoxic T-lymphocytes from CBA mice ($H-2^k$) would kill vaccinia-infected targets that exhibited $H-2^k$ Class I antigens, but not targets that had $H-2^b$ Class I antigens. A similar phenomenon has been observed by Shearer and co-workers using chemicals such as TNP attached to cells. This observation of "genetic restriction" for cytotoxic or killer cells has fostered two hypotheses in explanation,

which are schematically outlined in Figure 3–4. The first, termed altered self, assumes that the virus or chemical modifies the Class I molecule so that it presents a new antigenic determinant (neoantigen); i.e., self is altered. This hypothesis uses a single receptor on the cytotoxic cell to recognize the neoantigen, which then initiates killing of the virus-infected target.

The second hypothesis is called dual recognition and postulates that the cytotoxic cell has two separate receptors: one that recognizes the virus or chemical, and a second that is specific for the self–Class I molecules, "restricting determinant," such as H-2K or H-2D, the binding of both receptors being re-

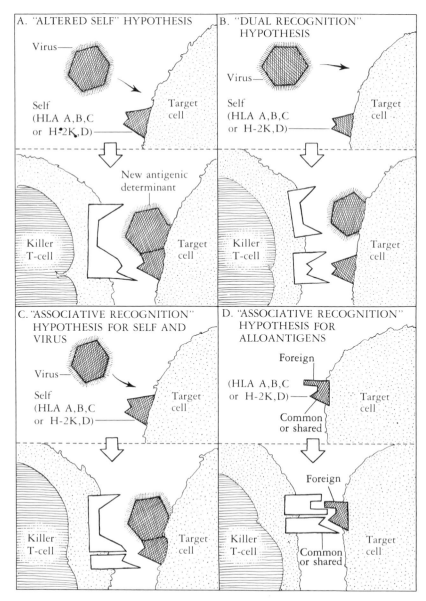

Figure 3–4. Schematic representation of the role played by Class I histocompatibility antigens in T-cell recognition of virally infected cells and allogeneic cells. Two major theories—"altered self" and "dual recognition"—are depicted. A third possibility—"associative recognition"— utilizes portions of both theories. Panel D depicts recognition of "foreign" HLA antigens, as might occur in transplantation rejection, using the "associative recognition" model of receptor interaction.

quired for cell killing. A third "hybrid" hypothesis, recently put forward by Reinherz and Schlossman, using human cytotoxic cells, favors the concept that the antigen-specific receptor displays two major recognition units; one recognizes viral antigen attached to a small, unique portion of self–Class I (altered self), while a second receptor recognizes a "shared" portion of the Class I molecule common to all Class I molecules. This is shown schematically in Figure 3–4, panel D. This associative recognition would account for killing of virus-infected and hapten-modified cells as well as HLA or H-2 incompatible cells, where the target antigen itself may be a Class I alloantigen, as described below.

The Class I antigens were originally defined as strong transplant antigens that serve as targets in graft rejection. Such rejection can be mediated either by antibody, as the foreign Class I antigens evoke a strong antibody response, or by cytotoxic cells that recognize the foreign Class I antigens (Fig. 3–4). Class II antigens can also serve as targets for antibody or cellular recognition and also play a role in graft rejection, as will be discussed later.

FUNCTION OF CLASS II ANTIGENS: MICE

The Class II antigens are coded for by genes located within the I (immune) region of the murine MHC complex (see Fig. 3–3). At one time it was thought that this region contained several sets of genes, some of which coded for products known as immune-associated or Ia antigens, and others that controlled immune responses, the histocompatibility or H-2–linked IR genes. More recently, it has been suggested that the IR genes and the Ia genes are the same, the Class II antigens then representing the IR gene products. The functional activities in which the Class II antigens are involved may be divided into several categories, including immune responsiveness, immune suppression, cellular recognition, and cellular interactions. Dr. Benacerraf, of Harvard University, recently received the Nobel Prize for his work in this field.

IMMUNE RESPONSIVENESS

Since the first studies by McDevitt and Tyan 15 years ago, showing linkage of immune responses to the MHC of mice, the number of immune functions ascribed to the H-2 I region genes has been substantial. The early studies, using inbred mouse strains and small synthetic polypeptides, showed clearly that certain autosomal dominant genes controlled the ability of an animal to initiate a cell-mediated or an antibody-mediated response to the peptide antigens. The immune responsiveness was usually relative, and strains were designated as "high" or "low" responders. In general, the responses were functionally measured by capacity to produce antibody, ability of the T-lymphocytes to proliferate, or delayed-type hypersensitivity reactions. A number of excellent reviews, listed at the end of the chapter, detail these studies, which will be briefly outlined here.

The initial step in immune responsiveness, whether measured by antibody production, cellular proliferation, or delayed-type hypersensitivity, requires that antigen be processed and "presented." The cells able to perform this function are those that exhibit surface expression of Class II (Ia) antigens (Chapter 7). In the murine system, presenting cells with Ia antigens include macrophages, dendritic cells, B-cells, and other cell types. The antigen must be "expressed" on the surface either attached to, or nearby, the appropriate Ia molecule. Certain animals that are "nonresponders" are unable to display or effectively "present" certain antigens. Whether the defect is in the type of Class II molecule or in the antigen processing is not clear.

The second step in immune responsiveness appears to be the recognition of the Ia molecule-antigen complex by T-lymphocytes. These T-lymphocytes have been termed helper cells, since they induce B-cells or other cell types into activity. The T-lymphocytes, which in murine systems do not have surface Class II antigens, must have a receptor(s) for the Ia molecule-antigen complex, which triggers proliferation and clone expansion. The structures that the T-cell uses to recognize the processed antigen are schematically shown in Figure 3–5.

The capacity to recognize the various antigens and the critical portions of the Class II molecules, in order to initiate activation, is selected for in the thymus during ontogeny. A nonresponder animal may have T-cells unable to recognize the antigen, the critical Ia antigen, or the complex. This gap in clonal repertoire may be responsible for certain nonresponsive states.

The transmission of information from T-

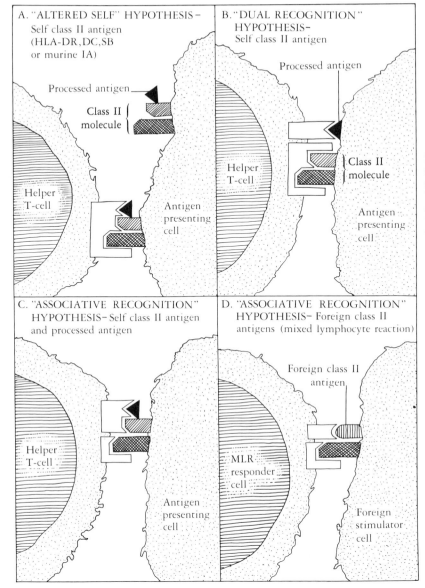

A. "ALTERED SELF" HYPOTHESIS –
Self class II antigen
(HLA-DR,DC,SB
or murine IA)

Processed antigen

Class II
molecule

Helper
T-cell

Helper
T-cell

Antigen
presenting
cell

B. "DUAL RECOGNITION"
HYPOTHESIS–
Self class II antigen

Processed antigen

Helper
T-cell

Class II
molecule

Antigen
presenting
cell

C. "ASSOCIATIVE RECOGNITION"
HYPOTHESIS– Self class II antigen
and processed antigen

Helper
T-cell

Antigen
presenting
cell

D. "ASSOCIATIVE RECOGNITION"
HYPOTHESIS– Foreign class II
antigens (mixed lymphocyte reaction)

Foreign class II
antigen

MLR
responder
cell

Foreign
stimulator
cell

Figure 3–5. Schematic representation of the role of Class II antigen in cellular interactions. The major theories of "altered self" and "dual recognition" as well as "associative recognition" can account for the recognition of antigen on the surface of antigen-presenting cells. The associative recognition concept has one receptor recognizing a public portion of the Class II molecule shared by all such molecules and another receptor that recognizes the antigen that is complexed or adjacent to the Class II molecule. Panel D depicts the model that might occur in recognition of foreign Class II antigens, as is seen in the mixed lymphocyte reaction (MLR).

cells to B-cells can occur by cell-cell contact or via "factors." The various augmenting factors, including "antigen-specific helper" factor and "allogeneic effect" factor, have, in some cases, been shown to contain portions of Class II molecules; others, such as "T-cell replacing factor," do not. How the interaction proceeds is unclear at present; however, it is apparent that the Class II molecules may play a regulatory role in this interaction.

In addition to the macrophage-T and T-B interactions, the early activation of cells that amplify the generation of cytotoxic or killer cells requires macrophages that express the Class II molecules (Chapter 7).

IMMUNE SUPPRESSION

Besides helper T-cells that augment the activities of other cells, there is another class of T-cells that manifest the opposite effect, i.e., the ability to suppress a specific immune response. Several types of T-suppressor cells have been identified and are grouped into those that suppress antibody responses by inhibiting T-helper cells and those that suppress other functional types. The early work with antigen-specific suppressor cells to the synthetic antigens GAT and GT provided information suggesting that the activity of these cells was controlled by genes in the I region. Further studies suggested that both the suppressor cells and the suppressive factors they secreted contained Class II determinants coded for by the functionally defined IJ subregion. The role of these IJ molecules in the suppressive event has not yet been clarified. It is apparent, however, that the generation of suppressor cells requires a complex series of cellular interactions.

Cellular Recognition

In several immunologic systems, cells recognize the presence of Class II antigens on other cells. These may include mixed lymphocyte culture, graft rejection, and graft-versus-host disease.

MIXED LYMPHOCYTE CULTURE

The mixed lymphocyte culture (MLR) represents a reaction in which lymphocytes from strain A are mixed with lymphocytes from strain B, the latter having been irradiated or treated with mitomycin C so that they cannot divide. Under this "one-way" mixed lymphocyte culture condition, strain B cells serve only as "stimulator cells," as they are unable to proliferate. During a five- to seven-day incubation, the strain A "responder cells" undergo blast transformation and cell division that can be measured by the incorporation of tritiated thymidine into new DNA. The stimulator cells in this situation express Class II antigens on their surface that are recognized by the responder cells. The strongest (most stimulatory) Class II antigens are coded for by IA genes, although other I region products and some non–MHC linked gene products (mls) induce significant stimulation. The cells bearing these Class II antigens are generally macrophages, dendritic cells, and B-cells. The recognition of foreign Class II antigens by the MLR responder cell is schematically shown in Figure 3–5D; it is discussed in human HLA-D region typing under Figure 3–10.

GRAFT REJECTION

Transplantation of organs or grafts between nonidentical strains of mice result in rejection. The strongest effect (shortest graft survival) is seen when grafts are exchanged between mice nonidentical at the H-2 locus. The use of H-2 recombinant mice has al-lowed investigators to map the most influential genes to the K, D, and I regions. It is thought that the MLR reaction is the initiator of the rejection process and that the MLR reactive cells amplify or help in the development of cytotoxic effector cells that are targeted for both the H-2K and D Class I antigens and the I region antigens. A similar event has been documented in human kidney transplantation, in which killer cells to Class I (HLA-A,B,C) and to Class II (HLA-DR) antigens have been observed.

GRAFT-VERSUS-HOST DISEASE

It has generally been assumed that the graft-versus-host disease represents an *in vivo* correlation of the MLR, with donor T-cells recognizing foreign Class II antigens on the macrophages and dendritic cells of the irradiated recipient. In mapping studies, the IA gene products appear to induce the strongest GVHD, although Class I antigens may also participate. As in graft rejection, the *in vivo* cellular events are complex, with the generation of proliferative and cytotoxic cells that may be targeted to cells carrying either Class I or Class II antigens.

Immune Response Genes

In the early 1960's, it was learned that certain autosomal dominant genes controlled the ability of an animal to develop antibodies to certain small synthetic peptide antigens. McDevitt found that the genes controlling the immune response in mice were mapped to the H-2 complex.

Subsequent studies using congeneic mice further mapped the genes to the I region within the H-2 complex. These genes were designated histocompatibility-linked immune response or H-2 IR genes. Sometime later, it was shown that the I region genes coded for Class II antigens, which were termed immune-associated or Ia antigens. Studies of immune responses have used antibody response or T-cell proliferation to characterize further the interactions, with the designation of "responder" or "nonresponder" based on immune reactivity to the particular antigen. How the IR genes function is not clear. At present, much of the cellular-restricting activity is mediated by Class II (I) antigens, as discussed above. The IR genes appear to control fine specificity of responses involving thymic-dependent antigens.

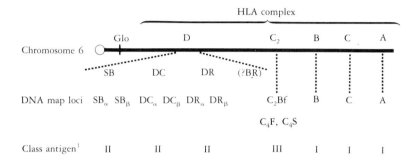

Figure 3–6. Schematic representation of the human HLA complex. The function of Class I molecules is to serve as target antigens for immune recognition and killing, while the function of the Class II antigens is to serve as restricting molecules in cellular regulation.

MHC OF HUMANS (HLA)

The human leukocyte antigen (HLA) system is best known as the typing method used to "match" recipients and donors for organ transplantation, most notably for kidney transplantation, although matching for other organs (heart, liver, pancreas, bone marrow, and so forth) is identical. The HLA typing system has also assumed prominence in paternity testing and is currently utilized to resolve legal questions of heredity. It has recently been shown that certain diseases are closely associated with unique HLA antigens; hence, in some cases the HLA type can be helpful in confirming the clinical diagnosis.

In addition to direct utility in clinical medicine, the HLA genetic system has received much scientific attention, as the genes in the HLA region code for the Classes I, II, and III transplantation antigens and also play a major regulatory role in cell interactions and immune responses, as will be discussed later.

A schematic map of the HLA genes that are located on chromosome 6 is shown in Figure 3–6.

The HLA complex is located on the short arm of chromosome 6, which also carries genes for several enzymes used in blood grouping, such as PGM_3 and GLO. The HLA genes are inherited in a codominant fashion as a group, in accordance with mendelian principles. Individuals receive one set or "haplotype" of the genes from each parent as diagrammatically shown in Figure 3–7 and Table 3–2.

Studies of various populations as well as large families, in which recombinant events can be detected, have made it possible to establish five major genetic loci: A, B, C, DR, and SB. However, several other Class II loci are under consideration as formal loci. The A, B, and C genes code for Class I molecules, whereas DR and SB code for Class II molecules. Each of the five genes has many alleles or alternate forms that represent small variations in the nucleotide sequence of the gene. These small changes result in cell surface glycoproteins with small variations, perhaps a change of one or two amino acids, or a small difference in three-dimensional structure. These variations in HLA antigen structure can be detected using HLA typing antisera, as schematically shown in Figure 3–8, or certain typing cells specific for Class II molecules. Those detected changes are called specificities and are used to assign the numerical alleles for the gene. The HLA-B gene has the largest number of detectable alleles (specificities) with 32, and is said to be the most polymorphic. The HLA-A genes have 17 alleles or specificities detected. The currently accepted list of alleles is shown in Table 3–3. Formal specificities for the SB loci will be determined in late 1984 at the International Workshop for HLA Genetics.

Parent	Haplotype designation	Sib 1 (a/c)	Sib 2 (b/d)	Sib 3 (a/c-d)
Father				
SB DR B C A				
◆-◆-◆-◆-◆	a	◆-◆-◆-◆-◆		◆-◆-◆-◆-◆
○-○-○-○-○	b		○-○-○-○-○	
Mother				
SB DR B C A				
△-△-△-△-△	c	△-△-△-△-△		
□-□-□-□-□	d		□-□-□-□-□	△-△-□-□-□

Figure 3–7. Diagrammatic sketch of the mendelian inheritance pattern of HLA antigens within a family. In general, the HLA gene group from either parent is inherited as a set or "haplotype." By convention, the father's haplotypes are designated by the letters a or b, each letter representing the HLA-A, B, C, DR, DC, and SB types on the inherited chromosome. The mother's haplotypes are designated by the letters c, d. The possible haplotypes for the children are then ac, ad, bc, or bd. Sib 3 is a recombinant between the maternal DR and B genes and hence will have the DR and SB type of the c haplotype and the B, C, and A types of the d haplotype.

Table 3–2. Haplotype Inheritance of HLA Antigens*

	A Series Specificities				B Series Specificities				Phenotype	Genotype	Haplotype Designation
	A1	A3	A9	Aw19	B5	B7	B12	B13			
Father	+		+		+		+		A1, A9; B5, B12	A1, B5; A9, B12	a/b
Mother		+		+		+		+	A3, Aw19, B7, B13	A3, B7; Aw19, B13	c/d
Sib 1	+	+			+	+			A1, A3; B5, B7	A1, B5; A3, B7	a/c
Sib 2			+	+			+	+	A9, Aw19; B12, B13	A9, B12; Aw19, B13	b/d
Sib 3	+	+			+	+			A1, A3; B5, B7	A1, B5; A3, B7	a/c

*In this series, the father's haplotypes are: a = A1, B5 and b = A9, B12; the haplotypes represent the transmission of that HLA gene segment to the offspring. The + signs indicate positive reactions (lysis) of the test lymphocytes with the specific antiserum (see Fig. 3–9).

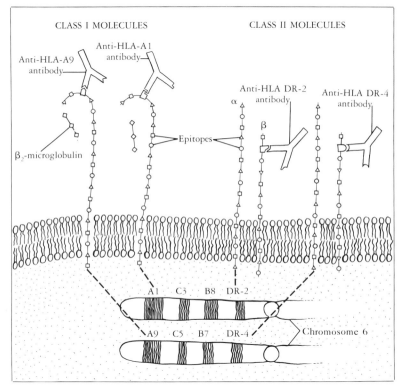

Figure 3–8. Schematic representation of HLA antibodies showing how serologic (allelic) specificities are detected. The small symbols in the schematic molecules represent areas with amino acid variations that can be recognized by specific antibodies. These variations recognized by antibody are known as epitopes.

Table 3–3. HLA Alleles Identified as Serum Specificities*

A HLA-A	B HLA-B	C HLA-C	D HLA-D	DR HLA-DR
A1	B7	Cw1	Dw1	DR1
A2	B8	Cw2	Dw2	DR2
A3	B13	Cw3	Dw3	DR3
A11	B14	Cw4	Dw4	DR4
Aw23 (A9)	B18	Cw5	Dw5	DR5
Aw24 (A9)	B27	Cw6	Dw6	DRw6
A25 (A10)	Bw35	Cw7	Dw7	DR7
A26 (A10)	B37	Cw8	Dw8	DRw8
A28	Bw38 (B16)		Dw9	DRw9
A29	Bw39 (B16)		Dw10	DRw10
Aw30 (Aw19)	Bw41		Dw11	
Aw31 (Aw19)	Bw42		Dw12	
Aw32 (Aw19)	Bw44 (B12)			
Aw33 (Aw19)	Bw45 (B12)			
Aw34	Bw46			
Aw36	Bw47			
Aw43	Bw48			
	Bw49 (B21)			
	Bw50 (B21)			
	Bw51 (B5)			
	Bw52 (B5)			
	Bw53			
	Bw54 (Bw22)			
	Bw55 (Bw22)			
	Bw56 (Bw22)			
	Bw57 (B17)			
	Bw58 (B17)			
	Bw59			
	Bw60 (Bw40)			
	Bw61 (Bw40)			
	Bw62 (B15)			
	Bw63 (B15)			

*Some of the early antisera contained antibodies that detected several alleles or specificities. In some instances, the original allele was "split" into several. A good example is Bw22, which is now known to contain three alleles: Bw54, Bw55, and Bw56. Alleles in parentheses represent the original allele that has now been split. The letter w indicates a workshop or temporary designation.

Detection of Class I Antigens

Class I molecules, described earlier in this chapter, are coded for by the HLA-A,B, and C genes. They are detected by using antisera that bind to the cell surface molecules bearing the particular specificity determinant.

The Class I antigens are present on all nucleated cells in varying amounts, although red cells and spermatozoa have few molecules on their surface. Antibodies against the HLA-A,B, and C specificities are commonly found in the serum of women who have had several pregnancies, or in individuals receiving an organ transplant or numerous transfusions. Most commonly, serum is collected from multigravida women. It is thought that lymphocytes from the fetus are released into the maternal circulation during the separation of the placenta. These fetal lymphocytes carry paternal HLA antigens that result in the immunization of the mother. Usually, more

than one sensitization is necessary to induce a level of circulating antibody that is useful for HLA typing; even then, the antisera are weak. In the case outlined in Table 3–2, the mother may make antibodies to the paternal antigens A1 or B5, with infant 1 and 3, as she does not have those antigens. To prepare an antibody that is monospecific for detecting A1, the maternal antisera must be incubated (absorbed) with cells that have B5 but not A1. The B5 antibody can thereby be removed, leaving an antiserum that detects only A1. Such operationally monospecific serum can then be used for detecting the A1 glycoprotein antigens, as demonstrated in Figure 3–9, which represents the format used for current HLA typing. Using a tray containing two to three antisera for each specificity enables the HLA typing serologist to type most individuals. Certain populations may have HLA antigens that are rare in Americans (of European descent). For example, about 33 per cent of Japanese have the antigen CW-1, which is seen in only 6 per cent of Caucasians. It is important, therefore, to make the serologist aware of the ethnic background prior to HLA typing.

Detection of Class II Antigens

The Class II DR antigens are identified serologically, whereas Dw and SB antigens are generally detected using the one-way mixed lymphocyte culture. In this assay, cells of two nonidentical individuals are mixed together, one cell (the stimulator) being irradiated so that it cannot proliferate. The other cell (the responder) recognizes the foreign Class II antigens on the stimulator cell and begins to proliferate. This proliferation is measured by the uptake of H^3-thymidine into new DNA over a five- to six-day period. The amount of new DNA made (measured as cpm of H^3-thymidine) is an index of the differences in Class II antigens between stimulator and responder. Two basic methods are currently used to type: the homozygous typing cell (HTC) method and the primed lymphocyte typing (PLT) method. These methods are schematically outlined in Figures 3–10 and 3–11, respectively. The recent production of IL-2–dependent populations of PLT cells, which can be continuously maintained, will increase the sensitivity of this assay system.

Using the PLT secondary stimulation type of assay, it is possible to show that primed

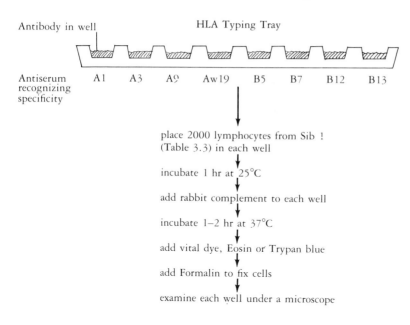

Antibody in well

HLA Typing Tray

Antiserum recognizing specificity   A1   A3   A9   Aw19   B5   B7   B12   B13

place 2000 lymphocytes from Sib 1 (Table 3.3) in each well

incubate 1 hr at 25°C

add rabbit complement to each well

incubate 1–2 hr at 37°C

add vital dye, Eosin or Trypan blue

add Formalin to fix cells

examine each well under a microscope

Figure 3–9. Diagram of the HLA serotyping procedures. Damaged or dead lymphocytes allow vital dye to enter the cell and appear dark under phase microscopy.

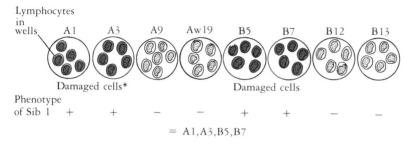

Lymphocytes in wells   A1   A3   A9   Aw19   B5   B7   B12   B13

Damaged cells*   Damaged cells

Phenotype of Sib 1   +   +   −   −   +   +   −   −

= A1,A3,B5,B7

HOMOZYGOUS TYPING CELL (HTC) METHOD:

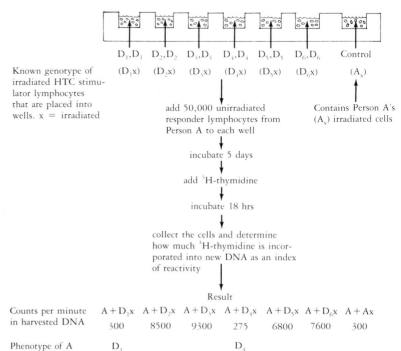

Known genotype of irradiated HTC stimulator lymphocytes that are placed into wells. x = irradiated

D_1,D_1 D_2,D_2 D_3,D_3 D_4,D_4 D_5,D_5 D_6,D_6 Control
(D_1x) (D_2x) (D_3x) (D_4x) (D_5x) (D_6x) (A_x)

add 50,000 unirradiated responder lymphocytes from Person A to each well

Contains Person A's (A_x) irradiated cells

incubate 5 days

add ³H-thymidine

incubate 18 hrs

collect the cells and determine how much ³H-thymidine is incorporated into new DNA as an index of reactivity

Result

Figure 3–10. Diagram of the procedures for cellular typing of Class II antigens. Since Person A's cells are D_1, D_4, they would respond by proliferation only to the foreign HLA-D types, which are D_2, D_3, D_5, and D_6, and not to D_1 or D_4.

	$A+D_1x$	$A+D_2x$	$A+D_3x$	$A+D_4x$	$A+D_5x$	$A+D_6x$	$A+Ax$
Counts per minute in harvested DNA	300	8500	9300	275	6800	7600	300
Phenotype of A	D_1			D_4			

Principles of cellular typing for Class II antigens.
Primed Lymphocyte Typing (PLT) Method:

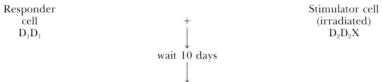

Responder cell D_1D_1	+	Stimulator cell (irradiated) D_2D_2X

wait 10 days

Harvest D_1 cells that are proliferating against the irradiated D_2 cells = primed lymphocyte typing (PLT) cells specific for D_2.

Responder PLT typing cell panel		Stimulator Irradiated cells from Person A		cpm in new DNA
anti-D_1		+		9500
anti-D_2		+		300
anti-D_3	incubated with	+	After 2–3 days	280
anti-D_4	stimulator cells	+	add ^{3}H-thymidine	8600
anti-D_5		+	and harvest cells	425
anti-D_6		+		318

Figure 3–11. Diagram of the procedures used for cellular typing of Class II antigens using the primed lymphocyte typing (PLT) methodology. The phenotype of Person A is D_1, D_4, as PLT's recognize and proliferate in response to D_1 and D_4 on Person A's lymphocytes.

cells can recognize and react to HLA-DR and HLA-SB molecules, although the latter determinants are just beginning to be studied systematically. The DC(DS) molecules are detected using antisera; however, they are not yet accepted as an allelic Class II gene.

The initial work suggests that the T-cell PLT clones recognize small antigenic determinants (epitopes) similar in size to those recognized by antibodies. It is felt that this technology will lead to a cellular typing system with specificity similar to that of serologic systems.

The detection of the DR antigens is routinely performed using serologic techniques similar to those for the detection of Class I antigens (Fig. 3–9). The serologic specificities generally follow the HTC-determined specificities, although exceptions are becoming more common. Alloantisera specific for DR molecules are somewhat more difficult to use because they are weak, and the DR molecules are normally expressed only on circulating B-cells, which constitute only 10 to 15 per cent of peripheral blood mononuclear cells; hence, B-cells must be separated from the peripheral blood in order to perform an effective typing. This is a time-consuming task and requires 20 to 30 ml of blood; hence, it cannot easily be applied to children. More sensitive techniques, such as two-color fluorescence, do, however, permit DR typing on small samples.

At present, it is thought that the DR antisera, the HTC's, and the PLT's all recognize essentially the same molecules; however, different determinants (epitopes) on the same molecule may be preferentially detected by the different methods. The HTC and PLT technologies can also detect Class II antigens for which only a few antisera exist, for example, the SB antigens. The correlation between serology and cellular typing has proved difficult, as each of the Class II antigens is made up of an alpha and a beta chain, and hybrid molecules may exist, as for the murine system.

Certain of the antisera against Class II antigens are cross reactive, allowing for the detection of "supertypic" groups of DR molecules, or groups that share some common (public) antigenic determinants. The MT1 supertypic group includes DR1, DR2, DRw6, and DRw10, while MT2 includes DR3, DR5, DRw6, DRw8, and MT3 (DR4, DR7, and DRw9). Other recently defined groups include MB1 (DR1, DR2, DRw6) MB2 (DR3, DR7), and MB3 (DR4, DR5). The relationship of these shared determinants with HLA-DR, SB, or DC(DS) loci is currently being worked out.

The distribution of Class II antigens in humans is of interest. Under normal circumstances, DR antigens are expressed on the surface of human B-cells, macrophages, and cells of the reticuloendothelial system, including Kupffer cells, Langerhans cells, and endothelial cells. They are also seen on spermatozoa and interstitial cells of the ovary. When activated, T-cells and other cells of the hemopoietic system, including myeloid cells, express the Class II antigens. In this capacity, the Class II antigens may serve as differentiation antigens. It has recently been demonstrated that gamma interferon is a powerful inducer of DR expression, even in some tissues that normally fail to exhibit DR. One theory, proposed by Feldmann and colleagues, suggests that the expression of DR, induced by gamma interferon, may permit and foster the recognition of self-antigens on certain tissues and may be the initiating event in certain types of autoimmunity.

Function of Class I Antigens: Human

The function of the Class I molecules in humans is thought to be similar to that in other mammalian systems. The murine models have provided the greatest insight, as discussed earlier in the chapter. Basically, they serve as determinants necessary for the immune recognition and the elimination of virally infected cells. It is thought that the $T8^+$ killer cell uses the T8 molecule to recognize self–MHC antigen and the T3 associated T-cell "idiotype" region to recognize and bind to antigen. In addition, the Class I antigens may serve as targets in graft rejection, which can be mediated by antibody or sensitized cells.

Function of Class II Antigens: Human

The Class II antigens are involved at many levels in immune interactions. Studies in animal systems, primarily the murine model, have provided us with insights into the various functions of the Class II antigens, as described earlier. Thus far, studies in humans have paralleled the observations in other mammals. This includes the need for sharing of certain Class II (HLA-DR or SB) molecules between macrophages and T-cells in order to obtain effective collaboration for the induction of T-helper cells. The human Class II antigens are detected in the MLC reaction. In some cases of kidney graft rejection, killer cells specific for HLA-D/DR region antigens have been identified. The Class II antigens are thought to play a major role in graft-versus-host disease, seen in bone marrow transplantation; however, the nature of this interaction remains to be resolved. As

for the $T8^+$ killer cell, it is thought that the T4 molecules on the $T4^+$ helper cell, with the T3-associated "idiotype" region, form the antigen-specific receptor.

HLA and Paternity Testing

The polymorphism of the HLA system and the reproducibility of the analysis make it ideal for studies of inheritance. One such area is the determination of paternity. The major question to be addressed is, "Can the paternity of the man be excluded?" If the child has none of the HLA haplotypes of the man, which happens in about one quarter of the cases, then paternity can be excluded. In most situations the child may share a few antigens with the putative father, and one must determine, based on haplotype frequencies in the particular ethnic population, the probability of that haplotype's originating from some other male.

HLA and Transplantation

NOMENCLATURE

Transplanted tissues are classified according to the relationship of the donor and recipient. Those terms in common usage are outlined below.

Autograft: A graft taken from one location on the same person and placed elsewhere.

Allograft: A graft taken from one member of a species and given to another member of the same species. There are several types of allografts.

Syngeneic allograft: Grafts between two genetically identical individuals, such as twins or HLA-identical siblings.

Semi-syngeneic allograft or semi-allogeneic allograft: A graft in which half of the HLA genes (one haplotype) are shared and half are different. This usually occurs in a parent-to-child graft, or grafts between siblings who share only one HLA haplotype.

Allogeneic allograft: A graft between two genetically unrelated individuals (non-HLA identical).

Xenograft: A graft taken from one species and placed in a member of another species.

Graft Rejection

It has been clearly shown that the HLA antigens serve as strong transplantation antigens by inducing a powerful immune response. The early events in allograft rejection include the production of T-cells that recognize the foreign HLA antigens. These cells may be of a variety that kill cells bearing foreign Class I or Class II antigens, or they may release mediators (lymphokines) that induce macrophages and neutrophils to enter the graft site, leading to graft destruction. Shortly after the initiation of cellular immunity, antibodies to the Class I and Class II antigens can be detected, which furthers the graft destruction.

Transplantation of organs into an individual with preformed circulating antibodies results in "hyperacute" rejection, as the antibodies immediately destroy the graft. Recent information has shown that matching of renal allografts for Class II antigens greatly improves graft survival. This matching is performed using DR typing and the mixed lymphocyte culture. Those recipients exhibiting high cellular proliferation to the donor cells are likely to manifest significant rejection reactions.

Linkage Disequilibrium

Assuming that the alleles at the HLA-A and HLA-B loci are independent of each other, one would expect them to occur together in proportion to the gene frequency in the population. Certain combinations occur in much higher frequencies than predicted, such as A1 and B8, and this unusual association is called linkage disequilibrium. The reason for this is unclear, unless it provides some selective advantage.

HLA and Disease Association

One area that has received great attention is the association of certain HLA antigens with various diseases. While the associations are primarily statistical in nature, it is generally agreed that they represent a biologically relevant finding and that the mechanism of this association will eventually be understood.

HLA and disease studies may be initiated in several ways. Most commonly, the HLA types of a group of patients with a particular disease are determined, and the types compared with the HLA types of a random panel of unaffected individuals from the same ethnic group and geographic area.

The most common statistical approach for evaluation is to establish a 2 × 2 contingency table.

		HLA antigen	
		Present	Absent
Disease	Present	a	b
	Absent	c	d

where a, b, c, and d are the number of individuals in each category. The X^2 is determined and the p value calculated. If the result is significant, one may wish to evaluate the strength of this observation. This is done by calculating the relative risk, which is the risk of developing a disease when an antigen is present, relative to the risk when it is lacking. It is calculated using the formula

$$\text{Relative risk} = \frac{ad}{cb}$$

A relative risk of greater than 1 indicates that the antigen is more frequent in patients than in controls.

Several difficulties arise in these types of analysis, one of the major ones being the ability to define clearly a clinical disease that may present as a broad spectrum. A good example is the various forms of arthritis that may vary from mild and nonsymptomatic to severe and disabling. There are, in addition, several statistical pitfalls, one being that associations can occur by chance in 1 of 20 observations (with p of <.05). This can be corrected for by multiplying each p value by the number of antigens typed for.

Dr. Arne Svejgaard, in Copenhagen, has established an international registry to evaluate HLA and disease associations. The results are periodically updated and published. A few of the more interesting examples are given in Table 3–4.

While the method described above uses populations with various diseases to develop a statistical association, it is also possible to perform formal linkage analysis between a gene disease and an HLA allele. This requires large families in which several members may have the disease. The information gained, however, is more powerful and may allow investigators to formally map disease-linked genes.

Table 3–4. **HLA and Disease Associations**

Disease Type	HLA Allele	Relative Risk
Rheumatologic Diseases		
Ankylosing spondylitis	B27	88
Reiter's syndrome	B27	37
Acute anterior uveitis	B27	10
Juvenile arthritis	B27, Dw5, or Dw8	4
Rheumatoid arthritis	Dw4(DR4)	4
Autoimmune/Endocrine Diseases		
Chronic hepatitis	Dw3(DR3)	14
" "	B8	9
Celiac disease	Dw3(DR3)	11
Graves' disease	Dw3(DR3)	4
Hashimoto's thyroiditis	Dw5(DR5)	3
Idiopathic Addison's disease	Dw3(DR3)	6
Juvenile-onset diabetes mellitus	Dw4(DR4)	6
" " "	Dw3(DR3)	3
Congenital adrenal hyperplasia (21-hydroxylase deficiency)	B47	15
" " "	B5	4
Myasthenia gravis	B8	4
" "	Dw3(DR3)	3
Multiple sclerosis	Dw2(DR2)	4
Systemic lupus erythematosus	Dw3(DR3)	6
Malignant Disorders		
Chronic myelocytic leukemia (CML)	A2	39
Chronic lymphocytic leukemia (CLL)	B18	5
Acute lymphoblastic leukemia (ALL)	A2	1
Hodgkin's disease	A1, A11, B8, B15	1–8

Investigators studying the DNA sequence of HLA antigens in individuals with these diseases have found restriction enzyme map patterns (restriction enzyme fragment length polymorphisms) that differ from those of normal individuals. This work would suggest that genes adjacent to the HLA "markers" may be unique in affected individuals, predisposing them to certain illnesses. Assuming that the disease associations are valid and represent a biologically relevant event, what hypothesis can be put forward to explain these observations?

A number of the rheumatologic, autoimmune, and endocrine disorders show an association with HLA alleles of the D/DR region. In many of these disorders, antibodies are found that have specificity for the target organ. One could postulate that the MHC-linked "immune response" alleles in these individuals permit an elevated or exaggerated response status to exogenous or endogenous antigens, which results in the production of autoantibodies. To account for some of the observations, one might anticipate that individuals who are homozygous for a particular allele may be more affected than a heterozygote would be; however, this is not the case, and it is necessary to include environmental factors as important in the initiation of the disease process. It was anticipated that strong "susceptibility" associations to infectious diseases would be found; however, this has not been the case, except with tuberculoid leprosy (Rr = 5).

Alternative explanations suggest that the MHC genes influence receptor binding for toxins, oncogenic viruses, bacteria, or other pathogenic materials, thereby opening the way for subsequent disease development and progression; however, this remains to be proved.

It is commonly held that the HLA alleles are not responsible for disease susceptibility but that they are markers in strong linkage disequilibrium with as yet undefined, but responsible, genes. Although these associations are of interest and occasionally are useful to support the clinical impression, the mechanism is poorly understood and awaits future definition.

T-Cell and B-Cell Receptors for Antigen

The cells of the immune system are unique in that the T-cells and B-cells carry surface glycoproteins that must be able to interact with antigen, either alone or complexed with histocompatibility antigens in some specific way.

It has been known for many years that the antigen-binding molecules on the surface of B-cells are immunoglobulin molecules. When the B-cell differentiates to become a plasma cell, the same immunoglobulin molecules that served as receptors for antigen are now secreted. The portion of the immunoglobulin molecule that binds to antigen is called the antigen-binding site or idiotype region (Chapter 5).

It is possible, under certain circumstances, to produce antibodies that recognize and bind to this idiotype region of the immunoglobulin molecule, so-called anti-idiotype antibodies. In several experimental systems it was demonstrated that certain anti-idiotype antibodies could bind to T-cells and T-cell factors; hence, it was suggested that T-cells used the same antigen-recognition system as B-cells, namely, the immunoglobulin variable regions (V_H). This hypothesis seemed reasonable, as the receptor system would then be conserved, and one need not postulate an entire new receptor system, with associated diversity, outside of the well-studied immunoglobulin regions. In a series of recent studies using c-DNA probes to various immunoglobulin regions, it has been demonstrated that antigen-specific T-(suppressor) cells fail to rearrange the immunoglobulin V_H genes, as would be anticipated if they were using those genes to code for receptors, and they fail to make m-RNA with V_H sequences. Furthermore, studies attempting to detect immunoglobulin allotype markers, or other immunoglobulin determinants on cloned T-cells, have been inconsistent. Recent studies by Reinherz, Meuer, and Schlossman, show a 43K and 49K complex associated with T3 that is not immunoglobulin yet appears to be the putative T-cell receptor. It is currently postulated that the T-cell receptor for antigen is coded for by a set of genes unassociated with the immunoglobulin or MHC genes. Such a set of genes might exhibit levels of genetic polymorphism similar to immunoglobulins, within the antigen-binding regions. This is supported by the recently published sequence of portions of the human T-cell receptor by Mak and colleagues as well as similar reports of murine T-cell receptors by Davies and coworkers. The studies indicate that the T-cell receptor has 30 to 60 per cent homology with immunoglobulin, undergoes somatic gene rearrangement during expression, and has "constant" and "variable" regions. The receptors are also likely to have a "hypervariable" region for binding antigen or MHC product. This development implies that, in addition to the immunoglobulin and MHC systems, the T-cell receptor genes form a third polymorphic genetic system that influences immune responsiveness.

GENETICS OF BLOOD GROUPS SYSTEM

One of the genetic traits that have been extensively studied using immunologic methods is the major blood group antigens, including the ABO and Rh systems. The erythrocytes carry a large number of antigenic determinants; however, only a few of them are clinically important, either because of their immunogenicity or because of their frequency in the population.

PRINCIPLES OF BLOOD GROUP DETECTION

The assignment of blood group antigens is made using alloantisera that have been procured from individuals who have been previously immunized by transfusions or pregnancy. In the future, monoclonal antibodies will certainly be utilized to obtain precise definitions of the blood group antigens; however, at present the serum from immunized individuals is rendered operationally monospecific by absorption with red cells of known specificity.

The most common assay used is hemagglutination, whereby the antibodies agglutinate the red cells. IgM antibodies, because they are pentavalent, agglutinate red cells more readily and at lower temperatures (18°C), while IgG antibodies agglutinate best at higher temperatures (37°C).

In saline, IgG antibodies often fail to agglutinate, since the red cell antigens are too distant for cross linking. Under such circumstances, the IgG is an *incomplete antibody*, and because it covers up sites that would permit IgM agglutination, the IgG antibodies are often termed *blocking* antibodies. The standard method to detect IgG antibodies is the indirect antiglobulin test or Coombs' test. This assay utilizes an antibody directed at the IgG bound on the erythrocytes, thereby forming a large lattice that agglutinates and permits detection.

The ABO Blood Group System

For centuries, it was known that recipients of blood transfusions often experienced serious or fatal transfusion reactions. The mechanism for these reactions was not understood until the classic work of Landsteiner, who, in 1900, defined the major isoantigens (alloantigens) of human red cells. He performed a very simple experiment, which is outlined below, using serum and red cells from six members of his laboratory staff, leading to the discovery of blood groups and antigens (Table 3–5).

From this experiment, Landsteiner was able to determine that there were two antigenic determinants present on human red cells, which he called A and B. Some (3 and 4) individuals possessed the A determinant and were A blood group; others (2 and 5) possessed B and were B blood group. A third group (1 and 6) had erythrocytes that failed to agglutinate with any of the sera and were called C. It was subsequently shown that the C group, now known as O, failed to express a unique antigen. Finally, the work of Landsteiner established that individuals have naturally occurring antibodies directed against the antigenic determinants absent from their own erythrocytes. Thus, individuals of blood group A possess anti-B antibodies and vice versa, while individuals with blood group O have both anti-A and anti-B antibodies. Some years later, students of Landsteiner discovered another group that had both A and B antigens and had no antibodies, now known as the AB type (Table 3–6). These original studies formed the foundation of the immunohematology system, for which Landsteiner was awarded the Nobel Prize in 1930.

GENETIC GROUP OF ABO ANTIGENS

The erythrocyte expression of the ABO antigens is controlled by a single gene with three alleles—A, B, and O. The alleles A and B are codominant and are dominant over the O allele, which is not expressed. The blood group antigens are known to be glycoprotein and glycolipid in nature, and their antigenic potential relates to the carbohydrate portions. It is now accepted that the A and B alleles code for enzymes that attach carbohydrate molecules to the basic glycoprotein (H substance).

The A allele codes for the enzyme N-acetyl

Table 3–5. Summary of Landsteiner's Original Experiment Leading to the Discovery of Blood Group Antigens

Sera	Erythrocytes						Designated Group
	1	2	3	4	5	6	
1	–	+	+	+	+	–	C
2	–	–	+	+	–	–	A
3	–	+	–	–	+	–	B
4	–	+	–	–	+	–	B
5	–	–	+	+	–	–	A
6	–	+	+	+	+	–	C

+ = agglutination

galactosaminyl transferase, which adds alpha-D-N-acetylgalactosamine to the H stem carbohydrate substance, thereby generating the A antigenic determinant and creating the A antigenic structures. The B allele codes for the enzyme galactosyl transferase, which catalyzes the attachment of an alpha-D-galactose molecule to the H substance, thereby creating the B antigen.

The O allele apparently fails to code for any enzyme and therefore fails to create any unique antigen.

The H Gene and its Alleles. The H gene codes for an enzyme known as fucosyl transferase, which catalyzes the attachment of alpha-L-fucose to the carbohydrate beta-galactosyl-N-acetylglucosamine disaccharide (Fig. 3–12). The latter disaccharide is a part of the stem glycoprotein that serves as the backbone structure for the A and B antigens. The addition of alpha-L-fucose to this glycoprotein converts it into H substance, which can then be modified to form the A and B antigens. The majority of the population is H/H or H/h, which enables them to synthesize H substance, as the H allele is dominant. Occasionally, an individual will be h/h and lacks the fucosyl transferase and hence, H substance and A or B antigens. These people phenotypically blood type as O blood group. This phenotype is known as the Bombay phenotype.

ABO SYSTEM AND ITS CLINICAL SIGNIFICANCE

The A, B, and H antigens are examples of substances whose antigenic expressions are influenced by small structural differences in single sugar residues that are under genetic control.

These antigens are of obvious importance in blood transfusions, in which the infusion

Table 3–6. Summary of Blood Group Typing

Genotype	Phenotypic	Red Cell Antigen	Antisera Reaction Anti-A	Anti-B	Serum Alloantibody
O/O	O	O	−	−	anti-A, -B
A/O, A/A	A	A	+	−	anti-B
B/O, B/B	B	B	−	+	anti-A
A/B	A/B	A/B	+	+	none

of blood cells carrying A or B antigens into a person with natural anti-A or anti-B antibodies (agglutinins) may result in a life-threatening transfusion reaction. Numerous other blood group antigens may also be involved in such reactions. This possibility has led to the development of a series of tests, called a major crossmatch, that analyzes for the presence of IgM and IgG antibodies in the serum of the recipient for the donor cells.

The presence of anti-A or anti-B antibodies in the serum may induce hemolytic disease of the newborn. In this case, the maternal IgG antibodies cross the placenta and bind to fetal erythrocytes, causing hemolysis. The ABO-induced hemolytic disease is usually milder than that induced by Rh incompatibility.

The ABO antigens are useful in paternity determinations, although testing for more polymorphic antigens, such as the HLA antigens, is usually superior. Forensic pathologists often use ABO antigens to determine the type of blood found at the scene of a crime, as these antigens are very stable. Finally, the ABO antigens, because of their wide distribution on many organs and their binding with natural antibody, are considered to be important in organ transplantation. An ABO-incompatible kidney graft, for example, may be rejected in a hyperacute fashion, if the individual has preformed natural antibodies.

Rh Blood Group Systems

The second red cell antigen system that is of clinical significance is the Rh system.

Levine and Stetson, in 1939, discovered an

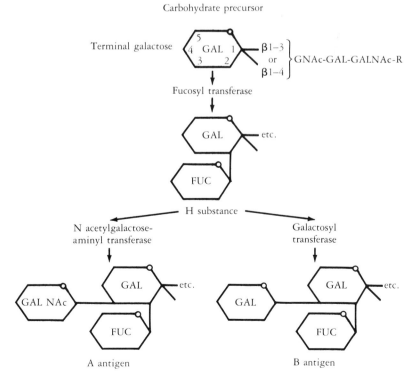

Figure 3–12. Schematic representation of H, A, and B blood group antigens. Shown is a representation of the proposed structure of the A and B blood group antigens. Type A blood cells carry Type A antigens; Type B cells have B antigens, while Type AB has both; and Type O has only H substance. The difference between Types A and B is the N acetylation of the terminal galactose. The sugars are linked to sphingomyelin (R) to form the red cell surface antigen. Linkage of this complex to certain peptides produces "secretory substances." G = glucose, GAL = galactose, FUC = fucose, NAc = acetyl group.

antigen that reacted with serum from a mother who had delivered a child with hemolytic disease of the newborn. This antigen was later shown to be detected by antibodies prepared by injecting rhesus monkey erythrocytes into rabbits or guinea pigs. The later observation, fostered by Landsteiner and Wiener, led to the name "rhesus factor" or Rh antigen.

GENETIC CONTROL OF Rh ANTIGENS

The immense complexity of the Rh system has been revealed over the past 30 years, with the discovery of many additional Rh antigenic types. Approximately 30 types have been identified; however, the original Rh antigen is by far the most important in terms of immunogenicity and clinical significance.

The lengthy interval between the discovery of the ABO and the Rh blood groups was due, in part, to the serologic properties of the anti-Rh antibodies. Unlike those of the ABO system, Rh antibodies do not occur naturally; rather, they are products of frank immunization either through pregnancy or transfusion. The serologic properties of these antibodies are described in Chapter 8.

Two theories have been proposed to explain the inheritance of the Rh antigens. The first of these, suggested by Fisher and Race, proposed that the system consists of three genes, C, D, and E, with paired alleles, coding for five antigenic determinants (D, C, E, c, and e). The three loci are considered to be so closely linked on the chromosome that crossing over is an infrequent event. It is thought that they are inherited, one set from each parent, as depicted in Figure 3–13.

The most important of these loci was called D, which controls the production of the most clinically significant Rh isoantigen, the D antigen. This isoantigen is the strongest im-

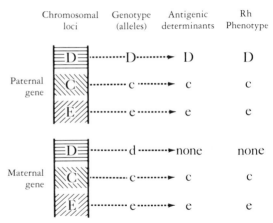

Figure 3–13. Schematic representation of the Fisher-Race Rh phenotype concept with three loci, each having two alleles. The C alleles are C and c, while the E alleles are E and e, these genes being codominant. The D locus has only one allele, D, which is expressed; no antigen for d has been found.

munogen and was responsible for the erythroblastotic infant described by Stetson and Levine, accounting for more than 90 per cent of cases of hemolytic disease of the newborn due to maternal isoimmunization. An alternate allele at this locus was called d (Fig. 3–13). To date, the antigenic product of this hypothetical allele has not been described, and there is considerable doubt that such an antigenic determinant actually exists. The symbol d is used to represent the absence of D, rather than the presence of any known antigenic determinant. A second locus, according to the Fisher-Race scheme, is the position at which one of two alleles, C or c, is located. These genes control the production of either the C or the c antigens. Alleles at a third locus, called E, are responsible for the production of the antigenic determinants E or e. These isoantigens occasionally account for isoimmunization. In order of immunogenicity, the antigens are $D > c > C > E > e$.

Table 3–7. Notation of Commonly Encountered Rh Isoantigens and Alleles

Genes			Expressed Antigens		
Fisher-Race Rh Haplotypes	Wiener Alleles	Wiener Agglutinogens	Fisher-Race	Wiener	Rh Type
Dce	R^0	Rh_0	D,c,e	Rh_0, hr', hr''	+
DCe	R^1	Rh_1	D,C,e	Rh_0, rh', hr''	+
DcE	R^2	Rh_2	D,c,E	Rh_0, hr', rh''	+
DCE	R^z	Rh_z	D,C,E	Rh_0, rh', rh''	+
dce	r	rh	− c,e	− hr', hr''	−
dCe	r'	rh'	− C,e	− rh', hr''	−
dcE	r''	rh''	− c,E	− hr', rh''	−
dCE	r^y	rhy	− C,E	− rh', rh''	−

Table 3–8. Partial List of Proposed Numerical Notation for Rh Antigens

Rosenfield et al.	Fisher-Race	Wiener
Rh1	D	Rh_O
Rh2	C	rh′
Rh3	E	rh″
Rh4	c	hr′
Rh5	e	hr″

If Rh-negative persons are given a unit of Rh-positive blood, over 50 per cent are immunized to D, while less than 5 per cent would form anti-E or e antibodies. In general practice, only compatibility for D is routinely established, except when blood is being transfused into an Rh-negative individual.

A second theory of inheritance, proposed by Wiener, differs to the extent that one locus is responsible for the production of several antigenic determinants. This theory utilizes the concept of "multiple complex alleles," in which a single locus on the chromosome controls the production of the Rh antigenic determinants found on the red cell. At this locus, however, there are a large number of alleles, each being responsible for the production of a single large antigenic structure that encompasses multiple smaller antigenic determinants. The original antigenic determinants were classified as Rh_O, rh′, rh″, hr′ and hr″, which corresponds to D, C, E, c, and e of the Fisher-Race scheme (Tables 3–7 and 3–8). Each allele is given a symbolic designation, such as R^O, to designate the antigenic specificity it controls. For example, Rh^O leads to the production of the

antigenic determinants Rh_O, hr′, and hr″ on the red cell. Figure 3–14 depicts the same examples used in Figure 3–13, using the Wiener scheme.

Tables 3–7 and 3–8 present some of the more commonly encountered Rh isoantigens, together with their controlling allelic forms, employing both systems of notation. Table 3–8 shows the newer nomenclature proposed by Rosenfield and colleagues, which simplifies this complex system.

According to the Fisher-Race scheme, the isoantigens are controlled by three linked loci. Since man is diploid, one set of these genetic loci is inherited from each parent. A person is said to be Rh-positive if he inherits D from either parent (DD or Dd). In either case, the father can transmit a D to one of his offspring's chromosomes.

For the physician, therefore, the determination of the genotype of an individual is an important consideration when sensitization due to D has occurred in a D-negative (Rho-negative) mother. For example, a father who is homozygous will transmit D to all the offspring, and each child could suffer from hemolytic disease of the newborn. If, on the other hand, the father is heterozygous, each child has a 50 per cent chance of being negative for D. Thus, by determination of the genotype of the father, the outcome of future pregnancies can be predicted.

Suggestions for Further Reading

Dausset, J., and Svejgaard, A.: HLA and Disease. 1st ed. Baltimore, Williams & Wilkins Company, 1977.

Festenstein, H., and Demant, P.: HLA and H-2, basic immunogenetics, biology and clinical relevance: No. 9. *In* Turk J. (ed.): Current Topics in Immunology. London, Edward Arnold, Ltd., 1978.

Fudenberg, H. H., Pink, J. R. L., Wang, A. C., et al.: Basic Immunogenetics. New York, Oxford University Press, 1978.

Hedrick, S. M., Cohen, D. I., Nielsen, E. A., and Davis, M. M.: Isolation of CDMA clones encoding T cell specific membrane associated proteins. Nature, *308*:149, 1984.

Hedrick, S. M., Nielsen, E. A., Kavaler, J., Cohen, D. I., and Davis, M. M.: Sequence relationships between putative cell receptor polypeptides and immunoglobulins. Nature, *308*:153, 1984.

Hood, L., Steinmetz, M., and Malissen, B.: Genes of the major histocompatibility complex of the mouse. Ann. Rev. Immunol., *1*:529, 1983.

Johnson, R. H., Hartzman, R. J., and Robinson, M. A.: HLA: The major histocompatibility complex. *In* Henry, J. (ed.): Clinical Diagnosis and Management by Laboratory Methods. Philadelphia, W. B. Saunders Company, 1984.

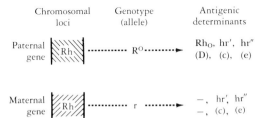

Chromosomal loci	Genotype (allele)	Antigenic determinants
Paternal gene	R^O	Rh_O, hr′, hr″ (D), (c), (e)
Maternal gene	r	—, hr′, hr″ —, (c), (e)

Figure 3–14. Schematic representation of the Wiener "one gene–multiple allele" theory. The Weiner concept suggests that a single "Rh" gene has eight alleles. Each allele codes for a cell surface molecule with two or three antigenic determinants or epitopes, which are recognized by the typing antisera. In this scheme, the Fischer-Race equivalents are in parentheses below the Wiener designations. The allele depicted by R^O code for a molecule with three epitopes, Rh_O, hr′ and hr″, which correspond to the Fisher-Race D, c, and e. The r allele codes for a molecule with only two epitopes hr′ and hr″, which correspond to c and e, as d is not expressed.

Kindt, T. J., and Robinson, M. A.: MHC antigens in fundamental immunology. *In* Paul, W. E. (ed.): Fundamental Immunology. New York, Raven Press, 1983.

Klein, J., Figueroa, F., and Nagy, Z. A.:Genetics of the major histocompatibility complex, the final act. Ann. Rev. Immunol., *1*:119, 1983.

Melief, C.: Remodelling the H-2 map. Immunol. Today, *4*:57, 1983.

Race, R. R., and Sanger, R.: Blood Groups in Man. 6th ed. Oxford, Blackwell Scientific Publications, 1975.

Reinherz, E. L., Meuer, S. C., and Schlossman, S. F.: The delineation of antigen receptors on human T lymphocytes. Immunol. Today, *4*:5, 1983.

Rosenfield, R. E., Allen, F. H., and Rubinstein, P.: Genetic model for the Rh blood group system. Proc. Natl. Acad. Sci., *70*:1303, 1973.

Schaller, J., and Hansen, J.: HLA relationship to disease. Hosp. Pract., *41*, 1981.

Schwartz, R.: Functional properties of I region gene products and theories of immune response (Ir) gene function. *In* Ia Antigens. Volume 1, Mice. Boca Raton, Fla., CRC Press, 1982, pp. 161–218.

Throwsdale, T., Lee, J., and McMichael, A.: HLA-DR bouillabaisse. Immunol. Today, *4*:33, 1983.

Yanagi, Y., Yoshikai, Y., Leggett, K., Clark, S. P., Aleksander, I., and Mak, T. W.: A human T cell specific cDNA clone encodes a protein having extensive homology to immunoglobulin chains. Nature, *308*:145, 1984.

Zaleski, M. B., Subiski, S., Niles, E. G., et al.: Immunogenetics. Boston, Pitman, 1983.

Chapter 4

Antigens and Immunogenicity

Anne L. Jackson, Ph.D.

DEFINITIONS

Immunogenicity may be defined as that property of a substance (immunogen) that endows it with the capacity to provoke a specific immune response. This consists of the elaboration of antibody, the development of cell-mediated immunity, or both. Antigenicity, on the other hand, is the property of a substance (antigen) that allows it to react with the products of the specific immune response, e.g., antibody or specifically sensitized T-lymphocytes. Substances that are immunogenic are always antigenic, but antigens are not necessarily immunogenic. For example, certain low molecular weight substances, referred to as haptens, e.g., penicillin, are not immunogenic unless coupled to a larger *carrier* molecule. Thus, a hapten functions as an antigen but not as an immunogen. Allergens refer to a specialized class of immunogens that induce hypersensitivity (allergic) reactions and include substances that function as immunogens or haptens.

Portions of the three-dimensional structure of every immunogen contain surface groupings, e.g., amino acids in a globular protein or protruding sugar side chains in polysaccharides. These structures are referred to as antigenic determinants or epitopes and represent exposed active areas of the molecule with which an antibody can combine. Most complex materials, such as red blood cells, tissues, and bacteria, contain numerous antigenic determinants. Because of its small size, an individual antigenic determinant may not be immunogenic and therefore may be considered a hapten. Thus, the immune response to a complex immunogen represents the collective immune responses to a number

of antigenic determinants. Of importance to clinical medicine is that new antigenic determinants may appear as a consequence of physical or chemical modifications of that material within the body. The significance of this finding is seen in certain immunologically mediated diseases of man, such as drug allergies, the autoimmune diseases, and neoplasia.

DEFINITIONS OF ANTIGENIC SPECIFICITIES

Broadly speaking, antigens may be classified into two major types: *exogenous* and *endogenous* (Table 4–1). This is an operational classification of antigens, based upon their applications in immunologically mediated diseases of man.

Exogenous Antigens

Exogenous antigens are those that are presented to the host from the exterior in the form of microorganisms, pollen, drugs, or pollutants (see Table 4–1). These antigens are responsible for a spectrum of human diseases ranging from the infectious diseases to the immunologically mediated diseases of man, such as bronchial asthma. There are also genetic mechanisms operating at the level of the exogenous antigens. Influenza virus, for example, which is a major cause of epidemic respiratory disease in man, exists in nature in many antigenic types recognized as A, B, and C. These types represent different mutations of the virus. A susceptible population will be infected by a given serotype.

Table 4–1. Classification of Antigens

Source	Type	Example	Clinical Significance
Exogenous	Several	Microorganisms, pollen, drugs, pollutants	Susceptibility to infection, immunologically mediated disease (asthma)
Endogenous			
Xenogeneic (Heterologous)	Xenoantigen (Heteroantigen)	Forssman antigen, certain tissue antigens that cross-react with exogenous antigens (e.g., renal and cardiac tissues and beta hemolytic streptococcus)	Pathogenesis of certain diseases, e.g., glomerulonephritis, rheumatic fever
Autologous	Autoantigen	Organ-specific antigens (e.g., thyroid antigen)	Autoimmune diseases, e.g., Hashimoto's thyroiditis
	Idiotype	Immunoglobulin-specific antigens	Switch of immunoglobulin classes
Allogeneic (Homologous)	Alloantigen (Isoantigen)	Blood group, histocompatibility antigens (HL-A)	Hemolytic disease of the newborn, transfusion reactions, transplantation immunity

Following recovery and establishment of immunity, the virus can no longer propagate, since there are insufficient susceptible individuals to establish continued infection. Owing to selective pressure, however, the virus is known to undergo mutation, following which new variants of influenza emerge. These newly acquired variants, when fully virulent, are responsible for new epidemics. Thus, man survives epidemics, and organisms mutate to re-create epidemics.

Endogenous Antigens

Endogenous antigens are those that are found within an individual and include the following: *xenogeneic* (heterologous), *autologous* and *idiotypic*, or *allogeneic* (homologous) antigens (see Table 4–1).

Xenogeneic antigens are those antigens that are found within a variety of phylogenetically unrelated species. These antigens are also known as *heterogeneic* antigens and are important in clinical medicine, since they give rise to antibody responses associated with or useful in the diagnosis of disease. For example, the cross-reaction of Group A beta-hemolytic streptococcal antigens and human heart tissue is an example of a relationship between the well-known incidence of rheumatic heart disease and infection. It is believed that tissue damage is due to the cross-reaction of antibody with these heterologous antigens. Other types of heterologous responses are helpful in diagnosis. The best known example of this is the Forssman antigen, which is found in the tissue of many

species and is closely related to other ubiquitous antigens such as the A blood group antigen. Because the Forssman antigen itself is not found in the tissues of man, it is possible that the great variety of other tissues or cells that contain this antigen could sensitize man. For example, following infectious mononucleosis, an infection caused by the EB virus, antibody responses develop, some of which are specifically directed against the EB virus and others against this heterogenetic antigen. This latter reaction, referred to as *heterophile antibody response,* is a useful test in diagnosing infectious mononucleosis.

Although generally nonimmunogenic within a species, antigens distinguishing various cell types (e.g., "helper" T-cells) are now being characterized by the use of monoclonal antibodies. Since a monoclonal immunoglobulin recognizes a single epitope, it is now possible to generate an antibody response to previously "weak" or nonimmunogenic antigens by hybridoma technology (Chapter 5).

Autologous body components are constituents of the host and are recognized as self-components. Under ordinary circumstances, they are nonimmunogenic. It is believed that a change in these body components may cause them to become immunogenic under certain circumstances, and the host mounts an immunologic attack against its own tissues. In some instances, human tissues contain antigens that normally can be recognized by the immune system of the host but are separated from the action of antibodies or immune cells by barriers, such as the basement membrane. In these situations, removal of the barrier, for instance, through the effects of inflammation or acute infection, may release the antigens in such a way as to produce an acute secondary immune response, stimulating the host to mount an immunologic attack against its own tissues. In either case, the final condition is referred to as autoimmunity.

By far the largest group of antigens significant to the clinician are those known as *allogeneic antigens*. Allogeneic antigens are those genetically controlled by antigenic determinants that distinguish one individual of a given species from another. In man, antigenic determinants of this variety are found on red blood cells, white blood cells, platelets, serum proteins, and the surface of cells making up the fixed tissues of the body, including histocompatibility antigens (Table 4–2). These antigens are known to be *polymorphic*. (Polymorphism is the existence of two or more genetically different forms in one interbreeding population due to an array of alleles at one locus of the chromosome. At any one locus, however, an individual has only two alleles of the entire array that exists in the population.) In Table 4–2 are listed some of the important isoantigens of man with their tissue distribution and clinical importance. Immunization with any of these antigens can occur and progress to disease. This results when an individual receives an incompatible blood transfusion or a solid graft containing antigenic determinants that are absent in the recipient host. When these specificities are lacking in the recipient, they are perceived as foreign and therefore lead to an immune response. In general, the intensity of the response is proportional to the degree of genetic disparity between immunogen and the host, i.e., the greater the disparity, the more intense the response. These reactions may take the form of a transfusion reaction, as in the case of an incompatible blood transfusion, or the rejection of a solid graft, as in the case of a kidney transplant. Alternatively, immunization can occur during the course of pregnancy when fetal cells (e.g., leukocytes, erythrocytes, platelets) or proteins gain access to the maternal circulation. The maternal production and transplacental transfer of antibody to any of these paternally acquired fetal antigens can lead to severe anemia, leukopenia, thrombocytopenia, or aberrations in gamma globulin production by the fetus (Fig. 4–1).

Within a single given immunoglobulin molecule, additional determinants, unique to that molecule, are found. These are called idiotypic determinants. They are found in all subclasses (isotypes), and antibodies to that epitope are specific for that particular immunoglobulin (anti-idiotype). Anti-idiotypes are thought to be of importance in the regulation of immune responses (Chapter 7).

Structure of an Antigen

A composite picture of an "antigen" may be seen in the case of the Group A streptococcus (Fig. 4–2). The bacterium is composed of several physically and chemically discernible structures, which vary in their immunogenicity. For example, the capsule, which is composed of hyaluronic acid, is relatively nonimmunogenic. This may be accounted for by its close structural similarity to hyaluronates present in animal tissues, and it may not be recognized as foreign by the host. This lack of immunogenicity may also account for the increased virulence of the organism. The surface antigens, M, T, and R, are found in the cell wall. Of these, the M proteins are the most important biologically since their presence impedes phagocytosis, and they are thought to be the major virulence factor of the Group A beta-hemo-lytic streptococcus.

Table 4–2. **Distribution and Clinical Significance of the Alloantigens of Man**

Type	Example of Alloantigens	Clinical Significance
Red blood cell	ABO, Rh_O, blood groups (called isoantigens)	Hemolytic disease of newborn, transfusion reactions
White blood cell	Histocompatibility (HL-A) and neutrophil (NA) antigens	Transplantation immunity
Platelets	Platelet (Pl) antigens	Transplantation, thrombocytopenia
Serum proteins	Gamma globulin	Immunologic deficiency
Fixed tissues	Histocompatibility antigens (HL-A)	Transplantation

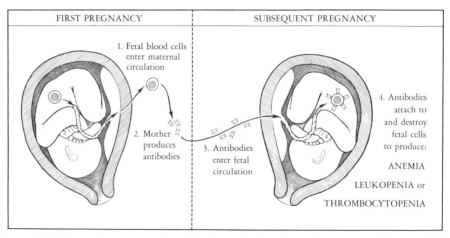

Figure 4–1. Schematic representation of isoimmunization due to feto-maternal incompatibility.

Bacteria that are coated with antibody are more readily taken up and destroyed by phagocytic cells. The M proteins are also important diagnostically because they determine the type specificity of the organism. The group-specific "antigens" (A through N) are carbohydrate in nature and are also found within the cell wall of the streptococcal organism. Antibodies to these carbohydrates are not protective but permit the classification of the streptococci into serologic groups, which were first described by Lancefield. In addition, immunogenic extracellular products are elaborated by the streptococcus. These include the erythrogenic toxins, the streptolysins S and O, and a variety of other toxins. Antibodies to these proteins can serve a protective function (e.g., antierythrogenic toxin in scarlet fever) and may also be of aid in diagnosis of that disease (e.g., antistrepto-

lysin O). When one considers that each of these immunogens has at least one, and probably more, antigenic determinants, the number of antibodies of different specificity that could be produced following immunization or infection becomes quite large. Not all immune responses are protective to the host, however. In assessing vaccines, it is important to determine the degree of protection produced in a patient by these immunogens.

GENERAL PROPERTIES OF IMMUNOGENS

Foreignness

The first and primary requirement for any molecule to qualify as an immunogen is that

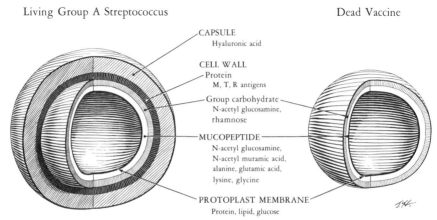

Figure 4–2. Schematic representation of living Group A *Streptococcus* and the dead vaccine prepared from it. (After Krause, R. M.: Factors controlling the occurrence of antibodies with uniform properties. Fed. Proc., *29*:59, 1970.)

the substance be genetically foreign to the host. In nature, an immune response will occur to a component that is not normally present in the body or normally exposed to the host's lymphoreticular system. On occasion, however, body constituents may be recognized as foreign, elicit an immune response, and become the adventitious target of injury, as seen in the autoimmune diseases of man. Under ordinary circumstances, the immune system discriminates between "self" and "nonself." However, not all foreign substances can induce an immune response. For example, exposure to carbon in the form of coal dust will not induce antibodies to these substances; only the phagocytic response is initiated.

In addition to the requirements for foreignness, there is a large body of evidence showing that the ability to elicit an immune response is under genetic control (Chapter 3). These controls operate both at the level of total immune response, e.g., responders versus nonresponders, and in the control of specific immune products, e.g., IgE antibody. Thus, there exists a genetic requirement with regard to both the immunogen in terms of genetic dissimilarity and the genetic controls of immune responsiveness.

The recognition of a specific immunogen and the commitment to respond to the stimulation by the production of either antibody or cell-mediated immunity or with tolerance also seem to depend on the physical and chemical properties of the immunogen. These responses are mediated by specific receptors on precommitted lymphocytes and will have an influence on the type of cells recruited (Chapter 7). For example, certain immunogens directly stimulate B-lymphocytes with the production of antibody without the requirement for T-cells (T-independent antigens); other types of immunogens require the interaction of T-helper and B-lymphocytes in the full expression of an immune response (T-dependent antigens). Another type of cell cooperation is probably mediated by macrophages (Chapter 7).

PHYSICAL PROPERTIES

Size

In order for a substance to be immunogenic, it must be of a certain minimum size; effective immunogens have molecular weights greater than 10,000. Although some smaller molecules, such as insulin (5000 MW) and glucagon (4600 MW), do function as immunogens, the immune response is minimal in most hosts, and these substances function as haptens after combining with tissue proteins. Haptens can induce a strong immune response if coupled to a carrier protein of appropriate size (greater than 10,000 MW). It should be noted that the response to a hapten-protein complex will be directed to (1) the hapten, (2) the carrier, and (3) an area of overlapping specificity involving the hapten and the adjacent carrier constituents. In the case of humoral immunity, specificity is directed primarily to the hapten; in cell-mediated immunity, reactivity is directed to both the hapten and the carrier protein.

Much of our understanding concerning the specificity of the immune reactions is derived from Landsteiner's studies of haptens. He was able to successfully distinguish antibody in animals immunized with l-tartaric acid from antibody produced in animals immunized with other isomers of tartaric acid (Table 4–3).

It is becoming increasingly clear that although immunogens are usually large in size, only restricted portions of the molecule are actively involved in the reaction with antibody. Recent studies employing peptide protein complexes have established that molecules of the size of a tetra-peptide participate in the binding of antigen with antibody. The subunits of that antigenic determinant appear to contribute unequally to this binding process. The degree to which these components of an antigen or antigenic determinant induce and are involved in the reaction with antibody is termed *immunodominance*.

Complexity

The factors that determine the complexity of an immunogen include both physical and

Table 4–3. **The Reactivity of Sera Prepared Against the Isomers of Tartaric Acid***

Antisera	Haptens		
	l-tartaric acid	d-tartaric acid	m-tartaric acid
Anti-l-tartaric acid	+ + +	±	±
Anti-d-tartaric acid	0	+ + +	±
Anti-m-tartaric acid	±	0	+ + +

*After Landsteiner, K.: The Specificity of Serological Reactions. Cambridge, Harvard University Press, 1956.

chemical properties of the molecule. The state of aggregation of a molecule, for example, influences immunogenicity. A solution of monomeric proteins may actually induce a refractory state or tolerance when present in monomeric form but is highly immunogenic in its polymeric or aggregated state (Chapter 10). Several immunogens that do not induce an immune response when isolated in pure form do so when they are a part of a larger particle. Some artificial particles, or adjuvants, such as bentonite or aluminum hydroxide, may also serve to enhance immunogenicity.

Conformation

There is no one molecular configuration that is immunogenic. Linear or branched polypeptides or carbohydrates, as well as globular proteins, are all capable of inducing an immune response. Nonetheless, antibody that is formed to these different conformational structures is highly specific and can readily discriminate these differences. When the conformation of an antigen has been changed, the antibody induced by the original form no longer combines with it. When a determinant group consists of a sequence of amino acids derived from different portions of a folded polypeptide chain, an antibody directed to it cannot, of course, recognize the extended chains when denaturation-unfolding takes place. Figure 4–3 schematically depicts the relationships of antibody-combining sites for antigenic determinants. It can be seen that antibody to the first antigen (A) will clearly accommodate its own antigen. Determinant B, which has an additional residue, may not be as easily accommodated with antibody to A.

Charge

Immunogenicity is not limited to a particular molecular charge; positive, negative, and neutral substances can be immunogenic. However, the net charge of the immunogen does appear to influence the net charge of the resultant antibody. It has been shown that immunization with some positively charged immunogens results in the production of negatively charged antibodies. These data suggest that the production of antibody may be influenced by the overall charge of an immunogen.

Accessibility

The accessibility of the determinant groups to the recognition system will determine the outcome of an immune response. Recent developments have allowed investigators to prepare synthetic immunogenic polypeptides that contain a limited number of amino acids and in which chemical structure can be defined. In Figure 4–4, three types of multichain branched synthetic polypeptides are shown. In the first example, alanine side chains are attached to the amino groups of polylysine backbone, and on the outside the immunodominant tyrosine and glutamic acid groups are added. An immune response will occur to these immunodominant groupings when this polymer is injected into a rabbit. In the center diagram, the immunodominant tyrosine and glutamic acid determinants are placed next to the polylysine backbone, and the alanine side chains or "whiskers" protrude into the outside milieu. No immune response occurs to this configuration. In the third example, however, the spatial configuration of the side chains has been modified by alternating alanine with lysine residues,

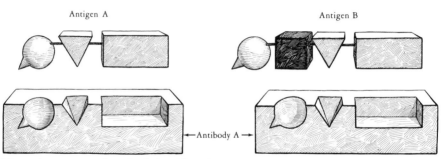

Figure 4–3. Schematic representation of relationships of antibody-combining sites for antigen determinations. (After Sela, M.: Antigenicity: Some molecular aspects. Science, *166*:1365, 1969.)

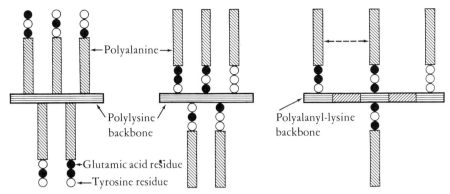

Figure 4–4. Three types of multichain-branched synthetic polypeptides. (After Sela, M.: Studies with synthetic polypeptides. Adv. Immunol., 5:29, 1966.)

forming a polylysine-polyalanine backbone structure. Since the side chains can be inserted only at the location of the lysine groupings, the space between them is greatly lengthened. When injected into an experimental animal, this polymer will induce an immune response. Thus, the accessibility of determinant groupings on an immunogen will influence whether an immune response will occur.

CHEMICAL PROPERTIES

Most organic chemical groupings, with the exception of pure lipids, can be immunogens. The most effective immunogens are those that display diverse chemical and structural characteristics. However, a single amino acid variation in a protein may give rise to a new antibody specificity owing to a profound change in conformation, which might occur as a result of this single substitution.

There are two kinds of chemical structures that appear to influence immunogenicity: (1) the sequential determinants whose specificity is determined by the sequence of subunits within the determinant, e.g., primary amino acid sequence in the case of a protein, and (2) the conformational determinants that are determined by secondary, tertiary, or quaternary structure.

Digestibility

In general, a potent immunogen is one that is capable of being phagocytosed and degraded within the host. Recent information has shown, however, that nonmetabo-lized or noncatabolized substances, such as polystyrene, can also be immunogenic in minute quantities. Moreover, it should be noted that the efficiency with which phagocytosis proceeds appears to determine whether an antigen is eliminated or persists. This outcome is of profound biologic significance, since the elimination of antigens will determine whether an immune response will be beneficial or harmful. With successful elimination of antigen, the outcome is beneficial; if antigen persists, the tertiary manifestations of immunity may result in tissue damage by any of the various mechanisms of immunologic injury.

Different Chemical Types of Immunogens

The overwhelming majority of immunogens in nature are protein. These may exist as pure proteins or may combine with other substances such as lipids (lipoproteins), nucleic acids (nucleoproteins), or carbohydrates (glycoproteins). Shown in Table 4–4 are some examples of different chemical classes of immunogens.

Some examples of foreign proteins that may be immunogenic include serum and tissue proteins, the structural proteins of viruses, bacteria and other microorganisms, toxins, plant proteins, and enzymes. Antibodies to these substances are sometimes used clinically in immunotherapy (antitoxins) and in the preparation of certain vaccines. On the other hand, when they lead to the production of antibodies that are deleterious, they may be responsible for some of the sequelae of the immunologically mediated

Table 4–4. Chemical Classes of Immunogens

Type	Source
Protein	Serum proteins, microbial products (toxins), enzymes
Lipoprotein	Serum lipoproteins, cell membranes
Polysaccharides	Capsules of bacteria (pneumococcus)
Lipopolysaccharides	Cell walls of gram-negative bacteria (endotoxins)
Glycoproteins	Blood group substances A and B
Polypeptides	Hormones (insulin, growth hormones), synthetic compounds
Nucleic acids	Nucleoproteins, single-stranded DNA

diseases. For example, following streptococcal infections, some antibodies that cross-react with cardiac tissue may be associated with some of the disease expressions of rheumatic fever. The lipoproteins are special types of protein immunogens that are found as part of many cell membranes.

Polysaccharides are another class of immunogens. They may occur as pure polysaccharide substances, as in the capsules of bacteria such as the pneumococcus, or they may be lipopolysaccharides occurring within cell walls of gram-negative bacteria (endotoxins). These substances are quite important biologically, since antibodies directed to them may provide protective immunity (antipneumococcal antibody). The lipopolysaccharides account for pathogenicity of certain gram-negative organisms, e.g., cholera endotoxin.

The best known examples of glycoprotein antigens include the blood group substances A and B and the Rh antigens (Chapter 3). The immunogenicity of these substances has been associated with transfusion reactions and with isoimmunization of pregnancy. In addition, the histocompatibility antigens (Chapter 3) are also composed of carbohydrate and protein. Polypeptide immunogens have been used experimentally in the form of synthetic polypeptides and have contributed to our understanding of many basic principles underlying immunogenicity. They are also used in clinical medicine, e.g., radioimmunoassay of insulin. Their immunogenicity is at times undesirable, in which case the production of antibodies is associated with refractoriness to therapy, e.g., insulin antibodies.

The nucleic acids were for many years considered nonimmunogenic; however, under certain conditions they may serve as immunogens, particularly when single-stranded. In patients with the disease systemic lupus erythematosus, circulating antibody to native DNA or other nuclear constituents can be demonstrated. The inflammatory response induced by these antibodies or complexes of DNA–anti-DNA is thought to be responsible for the tissue damage (to blood vessels, glomeruli, and so forth) associated with severe forms of the disease.

HOST-RELATED FACTORS

Immunogenicity has profound biologic implications. The response to any given immunogens not only is a function of the physicochemical properties of the substance but also is connected with several host-related factors, including genetic makeup of the host, age, nutritional status, and any of a number of secondary effects that are derived from disease processes (Chapter 1). It should also be clearly understood that the measurement of any immunologic reactant to an immunogen should not necessarily be equated to a protective function in the host. For example, it is known that the presence of circulating antibody in many types of localized viral infections does not prevent reinfection with these viruses Other factors of immunity also appear to be involved with the total host protection, e.g., secretory IgA antibody, as well as cell-mediated immunity.

It is now well established that live attenuated vaccines have greater clinical efficacy in the prevention of disease than do their killed or inactivated counterparts. Further, serum antibody levels appear to be of longer duration following the use of live replicating vaccines or natural infection. Possibly owing to the continued persistence of immunogen, replicating agents may provide a more sustained stimulation of the immunologic system through the recruitment of additional immunocompetent cells. The methods used in preparation of an antigen may also have an adverse effect on the immunogenicity of a vaccine. Figure 4–2 shows Group A streptococcus from which critical protective immunogens have been removed during processing. As can be seen, the dead vaccine contains neither the capsule nor the M proteins important in inducing protective immunity. The recent development of effective capsular polysaccharide vaccines has been made possible by a knowledge of principles of immunogenicity and has provided effective and safe vaccines for the prevention of serious infections caused by encapsulated bacteria, e.g., *S. pneumoniae, N. meningitides,* and *H. influenzae* Type B. Obviously, these are important considerations in the preparation of killed microbial vaccines that may lead to products that are more effective in inducing protective immunity.

Immunogenicity varies from species to species and, within a given species, from individual to individual (Chapter 3). For example, although nonimmunogenic in the rabbit, the isolated polysaccharide capsule of the pneumococcus can lead to a full immune response in the mouse. However, if polysaccharide is injected as part of a whole bacterial suspension, the rabbit will produce antibody to these polysaccharides. When all physical and chemical requirements for immunogenicity are fulfilled, the capacity of a given individual or inbred strain of animal to respond to various immunogens is genetically determined. The genes controlling the immune response in the mouse (Ir genes) are found within the same complex as the major histocompatibility (H-2) locus. "Responder" and "nonresponder" strains of mice and guinea pigs have demonstrated the exquisite sensitivity of the immune response to minor variations of immunogen (Chapter 3).

The amount of immunogen injected also influences the response. Studies of immunologic tolerance illustrate that a very low or a very high dose of foreign material can inhibit future responses to the subsequent injection of an otherwise immunogenic dose (Chapter 10). Dose and intervals between injections have also been shown to produce antibody populations of differing titer and avidity.

The route of injection can influence the nature of the immune response. For example, certain immunogens, when injected parenterally, e.g., intravenously, lead to the production primarily of circulating antibody; when given intradermally, the same immunogen may also provoke cell-mediated immunity, in addition to circulating antibody. When assessing the immunogenicity of a preparation, the type of test assay must also be evaluated since false negative reactions may occur when test procedures lack sensitivity or specificity.

Finally, an important biologic property of immunogens is the ability of certain antigens to evoke allergic or hypersensitivity responses. These reactions, which are expressions of the immune response, may either be cell-mediated or humoral. For example, when certain low molecular weight compounds, such as the catechols from poison ivy, contact the skin, a dermatitis will result that is mediated through sensitized lymphocytes (delayed hypersensitivity). On the other hand, penicillin, when combined with tissue proteins, will evoke an antibody response that may lead to anaphylactic shock or urticarial hives (immediate hypersensitivity). These allergic manifestations are biologic expressions of the immune response that are harmful— the immunologically mediated diseases.

ADJUVANTS

Certain substances, referred to as adjuvants, enhance the immune response when injected together with an immunogen (Chapter 10). Their function has been considered to increase the surface area of antigen (e.g., alum-precipitated diphtheria toxoid) or to prolong their retention in the body, allowing time for the lymphoid system to have access to the antigen (Freund's adjuvant). Recent evidence suggests that adjuvants may selectively expand T- and B-lymphocyte populations in addition to their classic granuloma-producing effects. The current use of adjuvants in immunotherapy of cancer is described in Chapter 10.

SUMMARY

The term "immunogen" has been proposed to define any substance capable of evoking an immune response. The properties of an immunogen are determined by the physical, chemical, and biologic properties of the substance, which are, in turn, related to its primary structure. Certain chemical groupings on the immunogen that determine specificity of the immunologic reaction are referred to as determinant groups, the most potent of which are termed immunodominant points. Implicit in immunogenicity is the requirement for genetic dissimilarity and recognition of foreignness by the host's surveillance system. Thus, immunogenicity represents the net interplay of the physicochemical properties of the immunogen as well as the response of several host-related factors such as age, genetic makeup, and the general state of the host.

Suggestions for Further Reading

Borek, F. (ed.): Immunogenicity. North-Holland Research Monographs. Vol. 25. Amsterdam, North-Holland, 1972.

Benjamin, E., Scibienski, R. J., and Thompson, K.: The relationship between antigenic structure and immune specificity. *In* F. P. Inman (ed.): Contemporary Topics in Immunochemistry. Vol. I. New York, Plenum Press, 1972, pp. 1–43.

Goodman, J. W.: Immunogenicity and antigenic specificity. *In* Stobo, J. D., Fudenberg, H. H., Wells, J. V., et al. (eds.): Basic and Clinical Immunology. 4th ed. Los Altos, Lange Medical Publications, 1982.

Kabat, E. A.: Structural Concepts in Immunology and Immunochemistry. 2nd ed. New York, Holt, Rinehart and Winston, 1975.

Milstein, C.: Monoclonal antibodies. Sci. Am., *243*:66, 1980.

Sela, M.: Antigenicity, some molecular aspects. Science, *166*:1365, 1969.

Sela, M.: Studies with synthetic polypeptides. Adv. Immunol., *5*:29, 1966.

Williams, R. C., Jr. (ed.): Lymphocytes and Their Interactions. Kroc Foundation Series. Vol. 4. New York, Raven Press, 1977.

Chapter 5

Antibody and Immunoglobulins: Structure and Function

George M. Bernier, M.D.

Immunoglobulins are a remarkable collection of protein molecules, which are the effector molecules of the humoral limb of immunity. These proteins share many antigenic, structural, and biologic similarities, but at the same time significant differences in primary amino acid sequence permit their antibody function and biologic activity to be highly specific for their role in bodily defense. Immunoglobulins are not simply molecules that combine with antigens in a "lock and key" fashion; they are very complex proteins with many highly specialized features in addition to their antigen-combining abilities. For example, to be effective, a human antibody to influenza virus might require several different structural capabilities: (1) a portion of the molecule that could combine specifically with the influenza virus and inhibit it; (2) another portion that could facilitate passage into the respiratory tract at the point of viral replication and permit a high concentration of such molecules in that region; (3) a mechanism to prevent the molecule from being degraded by the proteolytic enzymes that abound in the respiratory tree; and (4) a portion of the molecule that can combine with phagocytic cells. The human immune system has developed the kind of sophisticated specialization that permits this remarkable combination of properties to exist in a single molecular species known as secretory immunoglobulin A. Other equally distinctive features are associated with other kinds of immunoglobulins. As knowledge of the structure of immunoglobulins has developed, as the details of amino acid sequence have been revealed, and, in particular, as the genetic basis of antibody has been unraveled, the chemical basis of these and related phenomena has become more understandable.

HISTORY

The first real chemical information regarding the structure of antibodies was provided by Tiselius and Kabat in the early 1940's. These workers demonstrated that the fraction of serum proteins, the gamma globulins, that migrated most slowly in electrophoresis contained most of the serum antibodies. In the 1950's, Porter treated antibodies with papain, a proteolytic enzyme that split the antibody molecules into three fragments; two retained antibody activity and one possessed most of the antigenic features of gamma globulin. In the early 1960's, Edelman demonstrated that immunoglobulins were multichain structures, and a four-chain model of immunoglobulins was proposed by Porter. Putnam and Titani and Hilschmann and Craig initiated the studies of amino acid sequence of immunoglobulins using Bence Jones proteins, which are excreted in the urine of patients with multiple myeloma. Determination of the amino acid sequence of the first complete immunoglobulin, an IgG myeloma protein, was completed in 1969 by Edelman and coworkers. In the 1970's, the primary sequence of a great many immunoglobulin molecules, myeloma proteins as well as more normally occurring antibodies, was determined. During the late 1970's and early 1980's the remarkable developments in molecular biology, pioneered by Leder, have unraveled the gene sequences and genetic mechanism of immunoglobulin production and variability.

Just as studies into the chemical nature of immunoglobulins were extremely fruitful, investigations into the complex biology of immunoglobulins clarified the function of the various kinds or classes of immunoglobulins.

In all these studies, the proteins elaborated by plasma cell tumors of man and mouse have proved to be of tremendous value in understanding the biologic, chemical, and genetic features of immunoglobulins.

THE FAMILY OF IMMUNOGLOBULINS

In man, five different classes of immunoglobulins are known to exist, each with a distinct chemical structure and a specific biologic role. These classes are designated by the letters G, A, M, D, and E following the abbreviation Ig (indicating their immunoglobulin function) or, by some writers, following the symbol γ (indicating their electrophoretic mobility as gamma globulins). Table 5–1 lists some of the properties of each class of immunoglobulins.

IgG is the most abundant of the immunoglobulins. These molecules achieve significant concentrations in both the vascular and the extravascular spaces, have a relatively long half-life (23 days), cross the placenta, and are able to activate complement. This class of immunoglobulin is thought to contribute to immunity against many infecting agents that have a blood-borne dissemination, including bacteria, viruses, parasites, and some fungi. In addition, it provides antibody activity in tissues. Receptors for IgG exist on human monocytes, on polymorphonuclear leukocytes (polys), on reticuloendothelial cells in spleen and liver, and on some lymphocytes.

Although IgA is the second most abundant serum immunoglobulin, its most important contribution to the immunity of the individual is in the external secretory system. This important secretory immunoglobulin is produced in high concentrations by the lymphoid tissues lining the gastrointestinal, respiratory, and genitourinary tracts. In these secretions (e.g., saliva, tears) IgA is combined with a protein termed *secretory component* that appears to facilitate its transport into secretions and to endow the molecule with some protection against the effects of the proteo-

lytic enzymes normally found in these regions. The IgA molecules do not activate complement by the classic pathway but may do so via the properdin system. IgA does not cross the placenta; however, it contributes to the immunity of the newborn by virtue of its high concentration in colostrum. Receptors for IgA are found on lymphocytes, polys, and monocytes.

IgM is the largest of the immunoglobulin molecules and, because of its large size, is restricted almost entirely to the intravascular space. These macromolecules are highly efficient agglutinators of particulate antigens such as bacteria and red blood cells, and they fix complement with a high degree of efficiency (Chapter 6). This class of immunoglobulin seems to be of greatest importance in the first few days of the primary immune response. When a foreign antigen is introduced into a host for the first time, the synthesis of IgM antibodies precedes that of IgG. However, the level of IgM antibodies peaks within a few days and then declines more rapidly than the level of IgG antibodies (Chapter 7).

The fourth class of immunoglobulins, IgD, was discovered in the mid-1960's by Rowe and Fahey when they encountered a myeloma protein antigenically and chemically different from the then known immunoglobulins. To date, IgD has not been assigned a specific biologic role as a humoral antibody. Antibody activity has been associated with IgD globulin, for example, in cases of penicillin hypersensitivity in the human. This immunoglobulin class is found on the surface of lymphocytes, particularly in neonates, with a frequency that far exceeds its relative serum concentration. Hence, a role for IgD as a specific surface receptor in the initiation of the immune response is likely (Chapter 7).

The reaginic antibody, IgE, is an immunoglobulin present in only trace amounts in serum. It has the ability to attach to human skin (homocytotropic antibody) and to initiate aspects of the "allergic reaction" (Chapter 8). IgE was initially isolated by Ishizaka, who purified it from vast quantities of serum containing reaginic antibody. Subsequently, a few myeloma proteins of the IgE class have been identified. Like IgA, IgE is produced chiefly in the linings of the respiratory and intestinal tracts and is part of the external secretory system of antibody (Chapter 2). Deficiency of IgE has been inconstantly associated with deficiency of IgA in individuals

Table 5–1. Some Physical and Biologic Properties of Human Immunoglobulin Classes

Class	Mean Serum Concentration (mg/100 ml)	Molecular Weight	$S_{20 \cdot w}$	Mean Survival T/2 (days)	Biologic Function	Receptors on	Heavy Chain Designation	No. of Subclasses
IgG or γG	1240	150,000	7	23	Fix complement Cross placenta Heterocytotropic antibody	Polys, lymphocytes, monocytes	γ	4
IgA or γA	280	170,000	7,10,14	6	Secretory antibody Properdin pathway	Polys, lymphocytes, monocytes	α	2
IgM or γM	120	890,000	19	5	Fix complement	Lymphocytes	μ	1
IgD or γD	3	150,000	7	2.8	Lymphocyte surface receptor	—	δ	2
IgE or γE	0.03	196,000	8	1.5	Reaginic antibody Homocytotropic antibody	Mast cells Lymphocytes	ε	1

with impaired immunity who present with undue susceptibility to infection.

Subclasses

By antigenic analysis, it has been possible to detect relatively minor differences between molecules of a given class of immunoglobulin (Table 5–1). In this way, four different subclasses of IgG have been found and designated IgG1, IgG2, IgG3, and IgG4. In addition, two subclasses each for IgA and IgD globulins have been found and are termed IgA1 and IgA2 and IgD1 and IgD2, respectively. Subsequent chemical analysis has shown that subclass antigenic differences reflect substantial differences in amino acid sequence. As indicated below, important biologic distinctions have been correlated with the various subclasses. For example, IgG4 does not fix complement, whereas the other three IgG subclasses do, and IgG3 globulins have a half-life significantly shorter than that of the other three. A major chemical difference between subclasses is the location and number of interchain disulfide bridges.

Chain Structure of Immunoglobulin

The classification of immunoglobulins, as described above, was made on the basis of antigenic and structural considerations; the real basis for this classification is found in the chemical structure of the molecules. The IgG antibody molecule, for instance, is made up of four polypeptide chains held together by disulfide bonds (Fig. 5–1). Two of the chains are small, with molecular weights of 22,000, and are termed light chains. The other two, with molecular weights of 55,000 are called heavy chains. Each immunoglobulin molecule has two identical heavy chains and two identical light chains. A chemically different kind of heavy chain exists for each of the five classes of immunoglobulin and is responsible for the antigenic differences that have been observed between classes. More important, it is the heavy chain that is responsible for the observed biologic differences between the various classes.

Just as there are five kinds of heavy chains, two different *types* of light chains have been found to exist. The light-chain types are called kappa (κ) and lambda (λ) (for the pair of investigators who originally observed the two types—Korngold and Lipari). Each type of light chain occurs in association with each kind of heavy chain, i.e., in each of the five classes of immunoglobulins. There are ten possible combinations of heavy and light chains, and all ten are normally found in any individual. As indicated in Table 5–1, the five kinds of heavy chains are identified by the Greek-letter equivalent of their class name—γ, α, μ, δ, and ϵ. Any immunoglobulin may therefore be designated by its heavy- and light-chain composition, in a manner analogous to the hemoglobin nomenclature. An IgG molecule, for example, would have a formula $\gamma_2\kappa_2$ or $\gamma_2\lambda_2$.

This basic four-chain structural unit is the form in which IgG, IgD, and IgE exist. A four-chain unit is repeated in the higher molecular weight immunoglobulins; IgM generally exists as a pentamer of basic four-chain subunits with each of five subunits held together by disulfide bonds (Fig. 5–2). A relatively small molecule with high sulfhydryl content, the *J chain*, participates in the polymerization of IgM. The IgM subunits (180,000 daltons) are each made up of two heavy chains (67,000 daltons) and two light chains.

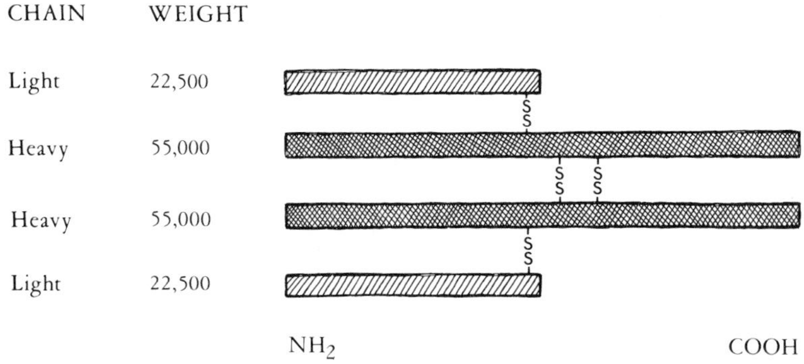

CHAIN	WEIGHT
Light	22,500
Heavy	55,000
Heavy	55,000
Light	22,500

NH$_2$ COOH

Figure 5–1. Schematic diagram of human IgG1 showing the location of interchain disulfide bonds. The molecule consists of two light chains and two heavy chains. The amino-terminal end is at the left and the carboxyl-terminal end is at the right. The structure depicted here is also applicable to other immunoglobulins with varying heavy-chain composition and polymerization.

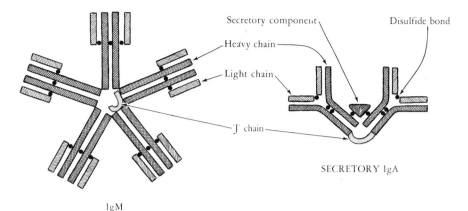

IgM

SECRETORY IgA

Figure 5–2. Models of IgM and secretory IgA. The former is shown in its usual pentameric form with a J chain involved in the pentamer formation. Secretory IgA is shown as a dimer attached to a secretory component. Note the absence of the light-heavy interchain bonds in the IgA. The IgA predominant in secretions is of the IgA2 subclass, which lacks such bonds.

IgA globulin, and occasionally IgG globulin, may also exist in a polymeric form in serum. Serum IgA, like IgM, may be polymerized through a sulfhydryl residue near the carboxyl terminus of the molecule, with the participation of J chain. In secretions, two IgA monomers are linked by J chain and *secretory component* (another non-immunoglobulin) to produce a complex of high molecular weight (Figs. 5–2 and 5–3).

As described before, it has been possible to classify IgA globulins into two subclasses, IgA1 and IgA2, based upon differences in antigenic structure and variation in the arrangement of interchain disulfide bridges. Whereas the IgA2 is a minor component of serum IgA, this subclass is the dominant form in secretions. Curiously, no covalent bonding exists between light and heavy chains in the common genetic variant of this subclass (Fig.

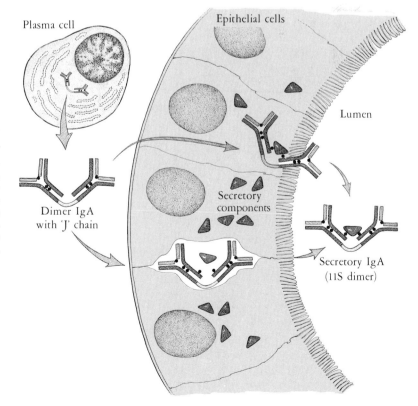

Figure 5–3. Representational drawing depicting the formation of secretory IgA. The IgA globulins are synthesized as monomers but are secreted from the plasma cells as dimers linked by the J chain. As the molecule passes through or in between the epithelial cells, it acquires the secretory component and enters the lumen as the secretory IgA molecule.

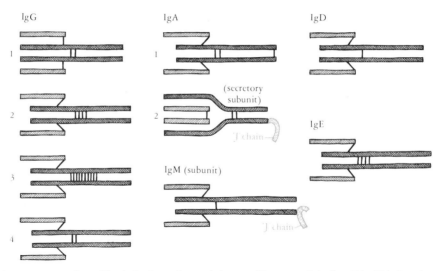

Figure 5–4. Arrangement of peptide chains in various subclasses of immunoglobulins. Disulfide bonds are represented by black bars. In the IgA and IgM subunits, the J chain, in gray, indicates where it would appear in the respective polymeric forms.

5–2). It has been noted that the IgA globulins are synthesized as monomers within plasma cells, which also synthesize J chain and are in contiguity with epithelial cells, containing the secretory component. After passage through the epithelium, IgA is recovered as a dimer, complexed with the secretory component (Fig. 5–3).

Just as the arrangement of interchain disulfide bonds is different in IgA subclasses, so too are there differences in the interchain bonds in the various IgG subclasses (Fig. 5–4). The biologic significance of these differences is not readily apparent, but they may account for some observed differences in such functions as life span or susceptibility to proteolytic degradation. For example, the IgG2 subclass has four heavy-heavy interchain bonds and is quite resistant to papain hydrolysis, as will be described below. Pathologically, the differences may be quite important, too. Myeloma globulins of the IgG3 subclass have an asymmetric structure because of the unusually long hinge region, and the abnormal viscosity this imparts to the blood of individuals with myeloma involving this Ig subclass may create serious problems.

ANTIBODY FUNCTION

An antibody produced in response to one antigen obviously must have structural features that are different from an antibody produced in response to any other antigen.

Antibody to tetanus, for example, must differ in some chemically definable way from antibody to diphtheria, since both antibodies can be shown to combine specifically with their homologous antigens. This property, known as *specificity*, is determined by the primary amino acid sequence of the antibody molecule. For example, reduction of disulfide bonds and disruption of all noncovalent forces by dispersing agents such as $8\ M$ urea will unfold the polypeptide chains of the molecule, with loss of antibody function. When the molecule is reconstituted by oxidation and removal of the dispersing agent, the antibody will re-form and regain its capacity for combination with its specific antigen.

The "antigen-binding site" or "antibody active site" of the immunoglobulin molecule is the region that combines with a specific antigen. In this region, the antibody specificity is determined by the amino acid sequence that permits its combination with the appropriate antigen. Both heavy and light chains share in this site; specifically, the first 110 amino acids from the amino-terminal end of each polypeptide chain are known to house antibody activity. In Figure 5–5, the IgG molecule is represented in a T-shaped configuration. The amino-terminal regions of variability on both the heavy and the light chains make up the antibody active sites. It is the amino acid sequence in these regions that dictates the specificity of the antibody. In IgG, IgD, and IgE, two antigen-binding sites

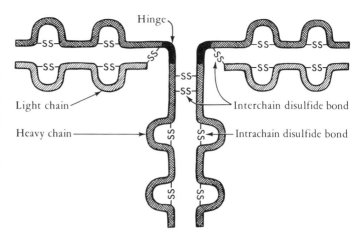

Figure 5–5. Schematic drawing of IgG in T-shaped model. The light chains are shaded by diagonal lines and the heavy chains marked with crosshatching. The hinge region is depicted in black. Disulfide bridges are represented by –SS–. The intrachain disulfide bonds pinch the chains into loops (domains). Extensive overall similarity is apparent in the placement of these loops between light and heavy chains and between the two portions of the heavy chains.

exist per molecule; in IgM, ten such sites exist; in dimeric IgA, such as is found in secretions, four combining sites are present.

A feature critical to the understanding of the overall structure of immunoglobulins is the symmetric arrangement of regions or *domains* for each of approximately 110 amino acids. These domains serve their own functions yet share some sequence homology. An immunoglobulin chain is composed of linked domains—two in light chains; four in the γ, α, and δ chains; and five in the μ and ε chains. In heavy chains, a nonhomologous stretch, the hinge region, separates the first two domains of the heavy chain from the other heavy-chain domains (Fig. 5–5).

Fragmentation of Immunoglobulins

Knowledge of the structure of the immunoglobulins has been greatly enhanced by the use of proteolytic enzymes, which degrade the molecule into definable fragments. *Papain* was shown by Porter to split the heavy chains of IgG in the hinge region, the area of the interchain disulfide bonds, yielding three fragments. One fragment, which can be crystallized, contains most of the IgG specific antigenic determinants of the molecule and is designated the Fc fragment; the other two fragments retain the ability to combine with antigen and are designated the Fab fragments (Fig. 5–6). Although of the same approximate size, the fragments differ strikingly in their function. Table 5–2 lists the composition and biologic activities associated with each. An attempt has been made in this table to describe the structure and function of the fragments in a format that is, if not memorable, at least mnemonic.

Another proteolytic enzyme, *pepsin,* acts upon the IgG molecule by degrading the heavy chain, beginning at the carboxyl-terminal end and proceeding to the region of

Figure 5–6. Schematic representation of the fragmentation of the IgG molecule by papain, which results in two Fab fragments and one Fc fragment. The Fab fragments possess one antigen-combining site each and can combine with, but may not give a visible reaction with, antigen. The Fc fragment lacks antigen-binding capabilities but retains many antigenic and biologic properties of IgG.

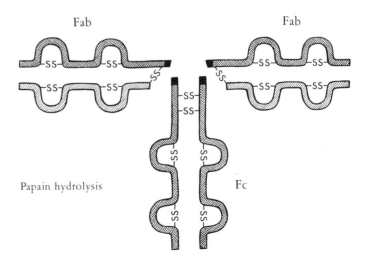

Table 5–2. Fragments of IgG Produced by Papain Cleavage

	Fab	Fc
Composition:	1. **A**mino-terminal half of heavy chain and one light chain 2. **A**berrated sequence	1. **C**arboxyl-terminal half of heavy chain dimer 2. **C**arbohydrate 3. **C**rystallizable (in some species) 4. **C**onstant amino acid sequence
Function:	1. **A**ntigen-binding or **a**ntib**o**dy active fragment	1. **C**omplement fixation 2. **C**ross placenta 3. **C**utaneous attachment (guinea pig skin)

the interchain disulfide bridge (Fig. 5–7). The splitting with *papain* produces univalent antibody fragments that can combine with antigens but not precipitate them; the *pepsin* treatment leaves a fragment that possesses two antigen-binding sites and can therefore still precipitate antigens. This fragment, termed F(ab′)$_2$, has lost most of the specific antigenic determinants of IgG, since most of these are located in the carboxyl-terminal half of the heavy chain (Fc fragment).

In addition to the Fab, F(ab′)$_2$, and Fc fragments, the term "Fd" is used to designate the amino-terminal half of the heavy chain, i.e., the half of the heavy chain located in the Fab fragment (Fig. 5–8). This region of the heavy chain is of great biologic importance, since it shares in the antigen-binding site and provides thermodynamically the lion's share of the binding affinity to antigen.

Trypsin has been employed in two different ways in the fragmentation of immunoglobulins. Prolonged digestion with trypsin results in cleavage of the peptide chain next to all arginine and lysine residues and the production of "tryptic peptides." These peptides may be examined by a combination of electrophoresis and chromatography, a technique called "fingerprinting" or "peptide mapping." This method has proved valuable in comparing the structure of two or more proteins, since it provides information about the comparative primary amino acid sequence without requiring exhaustive sequence analysis. The technique has been very useful in studies of variant human hemoglobins and in the study of human and animal immunoglobulins. Shorter periods of digestion of IgG and IgM with trypsin produce fragments similar to those derived by papain hydrolysis.

The other immunoglobulins can also be fragmented by proteolytic enzymes, but the fragments produced are not necessarily comparable to those derived from IgG. For instance, papain digestion of IgA often destroys the Fc portion of the molecule. However, in all immunoglobulin molecules, the regions are named according to the system described for the IgG, i.e., Fab, Fc, and Fd.

Enzymes produced by some bacteria, including the gonococcus and enteric streptococci, have been found to have proteolytic activity specific for the IgA1 subclass. This enzyme cleaves IgA1 molecules in the hinge region and produces fragments quite similar in size to the Fab and Fc fragments of IgG. While at first blush this is a tribute to the evolutionary adaptability of bacteria, in fact, the dominant form of IgA in the human intestinal tract is IgA2, a molecule impervious

F(ab′)$_2$

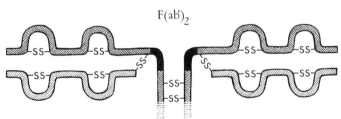

Pepsin digestion

Figure 5–7. Schematic representation of the degradation of IgG by pepsin. The Fc portion is hydrolyzed below the interchain disulfide bonds, leaving a single fragment with two combining sites intact, the F(ab′)$_2$.

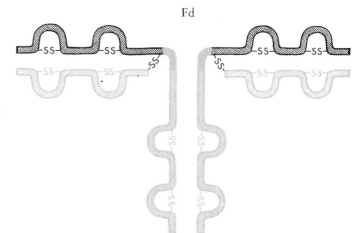

Fd

Figure 5–8. Molecular location of the Fd fragment of IgG is indicated in black. The light chains and the Fc portion of the heavy chain are represented in gray.

to the protease. Hence, it would appear that the human intestinal tract has emerged as victor in this particular evolutionary battle.

GENETIC FACTORS ASSOCIATED WITH IMMUNOGLOBULINS: GM, INV, AND AM FACTORS

Genetic markers have been found to be carried on immunoglobulin molecules (Chapter 7). The first two identified were designated Gm and Inv factors (Fig. 5–9) and were detected by the following indirect method.

The sera of some patients with rheumatoid arthritis agglutinate red blood cells coated with human gamma globulin. The anti–gamma globulin antibody contained in the sera of these individuals is called rheumatoid factor (RF). The reaction between the rheumatoid factor from a particular person and

gamma globulin–coated red cells was found to be inhibited by preincubation of the rheumatoid serum with serum from some normal persons. Some normal sera inhibited a particular rheumatoid factor reaction; others did not. The ability to inhibit a particular reaction was found to be inherited in a mendelian fashion, and the inhibitory substances in normal serum have been shown to be immunoglobulins. A number of hereditary factors reflecting different loci have been uncovered in this way and are associated with the various IgG heavy chains or with the κ-type light chain. Those factors associated with the heavy chain of IgG are termed Gm (for gamma) and those associated with the light chain are called Inv (the abbreviation of a patient's name) or sometimes Km (analogous to Gm). There are more than 20 recognized Gm factors and 3 Inv factors. As shown more recently (see Table 5–1), four different subclasses of IgG have been detected, and the various Gm factors are associated with one

Figure 5–9. In this drawing, the regions of sequence variability are depicted in gray. Note that the variable segment of the light chain is in apposition to the variable segment of the heavy chain—this is the region of antibody specificity. The antigenic markers Inv and Oz are indicated by ⊗. The Gm markers are localized in constant regions of the heavy chains and are the result of minor amino acid sequence variation.

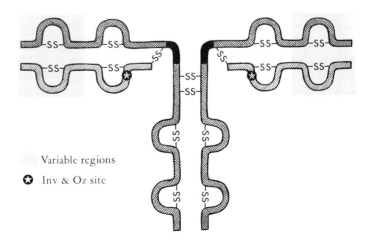

Variable regions

✪ Inv & Oz site

of these subclasses. The chemical basis for the Gm and Inv factors will be described later. It is important to point out that the Gm and Inv factors are nonallelic—that is, they are inherited independently of each other.

Another independently inherited group of genetic markers associated with IgA has been described. The reagents for identifying such factors have arisen as a result of transfusion. Some patients have been immunized in this way with an IgA genetically different from their own. Anti-IgA allotypic antibodies have thus been inadvertently produced, and their clinical manifestations have been transfusion reactions ranging from mild to severe. Different genetic factors have been found, and the term "Am" (referring to the IgA equivalent of Gm) has been applied to the system.

In all three systems (Gm, Inv, and Am), the detecting antibody is of human origin. In the first two it is frequently a rheumatoid factor, but, like the third factor, it is sometimes transfusion-induced. Since chemical differences between allotypes are minimal (one amino acid in the case of the Inv factor), detection has required antibodies generated in the same species. Allotypic differences between proteins of other species have been sought and detected immunologically by immunization within the species, under the assumption that the immunized animal's recognition system will detect minor differences between the immunizing antigen and its own proteins.

As might be anticipated, the various Gm factors are associated with specific subclasses of IgG, and the various Am factors are similarly associated with specific subclasses of IgA. To date, in the human system no allotypic markers have been found for the γ light chain or the μ, δ, or ε heavy chain.

PRIMARY STRUCTURE OF IMMUNOGLOBULINS

Heterogeneity

An aspect of antibodies that is of paramount interest to the protein biochemist paradoxically proved to be a major impediment to the understanding of immunoglobulins as protein molecules. This aspect is the unique situation of the extreme chemical heterogeneity of the gamma globulins occurring in the face of a degree of chemical constancy.

By way of illustration, albumin, transferrin, and most other serum proteins have a discrete electrophoretic mobility that is a manifestation of chemical homogeneity. Genetic variation in these serum proteins, as in the case of the human hemoglobins, often results in charge differences, which in turn are manifested as different electrophoretic forms. In contrast, the immunoglobulins of all individuals are spread over a very wide electrophoretic range. This electrophoretic variation is most apparent in the case of IgG and is readily illustrated by immunoelectrophoresis, which disperses the IgG molecules from the extreme cathodal end of the electrophoretic field almost all the way to the anode. The extreme electrophoretic heterogeneity of these molecules reflects a degree of variation in primary sequence that is remarkable among protein species. From what has been said before, this heterogeneity is obviously a manifestation of class, subclass, type, and genetic variation. More important, however, it reflects the chemical basis of antibody variability, i.e., of those differences, for instance, that distinguish an anti-tetanus antibody from an anti-diphtheria antibody.

Even when antibodies of a single specificity have been isolated, they too have been electrophoretically heterogeneous. It has been, therefore, most difficult to study the basis of chemical variability by analyzing antibodies themselves, because it is virtually impossible to establish the amino acid sequence in regions of variability. Instead, the problem has been approached by analyzing the homogeneous immunoglobulins produced in some malignant conditions that affect lymphocytes and plasma cells, notably in the human disease states of multiple myeloma and macroglobulinemia and in the mouse plasmacytoma system.

These disorders are characterized by the elaboration of large amounts of homogeneous immunoglobulins by proliferating cells. Such immunoglobulins are found in the serum or urine of affected individuals. The term "monoclonal" has been applied to the homogeneous immunoglobulin, implying that it is a consequence of the proliferation of a single clone of plasma cells. The proteins elaborated may be complete immunoglobulin molecules of IgG, IgA, IgM, IgD, or IgE class, or free light chains (Bence Jones proteins), or both. In very rare human conditions, such as the heavy-chain diseases, fragments or portions of immunoglobulin chains or molecules are produced.

Because of their homogeneity and their availability in great abundance, the monoclonal immunoglobulins are chemically suitable for amino acid sequence analysis. Much of the information relating to primary amino acid sequence derived from studies of such proteins has been applied to normal immunoglobulins. The rationale for using these abnormal immunoglobulins as models for normal antibody is based upon the following observations and suppositions.

1. Each complete monoclonal immunoglobulin appears to be one of the many normal immunoglobulins. The monoclonal proteins differ from pools of immunoglobulin in terms of restricted electrophoretic mobility, of biologic properties, of chain type, of genetic markers, and of physical properties. However, no unique pathologic features, such as novel amino acids, unusual prosthetic groups, or excessive lengths of peptide chains, have been found in any of the complete monoclonal immunoglobulins.

2. Many monoclonal immunoglobulins have been found to possess antibody activity. Indeed, the frequency of finding monoclonal immunoglobulins with antibody specificity seems proportional to the intensity of the search, and it is likely that all the monoclonal proteins would be *bona fide* antibodies, if only appropriate antigens could be found.

3. Monoclonal mouse and human antibodies have been produced using the hybridoma technology (see below). These antibodies have the characteristics of myeloma globulins: light and heavy chains of only one type and class, electrophoretic homogeneity, and restricted genetic markers.

Each monoclonal immunoglobulin possesses distinctive antigenic and chemical features. To date, complete identity has not been established between the monoclonal immunoglobulins produced by any two individuals. Even in the case of free light chains of one type (κ or λ) that have a molecular weight of only 22,500, no two have been identical. The chemical and antigenic differences are termed idiotypic markers, in contrast to the allotypic markers (Gm, Inv, and Am). If one assumes that one monoclonal immunoglobulin differs from another in the same way and to the same extent that one "normal" antibody molecule differs from another, then detailed examination of relatively few monoclonal immunoglobulins would be expected to provide information about the molecular location of variability, the extent of variability, and the genetic mechanisms responsible for the variability. It should be no surprise that the major antigenic and chemical differences that exist between myeloma proteins occur in that portion of the molecule in which variations between antibodies of different specificities occur.

The sequence of a wide variety of monoclonal immunoglobulins has been determined, and extensive amino acid sequence information is available to aid in the understanding of immunoglobulins. Moreover, the cells that produce these monoclonal Ig's have provided the DNA that has been useful in understanding the genetic basis of antibodies.

Hybridoma Technology as a Source of Monoclonal Antibody

One of the most important recent developments in immunology has been the development of a method for the *in vitro* production of large quantities of homogeneous antibody to a single antigenic specificity, i.e., monoclonal antibody. The source of this antibody is the hybridoma, which is the progeny of fusion between a normal antibody-secreting lymphoid (B) cell and a myeloma cell of animal or human origin. Since normal plasma cells usually die after a few cell divisions, there is a requirement to continue their cell divisions by fusion with a malignant myeloma cell. This technique therefore confers upon the progeny of the fusion the characteristics of both parental cells, namely the antigenic specificity of antibody secreted by the B-cell as well as the perpetuity of monoclonal immunoglobulin production by the myeloma cell.

The technique is schematically shown in Figure 5–10. Spleen cells obtained from mice that have been immunized with the desired antigen are the most commonly used source of antibody-secreting B-lymphocytes. These cells are exposed to an agent that promotes cell fusion, such as polyethylene glycol, while mixed with a suspension of myeloma cells in tissue culture. Following fusion a number of clones of hybrids appear, which are capable of producing various monoclonal antibody to any of the antigenic specificities found on the immunogen. Clones of hybrids of the desired antibody specificity are then selected from the pool and the antibody-producing cell lines are expanded by tissue culture techniques. Clones can be injected back into mice or into tissue culture and the purified

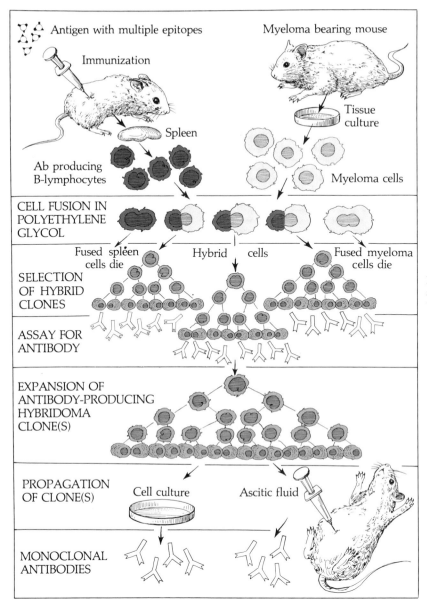

Figure 5–10. Schematic representation of the hybridoma technique for the production of monoclonal antibody.

monoclonal antibody then obtained from ascitic fluid or tissue culture supernatant fluid.

Monoclonal antibody produced by hybridomas is receiving widespread application as a source of diagnostic and therapeutic reagents. These include serologic reagents for identification of infectious agents, tumor antigens, histocompatibility antigens, and functional subpopulations of lymphoid cells, e.g., OKT3, OKT4, and OKT8.

Monoclonal antibodies have been employed in the treatment of lymphomas, acute and chronic leukemias, and T-cell malignancies and have virtually unlimited potential

use in tumor imaging and as vehicles for delivery of cytotoxic agents to tumor cells.

Light Chains

Bence Jones proteins (homogeneous free light chains) from myeloma patients and from mice with plasmacytomas were the first to be studied in appreciable numbers, and the following generalizations can be made. Two types of light chains exist throughout the vertebrate world: κ and λ. In various species one or the other is a predominant form. In man, approximately twice as many molecules have κ light chains as have λ chains. Light chains have been found to possess a region of constancy and a region of variability. The molecular topography of these regions is illustrated in Figure 5–11, and it is apparent that light chains are composed of two approximately equal halves—one constant and the other variable. The sequence of the carboxyl half of the molecule is virtually constant from one λ-type Bence Jones protein to another, or from one κ-type Bence Jones protein to another. Although a degree of homology is present (approximately 40 per cent), the κ chains are very different from the λ chains in this region, i.e., the constant region or domain.

In the amino-terminal half of the molecule, extensive variability is found between Bence Jones proteins of the same antigenic type. The transition from variable to constant region is an abrupt one. When larger numbers of Bence Jones proteins have been examined,

it has become apparent that subgrouping of κ and λ chains is possible, based on overall similarity in the amino-terminal half. The variability in this half within a given subgroup is considerably less and is of the kind that would result from changes in single base pairs. Approximately five different subgroups of each light-chain type have been determined on this basis.

There is one notable exception to the pattern of constancy in the carboxyl-terminal half of the light chains. In κ chains, either leucine or valine is found at position 191 and confers one of two genetic factors (Inv1 or Inv3, respectively). The great theoretical importance of this fact is that by inheritance of these markers the carboxyl-terminal half of the light chain can be shown to be transmitted according to mendelian principles. This will be described later as it applies to the genetic basis of antibody variability.

Another factor, called Oz, is found in an analogous position in the λ chain (position 190), where an arginine-lysine interchange

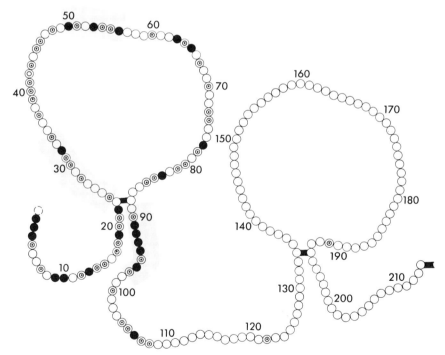

Figure 5–11. Composite drawing of human κ chain sequences illustrating variation in amino acid sequence among several different κ-type Bence Jones proteins. The amino-terminal end of the peptide chain is at the left, the carboxyl terminal at the right. Each circle represents one of the 214 amino acids of the chain. The *white* circles ○ indicate residues where only one amino acid was found. The *shaded* circles ◉ designate positions where two alternate amino acids were detected, and the *black* circles ● indicate positions where three or more different amino acids occurred. Disulfide bonds are indicated by black bars. The variable sequence is confined almost entirely to the amino-terminal half of the molecule. The carboxyl-terminal half is quite constant and the notable variation occurs at position 191, the site of the Inv genetic marker. The gray areas indicate the hypervariable areas that are apparent when sequences of human κ and λ chains and mouse κ chains are compared.

determines the presence or absence of an antigenic determinant. Unlike the Inv determinant, this is not a genetic factor, since all persons produce some λ chains with the Oz determinant and some λ chains without it.

Heavy Chains

The primary sequence of the heavy chains is different for each of the various immunoglobulin classes, but the amino acid sequence variation of the heavy chains is very similar to that observed in light chains. The amino-terminal end, comprising the first 110 or so amino acids, is the area of variable sequence and is termed the *variable domain* of the heavy chain or the V_H domain. The remaining residues represent regions of relative constancy and are termed constant regions or *constant domains* (Fig. 5–12). These are named according to the kind of peptide chain (γ, α, μ, δ, ϵ) and the relative position in the chain sequence (amino to carboxyl terminus). For example, in an IgG molecule, the domains would be identified in order as $V_H \ldots C\gamma_1 \ldots C\gamma_2 \ldots C\gamma_3$. In the heavy chain of IgM, which is larger by one domain, the order would be $V_H \ldots C\mu_1 \ldots C\mu_2 \ldots C\mu_3 \ldots C\mu_4$.

Each constant domain of each kind of heavy chain has a distinctive amino acid sequence. However, there exists a significant degree of homology from constant domain to constant domain within a peptide chain and between heavy chains of various classes. It is interesting, from an evolutionary view-point, that greater similarities exist between a given domain in different heavy chains than between two different domains in the same heavy chain. For example, the $C\alpha_2$ is more like the $C\gamma_2$ than the $C\alpha_3$. This would argue that class divergence occurred after basic immunoglobulin structure was established.

Two important points must be made concerning the V_H regions. These domains appear in every kind of heavy chain and are not distinctive for any class. The V_H of a particular IgG molecule may be more like the V_H of an IgM than that of another IgG. Also, just as subtypes of light-chain variable regions are evident from comparative amino acid sequence, so can the variable regions of heavy chains be subgrouped into V_{HI}, V_{HII}, $V_{HIII} \ldots$. Within a given subgroup, the variation in sequence is much less, as is true of the light chains.

Myeloma globulins have provided the prototype models for analysis in establishing these structural considerations. Although the chemical basis was determined by peptide mapping and amino acid sequence analysis, it has been possible to obtain a significant amount of information from immunologic analysis. It is possible, for instance, to recognize the unique variable region of a given myeloma globulin by immunizing rabbits with the monoclonal protein and absorbing the resultant antiserum with normal immunoglobulins. Antisera so prepared often (but not always) continue to react with the variable domains of the immunizing globulin and can distinguish this monoclonal globulin from all others. The antigens recognized in this way

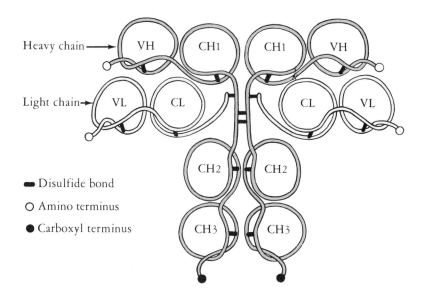

Heavy chain →

Light chain →

● Disulfide bond

○ Amino terminus

● Carboxyl terminus

Figure 5–12. Schematic drawing of IgG in a T-shaped model. Each peptide chain is drawn as a continuous line, and attachments between heavy and light chains and between the two heavy chains are indicated by solid bars. Note the two loops in each light chain and the four loops in each heavy chain. These loops are formed by intrachain disulfide bonds and are termed domains. In each chain, one domain (V) has a *variable* amino acid sequence depending on the antibody specificity of the molecule. The other domains (C) have a rather *constant* sequence common among molecules of the same class, subclass, and type. They are numbered in sequence from the amino-terminal end.

are called idiotypic antigens and the antisera are termed anti-idiotype.

By employing antisera made specific for the idiotypic markers of a monoclonal immunoglobulin, it is possible to identify the presence of similar idiotypic markers in cells, on cell surfaces, and in trace amounts in the serum of patients. Anti-idiotypic antibodies have been used to identify antibodies of a common specificity in inbred rabbits. Monoclonal anti-idiotypic antibodies have also been made using the hybridoma technique.

Three-Dimensional Structure

Immunoglobulins have been visualized by the negative staining technique of electron microscopy. X-ray crystallography has also been applied to the study of immunoglobulins, particularly crystallizable monoclonal immunoglobulins, and electron microscopy has been used in the study of sections of such crystalline IgG molecules. By a variety of physical methods, the IgG molecule appears to be composed of three principal units (one Fc and two Fab's). There appears to be a significant amount of flexibility in the hinge region between the Fc and Fab's, with the molecule able to assume a Y or T shape, depending on its association with antigen.

Each of the major fragments has dimensions of approximately 50 × 40 × 70 Å. Hence, the "wing span" of the molecule across the Fab's is approximately 130 to 140 Å (Fig. 5–13).

From hapten-binding studies, as well as physical measurements, the combining site would appear to be a crevice involving the light and heavy chain in the range of 15 Å deep.

Polymeric molecules, such as secretory IgA and pentameric IgM, have been observed by means of electron microscopy. The striking feature of the IgM molecules is their rosette-like structure, similar to that shown schematically in Figure 5–2.

Evolutionary Aspects

A feature common to both heavy and light chains is the location of the intrachain disulfide bonds. As described earlier, these are so situated that the peptide chains are "pinched" into a series of loops of approximately 60 amino acids each. Two loops are found in

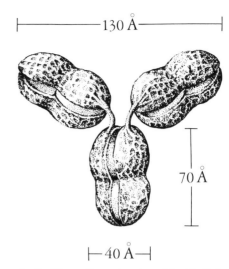

Figure 5–13. Three-dimensional model of IgG showing the close relationship between domains in each of the Fab fragments and in the Fc fragment. The compact areas are linked through the hinge region. This model is based on the studies of x-ray crystallography and electron microscopy.

each light chain, four are found in each IgG, IgA, and IgD heavy chain, and five are found in each IgM and IgE heavy chain. The loops are depicted in highly schematic fashion in Figures 5–11 and 5–12. The recurring periodicity of such loops or domains suggests that the complex immunoglobulin molecule has evolved from a primitive peptide chain approximately 110 amino acids long. A significant degree of homology is found among the various domains of light and heavy chains, and this gives credence to the concept of a common primitive progenitor. It is important to point out that as the particular peptide chains exist today, the differences are more pronounced between classes than between species. For instance, the κ chain of man is closer in sequence to the κ chain of the mouse than it is to the λ chain of man. From a phylogenetic point of view, a low molecular weight IgM class of immunoglobulin appears to be the most primitive of the extant immunoglobulins.

Of considerable interest along these lines is β_2 microglobulin, an 11,600 dalton cell surface protein associated with the HLA antigen system. This protein, which is also found free in body fluids, has the characteristics of a free domain in that it has a disulfide-bonded loop of 60 amino acids. The β_2 microglobulin has a homology of greater than 20 per cent with virtually every constant domain of every immunoglobulin. It is possible that the earliest forms of immunoglobulins were cell surface–associated protective molecules.

THE GENESIS OF ANTIBODY VARIABILITY

Under appropriate conditions, the introduction of a foreign antigen into a man or an animal results in the production of specific antibody. Two broad mechanisms were invoked to explain the phenomenon of specificity as it occurs in the immune response. The germ line theories held that cells already committed to production of a particular antibody were stimulated by the introduction of antigen to proliferate and elaborate their product. The germ line theories were predicated on the existence of myriad genes, representing all possible antibody specificities. In contrast, the somatic mutation theory postulated few germ line genes that underwent extensive somatic rearrangement and mutation.

In contrast to the "one gene–one polypeptide chain" concept that had been the keystone of molecular biology, new notions had to be invoked to explain the origin of antibody variability. A "two genes–one polypeptide chain" concept was proposed initially to account for the constant and variable portions of the immunoglobulin peptide chain. According to the concept, one gene (a "C" gene) would encode the constant portion of the peptide chain and another gene (a "V" gene) would encode the variable portion. During the selection process, the two genes would link up and the now completed DNA sequence would lead to synthesis of a complete polypeptide chain product. The germ line would contain relatively few "C" genes, one for each type of light chain (κ and the two kinds of λ) and one for each subclass or class of heavy chain (four for IgG, two each for IgA and IgD, and one each for IgM and IgE). A number of "V" genes, however, would have to be present to encode the variable portion of the peptide chain and thereby to confer antibody specificity.

Advances in molecular biology have greatly clarified many of the mechanisms underlying the genesis of antibody variability.

The germ line of an individual can indeed be shown to contain genes that code for the constant regions of immunoglobulins and other genes that encode for the variable segments. As can be shown for many other protein-synthesizing systems, intervening sequences of nonexpressed DNA (introns) separate genes and gene segments from each other. In the mouse the genes that encode for heavy chains are on chromosome 12, those for the κ light chain on chromosome 16, and those for the λ chain on chromosome 6. In each case, those chains responsible for the variable region are on the 5′ side (or "upstream") of the constant-region genes.

On chromosome 12, three distinct gene families that are involved in generating the variable region of heavy chains exist side by side. These three distinct gene families, variable (V_H), diversity (D), and joining (J_H), together generate the unique specificity of an antibody. During differentiation of the B cell, V_H, D, and J_H segments are linked, with a loss of the intervening sequences, to form a V-D-J gene. The process is termed rearrangement. Subsequently, the V-D-J gene and one constant-region gene are transcribed and the messenger RNA derived from this encodes for the complete immunoglobulin heavy chain (Fig. 5–14), deleting the introns.

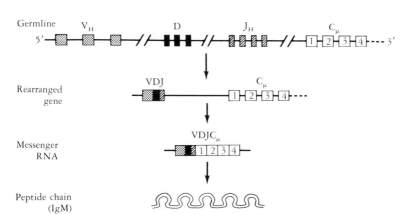

Figure 5–14. Schematic representation of the process whereby gene segments are linked and transcribed. One of many V_H region genes, one of several D genes, and one of several J_H genes are linked through rearrangement with loss of the other V_H, D, and J_H genes. This complex, which now codes the variable region of the antibody is transcribed along with the C region genes of the appropriate class into messenger RNA.

The temporal sequence in which the various immunoglobulins are expressed (μ, δ, γ, ϵ, α) follows the order of heavy-chain constant-region genes as they exist on chromosome 12. Following gene arrangement, a given heavy-chain constant gene is expressed and is transcribed with the variable-region gene. When a "switch" in Ig classes occurs, the previously expressed constant gene appears to be deleted and a subsequent constant gene is activated and transcribed. In this fashion a single cell can produce sequentially several different classes of immunoglobulin with the same antibody specificity.

A very similar process occurs with the assembly of the messenger for light chains, except that D genes do not exist in the repertoire, only V, J, and constant-region genes. Vλ and Jλ genes are transcribed with the Cλ DNA to produce λ chains, and Vκ, Jκ, and Cκ genes are transcribed for production of that kind of light chain. In the final assembly of antibodies, the heavy and light chains are themselves linked through disulfide bonds and secreted by the antibody-forming cell.

The diversity of the variable regions reflects (a) the V_H gene pool, (b) the D genes that provide frame shifts, (c) the J_H gene pools, and (d) the pairing of the heavy chain with one of many light chains. In addition, during the life of the cell, it appears that a significant degree of· somatic mutation occurs, which further defines and refines antibody specificity. Thus, elements of both the germ line and the mutational theories have been shown to be correct.

Suggestions for Further Reading

Edelman, G. M.: The covalent structure of human G-immunoglobulin XI. Functional implications. Biochemistry, *9*:3197, 1970.

Hood, L., and Talmage, D. W.: On the mechanism of antibody diversity: germline basis for variability. Science, *168*:325, 1970.

Ishizaka, T., and Ishizaka, K.: Biology of immunoglobulin E: molecular basis of reaginic hypersensitivity. Prog. Allergy, *19*:60, 1975.

Low, T. L. K., Liu, Y-S. V., and Putnam, F. W.: Structure, function, and evolutionary relationships of Fc domains of human immunoglobulins A, G, M, and E. Science, *191*:390, 1976.

Nisonoff, A., Hopper, J. E., and Spring, S. B. (eds.): The Antibody Molecule. New York, Academic Press, 1975.

Putnam, F. W. (ed.): The Plasma Proteins: Structure, Function and Genetic Control. New York, Academic Press, 1976.

Siebenlist, U., Ravetch, J. V., Korsmeyer, S., et al.: Human immunoglobulin D segments encoded in tandem multigenic families. Nature, *294*:631, 1981.

Chapter 6

The Complement System

Steven L. Kunkel, Ph.D., Peter A. Ward, M.D.,
Lynn H. Caporale, Ph.D., and Carl-Wilhelm Vogel, M.D.

INTRODUCTION

The complement system is an integral part of the body's immune system. Although the term "complement" was originally used to describe an auxiliary factor in serum that, acting upon an antibody-coated cell (such as a red blood cell or a bacterium), would cause cell death, the complement system is now known to involve at least 20 proteins that circulate in the plasma in an inactive form. These proteins can be activated by two independent pathways, termed the classical pathway and the alternative pathway.

Activation of the complement system results in a cascade of interactions of these proteins, leading to the generation of products that have important biologic activities and that constitute an important humoral mediator system involved in inflammatory reactions. First, coating of particles, such as bacteria or immune complexes, with certain components of complement facilitates the ingestion of the particle by phagocytic cells (opsonic function of complement). Second, the activation event generates many fission products of complement proteins for which specific receptors exist on a variety of inflammatory cells, such as granulocytes, lymphocytes, and other cells. Binding of these complement-derived products to such receptors results in biologic activities such as chemotaxis and hormone-like activation of cellular functions (inflammatory function of complement). Third, the late-acting proteins of the complement cascade form the macromolecular membrane attack complex, which causes death of target cells. This killing activity may be directed against viruses, bacteria, fungi, parasites, virus-infected cells and tumor cells (cytotoxic function of complement).

An intact complement system is essential to the maintenance of health. Moreover, it has been particularly useful to measure certain components of complement in clinical situations as indicators of disease activity. The importance of complement becomes evident in many patients with congenital defects of a complement protein, who present with recurrent infections or immune complex diseases. An understanding of the complement system is therefore important for diagnosis and management of patients who present with recurrent infections, allergic diseases, and autoimmune disorders.

PATHWAYS OF COMPLEMENT ACTIVATION AND THE COMPLEMENT PROTEINS

Activation of complement can occur by two separate pathways: the classical and the alternative pathways. Both pathways lead to a common terminal pathway referred to as the pathway of membrane attack. Twenty plasma proteins, listed in Table 6–1, are now known to be constituents of these pathways. These proteins can be divided into functional proteins, which represent the elements of the various pathways, and regulatory proteins, which exhibit control function. The concentration of the proteins in normal human plasma covers a broad range. They are synthesized in the liver but also by cells of the lymphoreticular system, such as lymphocytes and monocytes.

Both the classical and the alternative complement pathways can be organized into various operational units: initiation, amplification, and membrane attack (Fig. 6–1). Following an initial recognition event, which leads to initiation of the pathway, an ampli-

Table 6–1. **Proteins of the Complement System**

Protein	Molecular Weight	Plasma Concentration
Classical Pathway		
C1q	400,000	65 µg/ml
C1r	190,000	50 µg/ml
C1s	88,000	40 µg/ml
C4	200,000	640 µg/ml
C2	117,000	25 µg/ml
C3	185,000	1400 µg/ml
Alternative Pathway		
Factor B	93,000	200 µg/ml
Factor D	23,000	2 µg/ml
C3	185,000	1400 µg/ml
Membrane Attack Pathway		
C5	200,000	80 µg/ml
C6	128,000	75 µg/ml
C7	121,000	55 µg/ml
C8	154,000	55 µg/ml
C9	79,000	60 µg/ml
Regulatory Proteins		
C1 Inhibitor	85,000	20 µg/ml
C4b Binding protein	570,000	250 µg/ml
Carboxypeptidase N	310,000	50 µg/ml
Factor H	150,000	500 µg/ml
Factor I	80,000	35 µg/ml
Properdin	180,000 (heterogeneous)	25 µg/ml
S-Protein	71,000	600 µg/ml

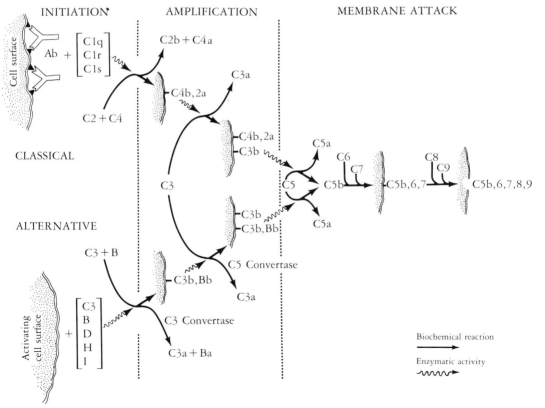

Figure 6–1. Schematic representation of the two pathways of complement activation.

fication phase takes place that involves the action of proteases and the recruitment of additional molecules; this is followed by a terminal phase of membrane attack during which the cell dies.

The recognition unit for the classical pathway, C1, is composed of three separate proteins, C1q, C1r, and C1s. The initiation of this pathway of complement typically involves the reaction of antibody with antigen, which may be soluble or on the surface of a target cell. This antigen-antibody reaction allows the binding of C1q to two or more Fc regions of certain IgG subclasses (IgG$_1$, IgG$_2$, IgG$_3$) or IgM. Activators of the classical pathway are listed in Table 6–2. The ultrastructure of C1q has been demonstrated by electron microscopy to consist of six subunits similar to a bouquet of six flowers. The central stalks of C1q resemble collagen in primary and secondary structure. Upon binding of one C1q molecule to the Fc regions of two or more antigen-bound antibody molecules, C1r proenzymes are activated. The chemical basis of this activation is the cleavage of a peptide bond by an autocatalytic mechanism, leading to the formation of activated C1r, a protease that subsequently cleaves the proenzyme C1s. Thus, the binding of C1q to an immunoglobulin in complex with the antigen represents the recognition event of the classical pathway, resulting in the activation of C1r and C1s. The final result is the generation of an enzymatically active component, C1s, which will cleave and thereby activate the next proteins in the cascade, leading to amplification of the recognition event.

The enzyme C1s has two physiologic substrates, C4 and C2. C4 is cleaved by C1s into C4a, one of the three anaphylatoxins (molecules that promote increased vascular permeability and smooth muscle contraction), and C4b, which binds to the target cell surface. C1s also cleaves C2 when C2 is in complex with C4b. Cleavage of C2 generates C2b, which is released, and C2a, which remains bound to C4b. The bimolecular complex C4b,2a is a protease that cleaves C3 and therefore is called C3 convertase. Cleavage of C3 by the C3 convertase generates two important biologically active peptides, C3a (another anaphylatoxin) and C3b, which attaches to target cell surfaces and can bind to C5. C5, when in complex with C3b, can be cleaved by the C3 convertase (then referred to as C5 convertase). The C5 convertase hydrolyzes C5, which generates the C5a ana-

Table 6–2. Activators of the Classical Pathway

Immunoglobulins
  IgG (human subclasses 1, 2, and 3)
  IgM

Nonimmunoglobulin Activators
  Bacterial lipopolysaccharide (lipid A portion)
  C-reactive protein bound to pneumococci
  Retroviruses
  Heart mitochondrial membranes
  Polyanions (e.g., polynucleotides)
  Urate crystals

phylatoxin and C5b. C5b is the nucleus for the formation of the membrane attack complex.

Immediately following their generation, C3b and C4b exhibit a unique transient ability to covalently bind to target cells ("metastable binding site"). This property has recently been shown to be due to an intramolecular thioester bond that is present between the sulfhydryl group of a cysteine residue and the gamma carbonyl group of a glutamine residue on C3 and C4 (Fig. 6–2). Upon activation of C3 or C4, this thioester becomes highly reactive and can react with a cell

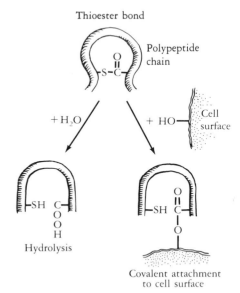

Figure 6–2. Schematic representation of the intramolecular thioester bond in C3 and C4, which upon cleavage to C3b or C4b, respectively, becomes highly reactive. Subsequent opening of this reactive bond by cell surface hydroxyl groups leads to covalent attachment of C3b or C4b to the cell surface. Prior opening of the bond by water (i.e., hydrolysis) prevents covalent attachment. In addition, slow hydrolysis of the thioester in native C3 is responsible for the activation of the alternative pathway (see text).

surface hydroxyl or amino group. This results in the covalent attachment of C3b or C4b to the target cell (Fig. 6–2). An additional function of the thioester bond is its hydrolysis by water, occurring during activation of the alternative pathway as described below.

The alternative pathway can be activated when a molecule of C3b is bound to a target cell. This C3b molecule combines with the plasma protein Factor B, which is a zymogen, and which, when bound to C3b, can be activated by the plasma protein Factor D by cleavage into two fragments, Ba and Bb. The Bb fragment, which contains the active enzymatic site, remains bound to C3b, as C3b,Bb. This complex, like C4b,2a in the classical pathway, is a C3 convertase (C3b,Bb); it is stabilized by the binding of another plasma protein, properdin. Thus, the alternative pathway used to be called the properdin pathway.

The presence of a single molecule of C3b generates many molecules of C3b,Bb, resulting in a tremendous amplification. The C3 convertase (C3b,Bb) cleaves C3, thereby generating more molecules of C3b, which can combine with other molecules of Factor B to give more molecules of C3b,Bb, which can, in turn, cleave more molecules of C3. Therefore, the central feature of the alternative pathway is a positive feedback loop that amplifies the original recognition event (Fig. 6–3). As in the classical pathway, attachment of many C3b molecules to the target cell will allow binding of C5 and its cleavage into C5a and C5b by the enzyme C3b,Bb, now referred to as C5 convertase.

Owing to the potential of this positive feedback loop to rapidly use up Factor B and C3, the positive feedback must be carefully regulated. There are two important regulatory proteins in plasma. The first protein, Factor H (formerly referred to as β1H), competes with Factor B for binding to C3b and also dissociates C3b,Bb into C3b and Bb. The second control protein, Factor I (formerly referred to as C3b inactivator), cleaves C3b that is bound to Factor H or to a similar protein found on the surface of the host cell. The resulting cleaved C3b, termed iC3b, can no longer form a C3 convertase. The action of these two control proteins prevents the consumption of Factor B and C3 in plasma; in addition, these two proteins inactivate C3b,Bb on host cell surfaces. In contrast, surfaces of many target cells, such as bacteria and other microorganisms, protect C3b,Bb

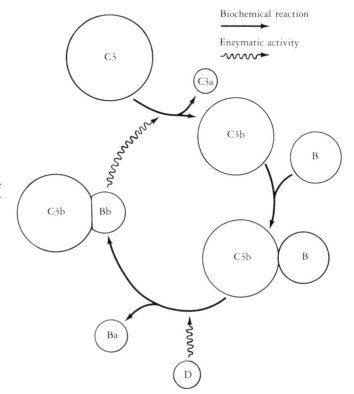

Figure 6–3. Schematic representation of the positive feedback loop of the alternative pathway.

Table 6–3. Activators of the Alternative Pathway

Polysaccharides (e.g., inulin)
Yeast cell walls (zymosan)
Bacterial cell wall components
    (lipopolysaccharide, peptidoglycan)
Influenza and other viruses
Schistosoma and other parasites
Cryptococci and other fungi
Certain tumor cells
Cobra venom factor
Nephritic factor (autoantibody
    that stabilizes C3b,Bb)
X-ray contrast media
Dialysis membranes

from inactivation by Factors H and I. This protection allows the positive feedback loop to proceed on the surface of the target cell, leading to the activation of the pathway and subsequent cell death. In other words, the alternative pathway is activated by those substances that prevent the inactivation of the positive feedback loop enzyme C3b,Bb. A substance is therefore treated as "foreign" if it restricts the action of Factors H and I and allows the positive feedback loop to continue. The chemical structures on surfaces of particles and cells responsible for activation or nonactivation of the alternative pathway have not been identified. There is some evidence that carbohydrate moieties are involved, particularly sialic acid. The alternative pathway protein(s) responsible for the recognition of these structures also remains to be determined. Table 6–3 lists known activators of the alternative pathway.

As pointed out earlier, the activation of the alternative pathway requires a C3b molecule bound to the surface of a target cell. An intriguing question is, "Where does the critical first C3b molecule come from?" Although it can be provided by the C3 convertase of the classical pathway or by cleavage of C3 by plasmin and certain bacterial and other cellular proteases, the alternative pathway can generate this first C3b molecule without these proteases. The intramolecular thioester, which is highly reactive in nascent C3b and is responsible for the covalent attachment to targets (see above), is also accessible in native C3 to water molecules (Fig. 6–2). Thus, spontaneous hydrolysis of the thioester bond occurs constantly in plasma at a low rate. The C3 molecules in which the thioester bond has been hydrolyzed behave like C3b, although the C3a domain has not been removed. C3 with a hydrolyzed thioester is called $C3(H_2O)$ or C3b-like C3. It can bind Factor B and

allow Factor D to activate Factor B, which results in formation of a fluid-phase C3 convertase, $C3(H_2O),Bb$. This enzyme is continuously formed and produces C3b molecules that can randomly attach to cells. Although these C3b molecules will be rapidly inactivated on host cells by Factors H and I, they will start the positive feedback loop on foreign surfaces, as outlined previously. In other words, the alternative pathway is constantly activated at a low rate, but amplification with subsequent cell death occurs only on foreign particles.

PRODUCTS OF COMPLEMENT ACTIVATION POSSESSING BIOLOGIC ACTIVITY

Activation of either the alternative or the classical pathway results in the generation of many important peptides involved in inflammatory responses (Table 6–4). The anaphy-

Table 6–4. Biologic Effects of Complement Activation Products

Substance	Biologic Activity
C3a	Smooth muscle contraction Increase of vascular permeability Degranulation of mast cells and basophils with release of histamine Degranulation of eosinophils Aggregation of platelets
C3b	Opsonization of particles and solubilization of immune complexes with subsequent facilitation of phagocytosis
C3e	Release of neutrophils from bone marrow resulting in leukocytosis
C4a	Smooth muscle contraction Increase of vascular permeability
C5a	Smooth muscle contraction Increase of vascular permeability Degranulation of mast cells and basophils with release of histamine Degranulation of eosinophils Aggregation of platelets Chemotaxis of basophils, eosinophils, neutrophils, and monocytes Release of hydrolytic enzymes from neutrophils
C5a-des-arg	Chemotaxis of neutrophils Release of hydrolytic enzymes from neutrophils
Bb	Inhibition of migration and induction of spreading of monocytes and macrophages

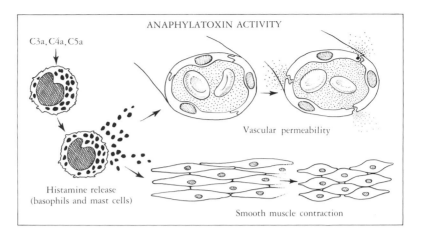

Figure 6–4. Anaphylatoxin activity of C3a, C4a, and C5a causing mediator release, e.g., histamine, from basophils and mast cells with subsequent smooth muscle contraction and alterations in vascular permeability.

latoxins C3a, C4a, and C5a are derived from the enzymatic cleavage of C3, C4, and C5 respectively. Historically, C3a and C5a were defined as factors derived from activated serum possessing spasmogenic activity. The anaphylatoxins are now recognized as having many additional biologic functions. Both C3a and C5a are known to induce the release of histamine from mast cells and basophils. As shown in Figure 6–4, both anaphylatoxins cause smooth muscle contraction and induce the release of vasoactive amines, which cause an increase in vascular permeability.

The effect of C5a anaphylatoxin on neutrophils is of considerable importance in the inflammatory response. Not only can C5a induce neutrophil aggregation, but this anaphylatoxin appears to be the main chemotactic peptide generated by activation of either complement pathway (Fig. 6–5). *In vitro,* na-

nomolar concentrations of C5a will induce the unidirectional movement of neutrophils. Other inflammatory cells, such as monocytes, eosinophils, basophils, and macrophages, have also been shown to exhibit a chemotactic response to C5a. The removal of the carboxy-terminal arginine from C5a by serum carboxypeptidase N, generating C5a-des-arg, inactivates the spasmogen, yet restoration of full chemotactic activity of C5a-des-arg may occur in the presence of serum. Therefore, C5a-des-arg may also be responsible for *in vivo* neutrophil chemotactic activity.

As described earlier, the cleavage of C3 by either the alternative or the classical C3 convertases results in the production of two major split products, the C3a anaphylatoxin and C3b. The larger C3b fragment can serve as an opsonin (promoter of phagocytosis) by binding to a target through the thioester

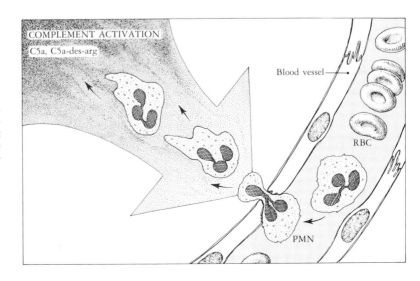

Figure 6–5. Schematic representation of unidirectional movement of neutrophils (chemotactic response) to C5a and C5a-des-arg generated by complement activation.

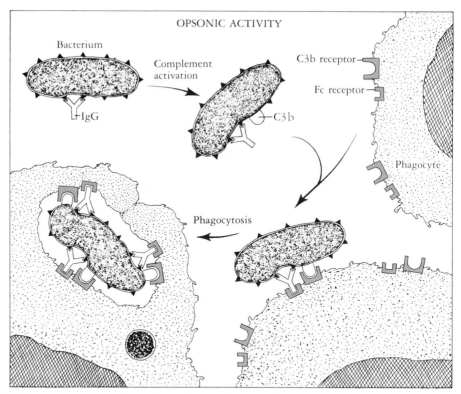

Figure 6–6. Schematic representation of the phagocytic-promoting activity (opsonin function) of complement, associated with the binding of C3b to cell surfaces.

mechanism. This renders the particle or cell immediately susceptible to ingestion by a variety of phagocytic cells that carry specific receptors for C3b (Fig. 6–6).

Many recent observations point to additional roles for complement fragments in regulating the activity of cells of the immune system. These observations include the presence of receptors on lymphocytes for various complement proteins, including C3 split products and Factor H, affecting B- and T-cell function. This is an important area for future research.

THE PATHWAY OF MEMBRANE ATTACK

The formation of C5b by the classical or alternative C5 convertase marks the initiation of the membrane attack pathway. Nascent C5b can bind to C6, resulting in the formation of the stable C5b,6 complex. Subsequently, C5b,6 reacts with C7 to form the trimolecular complex C5b,6,7, which exhibits a metastable binding site through which the complex can bind itself to the target cell membrane. Although the exact biochemical nature of this metastable binding site is unknown, it is believed that binding occurs through hydrophobic interactions with membrane lipids. Next, binding of C8 to the C5b,6,7 complex occurs on the cell membrane, which causes the transposition of C9 from the plasma into the target cell membrane by inducing a polymerization of C9. The polymerization of C9 in the membrane occurs typically in a circular fashion, inserting poly C9 cylinders consisting of about 12 to 16 C9 molecules. The poly C9 cylinders are responsible for the characteristic ring-like appearance of the complement lesions seen by electron microscopy (Fig. 6–7). The poly C9 with the attached C5b,6,7,8 complex is usually referred to as the membrane attack complex (MAC).

It has been established that the membranolytic action of the MAC is due entirely to physical interactions. The MAC is a hollow structure with an inner diameter of 100 Å; therefore, its insertion into the membrane results in transmembrane channels that are large enough to allow molecules the size of proteins to pass through. In addition, the

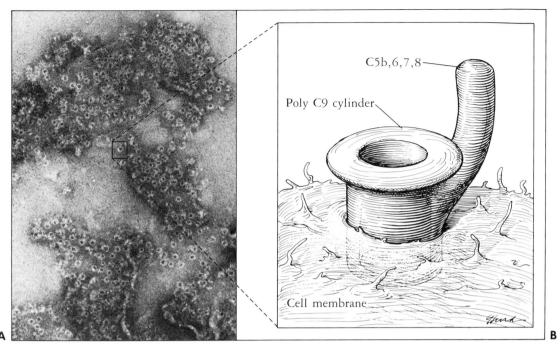

Figure 6–7. *A*, Electron micrograph of a membrane lysed by many membrane attack complexes (magnification approximately 130,000 ×). *B*, Schematic drawing of a MAC.

strong lipid-binding capability of the MAC results in disorganization of the phospholipid bilayer, causing impairment of membrane function. In the case of gram-negative bacteria, the peptidoglycan layer prevents MAC-mediated lysis. However, these bacteria are killed by the insertion of the MAC into the outer membrane. Lysis of these bacteria requires the presence of lysozyme, which can cleave the peptidoglycan.

REGULATORY MECHANISMS OF THE COMPLEMENT CASCADE

Activation of the complement cascade results in a complex series of molecular events with potent biologic consequences. Accordingly, modulating mechanisms are necessary to regulate complement activation and to control the production of biologically active split products.

The first mechanism by which the activity of many activated complement components is modulated is spontaneous decay. Examples of this mechanism are the transient stability of the activated thioester bond in C3b and C4b, and the short half-life of the enzymatically active complexes C4b,2a and C3b,Bb.

The second type of regulatory mechanism is the inactivation of certain components by proteolytic enzymes. For example, the plasma protease Factor I can, in the presence of certain cofactors (see below), inactivate C3b and C4b. A major mechanism for controlling the biologic activity of C3a and C5a anaphylatoxins is serum carboxypeptidase N, as described earlier. Another control protein that may exert a regulatory effect on the C5a anaphylatoxin is the chemotactic factor inactivator. Although the chemical basis of the inactivation is not known, this serum-derived factor appears to irreversibly inactivate many of the biologic activities of C5a.

A third mechanism of regulation involves specific binding proteins that modulate the activity of certain complement components. Examples are Factor H and C4b-binding-protein, which, when bound to C3b and C4b, respectively, make them susceptible to cleavage by Factor I. Another example is S-protein, which binds to the MAC if the MAC is assembling in plasma rather than on a target cell. Binding of the S-protein to the MAC abrogates its ability to attach to a cell membrane, thus limiting attachment of MAC to cells at the site of complement activation. Another important binding protein is C1 esterase inhibitor (C1 INA), which regulates activation of the classical pathway by forming irreversible complexes with C1r and C1s. Patients who lack C1 INA or who possess it in a nonfunctional form suffer from hereditary angioedema. They present with episodes of angioedema, which are life-threatening if they involve the larynx. Because C1 INA also inactivates activated kallikrein and Hageman factor, it is difficult to determine which of these enzymes causes the release of mediators most relevant in clinical episodes of angioedema in patients with deficiency of C1 INA.

Modulation of the activity of complement is also achieved by regulation of its synthesis. Cells that can synthesize these components are present at sites of inflammation, thereby helping to prevent complement depletion at the site of complement activation. The importance of complement in inflammation is further evidenced by the finding that certain complement proteins (e.g., C3 and C9) are acute-phase reactants; that is, their synthesis is increased during inflammation, resulting in higher plasma concentrations.

COMPLEMENT-DEPENDENT REACTIONS RESULTING IN TISSUE INJURY

Complement activation is responsible for tissue injury in the pathogenesis of certain diseases. Two major causes of complement-mediated pathogenesis are activation by autoantibodies and activation by immune complexes.

Autoantibodies may arise secondary to tissue damage or infection or by mechanisms that are not understood. The binding of an autoantibody will direct complement activation against the host's target tissue. This is the mechanism of tissue injury in Goodpasture's syndrome, in which autoantibodies to glomerular, tubular, and alveolar basement membranes are present. Autoantibodies to the acetylcholine receptor in the postsynaptic membrane of the motor end plate cause myasthenia gravis. Autoimmune hemolytic anemias and thrombocytopenias are caused by autoantibodies to erythrocytes and platelets. Autoantibodies to streptococcal antigens cross reacting with antigens of host tissues seem to be involved in the pathogenesis of rheumatic myocarditis and endocarditis. Activation of complement in the walls of the small vessels and capillaries by immune complexes, either locally formed or deposited from the circulation, leads to tissue injury

and inflammation causing vasculitis. This immunopathologic mechanism is known as the Arthus reaction and has been shown to be the pathogenesis of serum sickness and hypersensitivity pneumonitis. Circulating immune complexes are found in a variety of diseases, including infections, neoplasms, and autoimmune disorders. In rheumatoid arthritis, immune complex deposition in the synovial membranes causes polyarthritis. In patients with systemic lupus erythematosus, skin lesions, polyarthritis, myocarditis, polyserositis, and glomerulonephritis are the clinical manifestations of immune complex deposition. The renal glomeruli are the most common site of immune complex deposition causing glomerulonephritis. This is the mechanism of renal injury in Schönlein-Henoch purpura, in poststreptococcal glomerulonephritis, and in other acute glomerulonephritides.

In a form of membranoproliferative glomerulonephritis associated with low levels of C3, the nephrotoxic effects seem to be due to an autoantibody, called nephritic factor, which stabilizes C3b,Bb, resulting in chronic activation of the alternative pathway, which leads to tissue injury.

In paroxysmal nocturnal hemoglobinuria, an acquired alteration in the erythrocyte membrane leads to a slower decay of C3b,Bb on the surface of these cells. The erythrocytes therefore exhibit an increased susceptibility to complement-mediated lysis.

Among substances that have been found to provide activating surfaces for complement are nylon fibers and membranes used in hemodialysis and cardiopulmonary bypass. The released anaphylatoxins are thought to contribute to adverse reactions frequently seen in patients after extracorporeal circulation.

Finally, cobra venom contains a protein called cobra venom factor (CVF), which activates the alternative pathway by a unique mechanism. CVF is an analog of C3b. Like C3b, it forms a C3 convertase, CVF,Bb. This C3 convertase is resistant to inactivation by Factors H and I. Consequently, the enzyme will continuously activate C3 and thereby consume complement.

COMPLEMENT AND INFECTION

The bactericidal power of the complement system was demonstrated by the killing of laboratory strains of *E. coli* by a mixture of the purified complement proteins of the alternative and membrane attack pathways. The ability to destroy such organisms, without waiting for the synthesis of specific antibody, provides an immediate mechanism of defense. However, bacteria have evolved ways to protect themselves against the complement system. For example, most clinical isolates of *E. coli* (e.g., from neonatal coliform meningitis) are not killed by the alternative pathway. The resistance of these bacteria is due to the fact that their lipopolysaccharide coat, which would otherwise activate the alternative pathway, is hidden under a capsular polysaccharide. This capsular polysaccharide does not provide an activating surface. Thus, the classical pathway, activated by antibody that binds to the capsular polysaccharide, is needed to kill these organisms.

Similarly, viruses can activate, and be inactivated by, complement in the presence or absence of antibody. For many viruses, inactivation requires only the early complement components C1, C4, and C2, whereas other viruses are inactivated by MAC-mediated lysis.

Parasites, such as schistosomes, can activate complement by the alternative pathway in the absence of antibody. The resultant coating of these organisms by C3b has been found to greatly stimulate their killing by eosinophils.

Tumor cells have been shown to be susceptible to killing initiated through the alternative and classical complement pathways. C3b can be demonstrated on tumor cells *in vivo*.

All microorganisms can activate complement through the classical pathway once specific antibody of the appropriate class is available. A representative list of non–antibody-dependent methods of activation by a variety of organisms is given in Tables 6–2 and 6–3.

COMPLEMENT DEFICIENCIES

Deficiencies of complement components can be divided into congenital and acquired deficiencies of complement components and their inhibitors. Acquired multicomponent deficiencies are associated with circulating immune complexes, such as in systemic lupus erythematosus. This disease is characterized by low C1, C4, C2, and C3 levels in the early stages, with a return toward normal levels as the disease activity diminishes. As described earlier, low levels of C3 are seen in hypocomplementemic membranoproliferative glomerulonephritis. Genetic deficiencies of most complement components have also been described. The most common defect found in humans is a deficiency in C2. Although rare, deficiency states of other complement components have been reported (Table 6–5). Patients with a deficiency of an early component of the classical pathway often possess symptoms associated with connective tissue disease. Patients with a genetic deficiency in one of the terminal components (e.g., C8) have an increased susceptibility to *Neisseria* infections, while patients deficient in C3 or C5 present mainly with pyogenic infections. This points to different mechanisms of complement-dependent control of these organ-

Table 6–5. Genetic Complement Deficiencies

Component	Clinical Appearance
C1q	Systemic lupus erythematosus–like syndrome
C1r	Systemic lupus erythematosus–like syndrome
C1s	Systemic lupus erythematosus–like syndrome
C4	Systemic lupus erythematosus–like syndrome
C2	Systemic lupus erythematosus–like syndrome
C3	Severe recurrent pyogenic infections
C5	Recurrent infections (pyogenic, neisserial, and others), Leiner's disease, systemic lupus erythematosus–like syndrome
C6	Recurrent neisserial infections
C7	Recurrent neisserial infections
C8	Recurrent neisserial infections
C9	Apparently healthy
Factor H	Hemolytic uremic syndrome, infections
Factor I	Recurrent infections
Properdin	Recurrent neisserial infections
C1 Inhibitor	Hereditary angioedema
Carboxypeptidase N	Recurrent angioedema

isms. As described previously, a genetic deficiency of C1 esterase inhibitor manifests itself as the syndrome called hereditary angioedema. During an episode of angioedema, activated C1 is found in serum accompanied by a decrease in C4 and C2, while serum levels of C3 and the terminal complement components remain in the normal range.

AN OVERVIEW

The complement system has evolved essentially for protective functions. The complement system fulfills three major roles in host defense: first, coating of pathogenic organisms or immune complexes with opsonins, resulting in their removal by phagocytes; second, activation of inflammatory cells; third, killing of target cells. Activation of these biologic functions can occur by the classical or the alternative pathway. Both pathways exhibit a similar molecular organization: An initial recognition event is amplified, resulting in the generation of many effector molecules. Owing to the potentially destructive consequences to the host of uncontrolled complement action, this system is tightly regulated. Regulatory mechanisms include the inherently transient stability of certain activated complement components (generation of metastable binding sites, rapid decay of the convertases) and modulation of activities by regulatory proteins (binding to or limited proteolysis of activated components). All regulatory mechanisms are directed toward a common goal: to confine the effects of complement to the site of activation, thereby preventing generalized activation with potentially harmful effects on host cells. Just as the coagulation system may suddenly proceed through its activation sequence in an unchecked manner, resulting in the serious consequences of intravascular coagulation, the complement system, although tightly regulated, is involved in the pathogenesis of disease. Complement activation due to recognition of autoantibodies or tissue deposits of immune complexes will direct the response against the host's own tissues. Both acquired and inherited deficiencies of complement have been described. Common clinical manifestations of inherited complement deficiencies are recurrent infections and immune complex diseases; this demonstrates the importance of complement in the control of pathogenic organisms and in the removal of immune complexes.

Thus, complement can be considered as an array of proteins composing a tightly regulated system that is centrally involved in the initiation and coordination of the molecular and cellular response of a host to invasive foreign substances.

Suggestions for Further Reading

Esser, A. F.: Interactions between complement proteins and biological and model membranes. *In* Chapman, D. (ed.): Biological Membranes. Vol. 4. New York, Academic Press, 1982, pp. 277–325.

Fearon, D. T., and Austen, K. F.: The alternative pathway of complement—a system for host resistance to microbial infection. N. Engl. J. Med., *303*:259, 1980.

Hugli, T. E.: The structural basis for anaphylatoxin and chemotactic functions of C3a, C4a, and C5a. CRC Crit. Rev. Immunol., *1*:321, 1981.

Müller-Eberhard, H. J., and Schreiber, R. D.: Molecular biology and chemistry of the alternative pathway of complement. Adv. Immunol., *29*:1, 1980.

Porter, R. R.: Interactions of complement components with antibody-antigen aggregates and cell surfaces. Immunol. Today, *2*:143, 1981.

Reid, K. B. M., and Porter, R. R.: The proteolytic activation systems of complement. Annu. Rev. Biochem., *50*:433, 1981.

Ward, P. A.: Leukotaxis and leukotactic disorders. Am. J. Pathol., *77*:519, 1974.

Chapter 7

Immunophysiology: Cell Function and Cellular Interactions in Antibody Formation

Herbert B. Herscowitz, Ph.D.

INITIATION OF THE SPECIFIC IMMUNE RESPONSE

Individuals may acquire specific immunity either (1) through natural exposure by infection or immunization with specific agents or their products (*active immunity*); or (2) by the passive acquisition of preformed antibody, specifically sensitized lymphocytes, or their products, e.g., transfer factor (*passive immunity*). The fundamental differences between active and passive immunity are shown in Table 7–1.

Active Immunity

The acquisition of active immunity depends upon the participation of host tissues and cells after an encounter with the immunogen. It involves differentiation and proliferation of immunocompetent cells in lymphoreticular tissues, which lead to synthesis of antibody or the development of cell-mediated reactivity, or both. This type of immunity appears only after a specified time lapse subsequent to exposure to the immunogen. The duration of active immunity is relatively long and can be measured in terms of months or years, in some cases. This type of immunity results from natural exposure to immunogens by infection or through the use of vaccines.

Passive Immunity

Passive immunity may result from the transfer of serum-containing antibodies or products from specifically sensitized cells obtained from an immunized host to a nonimmune individual. Since this type of immunity

Table 7–1. **Comparison of Active and Passive Immunity**

	Active	Passive
Genesis:	Active host participation after exposure to immunogen either naturally (subclinical or clinical disease) or by immunization (vaccine)	No host participation; transfer of pre-formed substances (antibody, transfer factor, thymic graft, interleukin-2) from an actively immunized host to a nonimmune host
Components:	Humoral and cell-mediated immunity	Humoral and cell-mediated immunity
Onset of action:	Only after a latent period	Immediate
Duration:	Long-lived	Transitory
Application:	Vaccination	Immune deficiency, prophylaxis

involves the transfer of preformed substances, the onset of its action is immediate; however, because there may be no stimulus for continued production, its effect is usually of short duration. The passive transfer of immunity (specific IgG antibodies) from mother to fetus and the use of transfer factor in immunotherapy are examples of passive immunity. Prior to antibiotic therapy it was common practice to transfer pooled serum from individuals containing specific antibodies to certain infectious agents to susceptible hosts. Although this is generally no longer practiced, passive transfer of preformed antibodies against venoms and toxins is still used in some situations.

RESPONSE OF THE HOST: THE FATE OF IMMUNOGEN

Foreign substances either may enter the body naturally or may be introduced artificially. Most frequently, they gain entrance through the respiratory or gastrointestinal tract, although they may enter naturally through any body surface, including the mucous membranes and skin, or by transplacental passage. Artificial introduction of foreignness occurs by injection (e.g., vaccination) or by surgical intervention (e.g., transplantation).

An interesting and potentially clinically important observation has been made in animals given large amounts of protein antigen by the oral route. Animals treated this way do not produce specific antibodies after systemic challenge with the same antigen. This induced lack of ability to respond, called *tolerance* (Chapter 10), is thought to be due to the appearance of antigen-specific suppressor T-cells in the Peyer's patches. The suppressor cells or soluble suppressor factors exert their influence in peripheral lymphoid tissue (e.g., spleen), where they inhibit the production of IgM and IgG antibodies without affecting the secretory IgA response. These cells also appear to inhibit the development of delayed-type hypersensitivity to the same antigen. These observations served as the basis for the design of a protocol to treat severely Rh-immunized pregnant women in an attempt to save their fetuses. A group of women were given daily oral administration of extracts of Rh+ erythrocyte membranes. In all cases, the anti-Rh antibody titers of the women did not increase during gestation and all of them delivered live-born infants, whereas each had previously experienced stillbirth or intrauterine fetal death secondary to Rh sensitization. Thus, a potentially clinically useful modality can be achieved by manipulating the mode of antigen administration.

Metabolic Fate

The *in vivo* fate of an immunogen can be followed by the use of radioactively labeled materials. Following intravenous injection of the foreign substance (e.g., human serum albumin) into a rabbit, three phases of antigen disappearance are distinguishable (Fig. 7–1). The first phase involves the *equilibration* of the foreign material between the intravascular and the extravascular space by a process of diffusion. This phase is relatively rapid for a diffusible substance and is of similar duration whether the injected material is autologous or foreign. Particulate immunogens (e.g., bacteria or erythrocytes), when injected into animals, are ingested by phagocytic cells and do not diffuse into the extravascular space. Thus, there is no initial equilibration phase.

The second stage of antigen clearance, referred to as *catabolism,* occurs over a period of several days and involves the gradual degradation and digestion of the material. The actual duration of this phase is determined

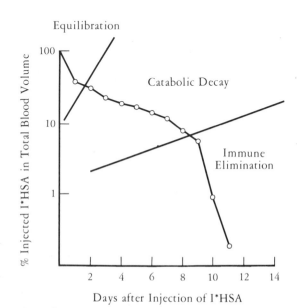

Figure 7–1. Rate of elimination of radiolabeled immunogen from blood.

by both the biologic half-life of the material and the enzymatic capabilities of the host for the particular type of substance. Certain substances will remain in the circulation for fairly long periods of time if the host is deficient in the metabolic machinery required for their degradation (e.g., poly D-amino acids, polysaccharide).

In the third phase of clearance, there is a further rapid removal of the antigen, referred to as *immune elimination*. This stage results from the appearance of newly synthesized antibody that combines with the circulating antigen, leading to the formation of antigen-antibody complexes that are phagocytized and degraded. These antigen-antibody complexes, particularly when formed in antigen excess, have clinical significance, since they may induce tissue injury. Following the third phase, free antibody appears in the serum. Although the curve shown in Figure 7–1 reflects almost complete elimination of the immunogen, absolute removal may take weeks, months, or years, if it ever occurs. Thus, persistence of a portion of the immunogen may provide continued stimulus to the cells involved in the immune response.

Organ Distribution of Immunogen

When injected intravenously, the immunogen is initially found at sites where fixed phagocytic cells are numerous, e.g., liver, spleen, bone marrow, kidney, and lung. When injected by other routes (e.g., intradermally), the major portion of the material either remains at the site of administration or is localized in the draining lymph node. The physicochemical properties of the injected material determine the degree of localization in the lymph node. For example, particulate materials (e.g., viruses) are more effectively retained in the lymph node than are soluble substances (e.g., human serum albumin).

Foreign substances most frequently enter the body via the gastrointestinal and respiratory tracts, where they become localized in lymphoid tissue, resulting primarily in the production of IgE and secretory IgA antibodies.

Cellular Distribution of Immunogen

Most immunogens are readily taken up by the endocytic processes (*phagocytosis* or *pinocytosis*) of the cells of the *mononuclear phagocyte system* within the body. Macrophages in the medullary cords of lymph nodes and in the red pulp of the spleen remove much of the injected material in animals that have not previously been exposed to the foreign substance. In previously immunized animals, the immunogen can be found associated with dendritic cells located in the follicles of the lymph node cortex. The immunogen appears to be retained, to a large extent, extracellularly between the membranes of dendritic cells. The ability of these cells to retain the immunogen appears to be dependent upon the presence of antibody.

There is conflicting information regarding the precise cellular location of endocytosed material because of the breakdown of internally labeled proteins used in these studies and the reutilization of the radiolabeled amino acids into new cellular components. Immunogenic material has been reported to be localized within the cytoplasm in small or large lysosomal granules, on the cell membrane, and in association with ribonucleic acid. It should be pointed out that there is still some controversy about the phagocytic function of macrophages in the immune response. While some investigators feel that the major function of the macrophage is to degrade and eliminate the foreign configuration, there is compelling evidence to indicate that this cell is necessary for the "processing" of foreign substances for presentation to lymphocytes in a form that will initiate the immune response.

ANTIBODY FORMATION IN THE INDIVIDUAL

Primary Response

The injection of a single dose of a foreign substance into an immunocompetent animal will cause specific antibody to appear in the serum after a definite time lapse. First exposure to an immunogen evokes the *primary response* (Fig. 7–2). Immediately after introduction of the immunogen, little or no anti-

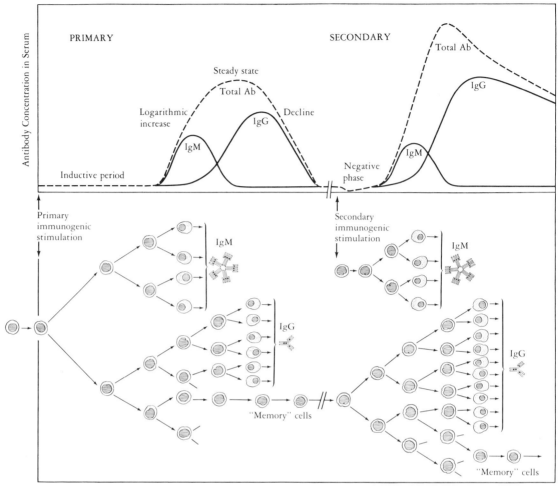

Figure 7–2. Schematic representation of humoral and cellular events in the primary and secondary (anamnestic) antibody responses.

body is detected in the serum. This period is referred to as the *inductive* or *latent* period. It is during this time that the immunogen is recognized as foreign and is processed, and an unknown signal is transferred to the appropriate cells destined to make antibody. This period is characterized by cellular proliferation and differentiation. The duration of this period is variable and depends upon (1) the immunogenicity, quantity, form, and solubility of the stimulant; (2) the animal species into which it is injected; (3) the route of immunization; and (4) the sensitivity of the assay used to detect the newly formed antibody. For example, antibodies can be detected three to four days after the injection of foreign erythrocytes (e.g., transfusion reaction), five to seven days after soluble proteins, and 10 to 14 days after bacterial cells.

Following the appearance of the first anti-

body at the end of the induction period, there is a time of active biosynthesis of antibody that can be further subdivided into three phases. In the first, the *logarithmic* phase, the antibody concentration increases logarithmically for four to ten days, again depending upon the nature of the immunogen, until it reaches a peak. During this phase the doubling time (that time required to achieve a twofold increase in serum antibody concentration) has been reported to be as short as five to eight hours. Peak antibody titers against heterologous erythrocytes are usually attained in four to five days; against soluble proteins, in 8 to 12 days; and against toxoids prepared from toxins of gram-positive bacilli (e.g., *Corynebacterium diphtheriae*), in as long as two to three months. On a cellular basis, the number of differentiated plasma cells increases soon after immunization, while peak cellular synthesis of antibody precedes the peak serum antibody response by several days.

The level of circulating antibody attained after primary immunization is a reflection of the difference between the antibody's rates of synthesis and catabolism. When these rates are the same the serum antibody concentration is constant, as shown in Figure 7–2 as a *plateau* or *steady state*. This phase of the response is highly transitory and in some cases almost nonexistent. The rate of antibody synthesis is dependent upon the number of antibody-forming cells, which can be influenced by the conditions of immunization. The rate of antibody catabolism, however, is a reflection of the half-life of the class of immunoglobulin (Chapter 5).

Finally, a *decline* phase is observed, in which the rate of antibody catabolism is greater than that of its synthesis. The duration of this phase is also variable, since there may be varying degrees of difference between rates of synthesis and catabolism.

The early primary response to most immunogens is characterized by the predominance of IgM antibody; the IgG class of antibody appears somewhat later. IgM antibody production is usually transient, and within two weeks after the initiation of the immune response, IgG antibody predominates. Whether or not IgM antibodies are always produced in greater quantity before their corresponding IgG counterparts is subject to question. The basis for this controversy is the fact that the IgM antibody is more readily detectable because of the greater sensitivity of the IgM assay methods. Administration of the immunogen in adjuvant (Chapter 10) usually results in the continued synthesis of both IgM and IgG antibodies for several months.

The antibodies formed early in the immune response usually have a low *affinity* (the attractive force between complementary conformational sites on the antibody and antigen that causes them to combine); the affinity of late antibodies is usually greatly increased. Differences in affinity are readily observed with IgG antibodies since such changes can be a thousand fold. In addition to increases in affinity with the passage of time, there is also an increase in *avidity* (the strength of the binding of antibody to antigen); in other words, antigen-antibody complexes formed with late antisera are less dissociable. These changes are related to the diverse antigenic determinants on the immunogen that give rise to a variety of antibody specificities, which appear after different latent periods. As a consequence of these changes, the *cross reactivity* of a given antiserum also increases with time, probably owing to the fact that high-affinity antibodies can react with closely related antigenic determinants more readily than their low-affinity counterparts can. The compilation of all of these changes exemplifies the fact that the humoral immune response is *heterogeneous*, the manifestation of a population of antibodies with differences in Ig class, affinity, avidity, and specificity.

Secondary Response

Upon a second exposure to the same immunogen, weeks, months, or even years later, there is a markedly enhanced response that is characterized by the accelerated appearance of immunocompetent cells and antibody (Fig. 7–2). If antibody is still present in the serum at the time of the second injection of immunogen, it disappears at a faster rate than in the decline phase of the primary response. This *negative phase* is due to the immediate reaction of pre-existing antibody with newly injected immunogen, resulting in the formation of antigen-antibody complexes. If the second dose of immunogen is very small, an enhanced immune response may not occur, possibly because all of the newly injected immunogen is consumed in antigen-antibody complexes, phagocytized, and effectively removed, so that the antibody-forming cells are deprived of a stimulus. However, if the dose of immunogen is sufficient to allow the material that remains after complex formation to stimulate the immune system, then a typical *secondary* (*anamnestic* or *recall*) response is initiated. This enhanced response serves as the principle for giving booster doses of vaccines.

The differences between the primary and secondary responses are summarized in Table 7–2. In contrast to the primary response, the secondary response is characterized by a shorter latent period, a more rapid rate of antibody synthesis, and a higher peak titer of antibody that persists for a longer period of time. The shorter latent period and more rapid rate of antibody synthesis, in spite of the fact that doubling times are similar in primary and secondary responses, are related to the number of antigen-sensitive cells,

Table 7–2. **Relative Differences Between Primary and Secondary Response**

	Primary	Secondary
Latent period	Long	Short
Rate of antibody synthesis	Low	High
Peak antibody titer	Low	High
Persistence of antibody titer	Short	Long
Affinity of antibody	Low	High
Crossreactivity of antibody	Low	High
Presence of memory cells	Few (?)	Many
Predominating Ig class	IgM	IgG
Dose of immunogen to elicit	High	Low

called *memory cells*, present at the time of secondary stimulation. The scheme presented in Figure 7–2 shows that upon primary stimulation the precursor cell divides and differentiates into a number of antibody-forming cells producing either IgM or IgG immunoglobulins. During this process, a small number of memory cells are also produced. Following secondary challenge the proliferative events appear qualitatively similar, but the number of antigen-sensitive cells is greatly increased over that present in the primary response; the result is a greater pool of antibody-forming cells, and thus an increased amount of antibody is synthesized. Serum antibody formed in the secondary response may reach levels as high as 10 to 12 mg per ml and is predominantly of the IgG class, although some IgM is also expressed.

The dose of immunogen required to elicit a secondary response is far less than that required for the initiation of the primary response. Again, this is related to the number of antigen-sensitive cells bearing high-avidity receptors available for secondary stimulation and to the presence of circulating antibody remaining from the primary response. This circulating antibody will form complexes with the newly introduced material; antigen-antibody complexes formed in antigen excess are extremely immunogenic. The magnitude of the secondary response depends on other factors, including the interval between stimuli. Both short and long intervals result in decreased responses, the former because of the complete removal of immunogen and the latter possibly as a result of cell senescence. Immunologic memory may persist for many years and thereby provide long-lasting immunity against infection. Indeed, in the case of some bacterial and viral infections, immunity to reinfection may be lifelong. It is postulated that this immunity is related to the restimulation of long-lived memory cells by persisting antigen or newly introduced antigen. As in the primary response, antibody produced late in the secondary response has higher avidity and affinity for antigen than does that synthesized earlier. Late antibodies also appear to exhibit broad specificity. This may be attributed to the appearance of antibodies against certain antigenic determinants that do not stimulate antibodies early in the response (e.g., minor antigenic determinants). Therefore, the apparently broader specificity occurs because late antibodies exhibit a greater degree of *cross reactivity* with structurally related substances than do early antibodies.

A secondary response can be initiated by an immunogen that is closely related to the primary stimulating agent. In this case, the major portion of the antibodies produced will react more effectively with the first than with the second immunogen. This phenomenon, referred to as *the doctrine of original antigenic sin,* was first noted in studies of the response to influenza virus. It was observed that booster immunization with influenza vaccines induced antibodies that were directed mainly against strains of the virus that the individual had previously experienced, and the immune response to the booster vaccine was weaker. A possible explanation for this phenomenon is that the high-affinity antibody-forming cells are selectively stimulated in a population consisting of both low- and high-affinity antibody-producing cells.

Immunologic Memory

It appears that both B- and T-cells display immunologic memory. This finding was obtained from studies of cell cooperation in the immune response to hapten-carrier complexes. Although the hapten-carrier conjugates used in these studies may be considered unnatural immunogens, they are, in fact, true analogs of antigens that occur in nature, since the latter are also composed of multiple antigenic determinants, each of which can be considered a hapten. Under ordinary circumstances, when an animal is given a primary immunization with a hapten-protein conjugate, e.g., dinitrophenyl coupled to bovine serum albumin (DNP-BSA), and then is given a second injection of the same immunogen at a later time, antibodies against the hapten

(DNP) are formed at a rate typical of the secondary response (Fig. 7–3A). If the second injection is given with DNP coupled to a non–cross-reacting protein carrier, e.g., ovalbumin (OA), a secondary anti-DNP response is not usually manifested (Fig. 7–3B). However, if the animal that receives the second injection of DNP-OA has been previously primed with OA itself, then a substantial anti-DNP response will be elicited (Fig. 7–3C). This phenomenon, referred to as the *carrier effect*, suggests that recognition of both hapten and carrier is required for the secondary response. Further experiments have shown that T-cells recognize the carrier determinant and B-cells are responsible for recognition of the hapten.

The carrier effect is not always operative in secondary anti-hapten responses. In some cases, up to two years after animals have been given a primary injection with DNP-BSA, a potent secondary anti-DNP response can be induced with DNP coupled to a non–cross-reacting carrier, such as hemocyanin. This suggests that memory resides in B-cells. Evidence for T-cell memory comes from the inability of the so-called T-independent antigens (e.g., lipopolysaccharide, pneumococcal polysaccharide) to induce a secondary IgG response. Further, data obtained from studies with the congenitally athymic mouse strain (nude, nu/nu) suggest that T-cells regulate secondary responses of the IgG class.

Secondary stimulation of the immune response is not entirely without untoward effects, especially when soluble immunogens or haptens capable of binding to autologous substances are used. A portion of the anti-

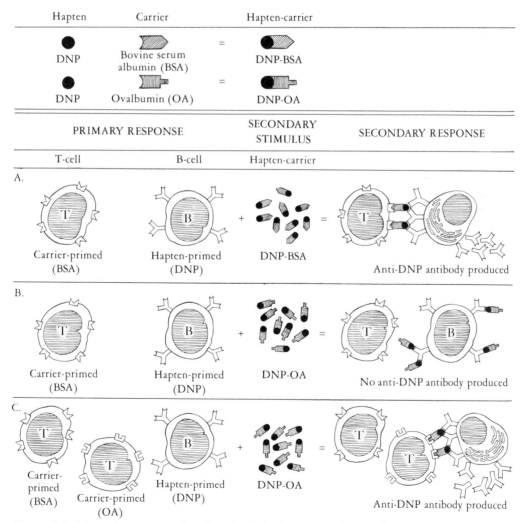

Figure 7–3. Schematic representation of carrier effect in the secondary antihapten antibody response.

body produced, as well as certain classes of antibody (e.g., IgE) made following primary stimulation, has the ability to fix to tissue cells. These cell-associated antibodies can bind the secondarily injected antigen, and, in some instances, this event can initiate a series of reactions that may be injurious or lethal to the individual. This antibody-mediated tissue injury is based on a secondary response.

CELLULAR EVENTS INVOLVED IN THE SPECIFIC IMMUNE RESPONSE

Functional Cells

Much of our current information regarding the nature of cells and cellular interactions involved in the immune response has been obtained from studies of the "experiments of nature" that take the form of human immune deficiency diseases. The results of these studies have shown that there is a functional division of the immune system involving two lines of immunocompetent cells, one concerned with humoral immunity and the other with cell-mediated immunity. Although the early events occurring in the *afferent* arm of both divisions are essentially similar, as depicted in Figure 7–4, the products of the *efferent* arm are different; specific antibody is the product of *humoral immunity,* and specifically sensitized lymphocytes and their lymphokines are the products of *cell-mediated immunity* (Chapter 9).

According to our current knowledge, both lymphocytes and macrophages are involved in the immune response. There are two major types of lymphocytes that are morphologically indistinguishable. These antigen-specific cells, which act upon stimulation of surface membrane receptors, have been classified on the basis of their site of differentiation into *thymus-derived* (*T-cells*) and *bursa- or bone marrow–derived* (*B-cells*) (Chapter 3). In addition to there being differences in functional capabilities between the two major classes of lymphocytes, there is also functional diversity among lymphocytes of the same class. For example, T-cells in both humans and mice can be further classified into *helper* and *suppressor* or *regulatory* and *effector* subpopulations. Similarly, B-cells exhibit functional diversity based on the different classes of immunoglobulin that they synthesize.

Macrophages have a wide variety of functions in the immune response that are also thought to be associated with distinct functional subpopulations. These cells, which function as *accessory cells (A-cells),* are not specific for a given immunogen. In addition to their function as "antigen-presenting cells," macrophages secrete a variety of biologically active mediators (*monokines*), which regulate the response of both B- and T-cells either by augmenting or by suppressing cell division and/or differentiation. Tables 7–3 and 7–4 summarize some of the major properties of these cell types.

Lymphocytes

Lymphocyte precursors arise in the bone marrow from pleuripotent stem cells, pass through the blood stream, and enter the central lymphoid organs where further development takes place (Chapter 2). Those cells that enter the thymus (thymocytes) may be modified therein or may pass through the organ and be eliminated. It has been suggested that maturation of T-lymphocytes in the thymus may be influenced by one of several soluble hormones elaborated by the epithelial cells of the thymus, e.g., *thymosin.* It has also been suggested that macrophages or their soluble products have an influence on lymphocyte differentiation in the thymus. Evidence for a thymic humoral factor is derived from experiments in which animals made immunologically deficient by removal of the thymus were rendered immunologically competent after transplantation of fetal thymus tissue contained within a cell-impermeable chamber. Attempts have been made to use thymic factors to reconstitute immunologic competence to humans having congenital T-cell defects, with some reported success.

Precursors of B-lymphocytes, which are also of bone marrow origin, may go directly to the peripheral lymphoid tissue or may first pass through or be influenced by the liver, bone marrow, appendix, intestines, or tonsils in order to develop into functional B-cells. Evidence for the existence of an organ analogous to the bursa of Fabricius of birds is missing in mammalian species (Chapter 2).

In spite of their different maturation pathways, only in recent years, through the de-

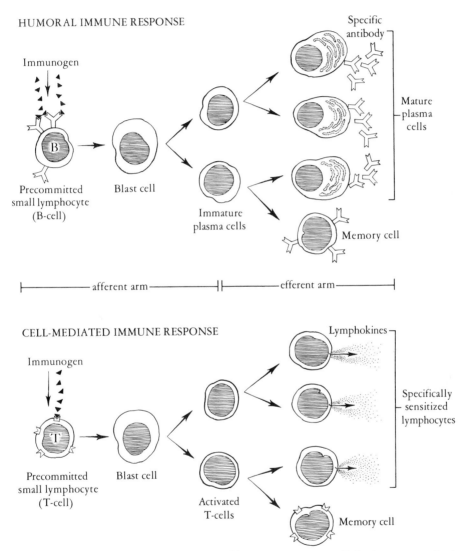

Figure 7–4. Schematic representation of the activation of immunocompetent cells by immunogen for humoral and cell-mediated immune responses.

Table 7–3. **Characteristics of Human Lymphocytes and Macrophages**

	T-Cells	B-Cells	Macrophages
Site of Differentiation	Thymus	Bone Marrow	Bone Marrow
Surface markers			
Specific surface antigen	OKT and Leu series*	HBLA (?)	OKM1
Antigen-binding receptor	V region idiotype	Immunoglobulin	−
Receptors for:			
SRBC (E-rosette)	+	−	−
IgG Fc (EA-rosette)	+(Suppressor)	+	+
IgM Fc (EA-rosette)	+(Helper)	−	−
C3b (EAC-rosette)	−	+	+
Measles virus	+	−	−
Epstein-Barr virus	−	+	−
HLA alloantigens: A,B,C,	+	+	+
HLA alloantigens: D/DR	±	+	+
Location: per cent lymphocytes			
Peripheral blood	55–75	15–30	2–12
Thoracic duct	<75	<25	<10
Lymph node	75	20	5
Spleen	35–45	50–60	5–10
Bone marrow	<10	<75	10–15
Thymus	<75	<10	<10
Tissue location	Cortex	Germinal center	Sinuses
Life span	Both long- and short-lived	Most are short-lived	Long-lived
Traffic	Recirculate	Little recirculation	Little, if any, recirculation
Blast transformation induced by:			
Phytohemagglutinin (PHA)			
soluble	+	−	−
insoluble	+	+	−
Concanavalin-A (Con-A)			
soluble	+	−	−
insoluble	+	+	−
Lipopolysaccharide (LPS)	−	− (?)	−
Pokeweed mitogen (PWM)	+	+	−
Anti-immunoglobulin	−	+	−
Specific antigen	+	+	−
Susceptible to inactivation by:			
Corticosteroids	+	+ +	−
X-irradiation	+ +	+ + +	−
Anti-lymphocyte serum (ALS)	+ + +	(+)	−
Immunosuppressive drugs:			
Cyclophosphamide	+(Suppressor)	+ + +	+
Azathioprine	+ + +	+	+

*The Leu series of monoclonal antibodies is a trademark of Becton Dickinson Company, Sunnyvale, California. The OK series of monoclonal antibodies is a trademark of Ortho Pharmaceutical Corporation, Raritan, New Jersey.

Table 7–4. Immunologic Functions of T-Cells, B-Cells, and Macrophages

	T-Cell	B-Cell	Macrophage
Humoral response	Helper Suppressor Regulator	Differentiate into anti-body-secreting cells	Accessory cell for in-duction
Cell-mediated re-sponse	Helper Suppressor Regulator	?	Accessory cell for in-duction Effector cell
Specificity	Clonally restricted	Clonally restricted	Nonspecific
Products elaborated	Lymphokines Helper factors Suppressor factors	Immunoglobulins	Monokines (e.g., inter-leukin-1) Regulatory factors
Memory	Antigen-specific	Antigen-specific	None
Can be made tolerant?	Yes	Yes	No

velopment of sensitive immunologic techniques (e.g., immunofluorescence, rosette analysis), has it become possible to describe characteristic markers useful for the identification of morphologically indistinguishable B- and T-cells.

SURFACE MARKERS

In murine systems, some of the lymphocytes that enter the thymus acquire a surface alloantigen formerly called *theta* (θ) that occurs in two allelic forms now referred to as *Thy 1.1 and Thy 1.2*. This antigen is found on lymphocytes that leave the thymus (thymus-derived or T-cells), on brain cells, and on skin and fibroblast cells in very small amounts, but it is absent from B-cells. The presence of the Thy 1 antigen is detected by an antiserum prepared by immunizing mice not carrying the specific antigen with thymus cells from mice that do. This antiserum, in the presence of complement, can be used to deplete lymphocyte populations of Thy 1–bearing cells. T-cells express different concentrations of the Thy 1 alloantigen on their surface at different stages of their maturation. In the cortex of the thymus, thymocytes express the greatest amount of Thy 1. The more mature thymus medullary lymphocyte expresses a lesser amount of the Thy 1 antigen, and even less is expressed on circulating (peripheral) T-cells. An analogous thymus alloantigen in humans, called *human thymus lymphocyte antigen* (HTLA), has been used for the preparation of a cytotoxic antiserum that has immunosuppressive capabilities. This reagent has been used clinically to prevent the immunologic rejection of organ or tissue transplants.

Other alloantigens have been detected primarily on the surface of T-cells. Among these

is the *TL alloantigen*, which is expressed on the surface of lymphocytes within the thymus of genetically TL$^+$ mouse strains and is lost as the cells mature into T-cells. The TL antigen also appears on T-cells of leukemic mice in TL$^-$ strains, suggesting that de-repression of a previously existing gene occurs. In humans, alloantibodies against T-cells are found in the sera of patients with infectious mononucleosis and systemic lupus erythematosus, which suggests antigenic modulation of the cell surface or derepression of genetic information for expression of the given antigen.

The *Ly antigens* constitute a group of cell surface markers that are differentially expressed on murine T-cells (Lyt) and B-cells (Lyb). Further differential expression of Lyt antigens delineates functionally distinct subpopulations of T-cells (to be described later in this chapter). Functional subsets of murine T-cells can also be identified by the presence of Qa and Ia antigens (described later).

The development of flow fluorocytometry technology and hybridoma methodology for the production of monoclonal antibodies has led to the analysis of human lymphocyte subpopulations. Monoclonal antibodies that define various functional subsets of human T-cells have been developed. These monoclonal antibodies also react with human T-cells at different stages of maturation (see Chapter 2, Fig. 2–21). The earliest thymocytes bear the T10 marker alone or in combination with T9. During maturation, the cells acquire a unique thymocyte antigen, defined as T6. These cells also express the T4 and T5/T8 markers, which are also found on peripheral T-cells. Anti-T6, anti-T9, and anti-T10 monoclonal antibodies react almost exclusively with thymocytes and not with peripheral T-cells. Cells bearing the T10, T6,

T4, and T5/T8 markers account for 70 to 75 per cent of total thymocytes. As the cells undergo further maturation within the thymus, they lose T6, acquire T1 and T3 markers, and segregate into the T4 and T5/T8 subsets. Upon leaving the thymus to populate the peripheral T-cell compartment, the cells lose the T10 marker. Monoclonal anti-T1 and anti-T3 antibodies react with virtually 100 per cent of peripheral T-cells but with only about 10 per cent of mature thymocytes. Anti-T4 reacts with 75 per cent of thymocytes and 60 per cent of peripheral T-cells, identifying the *helper or inducer* subset of human T-cells. Anti-T5 and anti-T8 react with 80 per cent of thymocytes and 20 to 30 per cent of peripheral T-cells, identifying the *suppressor or cytotoxic* subset of human T-cells. Table 7–5 summarizes the functional properties of these cells. Monoclonal antibodies with specificities similar to those described above are commercially available and are readily applicable to quantitating lymphocyte subpopulations in clinical disease states in hospital laboratories.

Alloantigens on B-cells with a relationship similar to that which Thy-1 (theta) has for T-cells have not yet been described. In murine species, a *mouse B-lymphocyte antigen* (MBLA) has been used for the preparation of a heterologous anti-B cell antiserum. This reagent was used in studies of B-cell function only after it had been absorbed extensively with mouse tissue to remove cytotoxic activity against thymus cells. Another murine alloantigen, referred to as *PC.1*, is present on the surface of plasma cells, the terminally differentiated product of the antigen-stimulated B-

cell, and on certain mouse myeloma cells. This surface marker is thought to be a differentiation antigen. Although several attempts have been made to generate antisera against human B-cells, they have been unsuccessful for the most part because of the lack of identification of a unique B-cell alloantigen. The most useful marker to aid in the identification of B-cells to date is the presence of immunoglobulin on the cell surface. It is highly likely that in the not too distant future a collection of antibodies that define B-cells at various stages of maturation will also be available, as is the case for T-cells.

Macrophages, which also arise from bone marrow progenitor cells, find their way into the blood stream as monocytes (Chapter 2). The monocytes wander through tissues and, together with their fixed-form counterparts, serve both phagocytic and immunoregulatory functions. In recent years, monoclonal antibodies that react with surface antigens on both rodent and human mononuclear phagocytes have been described. At present there are more than 15 reagents that appear to be specific for antigens on human monocytes/macrophages. While none of these monoclonal antibodies, as yet, defines a molecule of known function (e.g., Fc receptors), some of the marker-bearing cells have distinct immunologic function (e.g., antigen-presentation). Several mouse anti-human monoclonal antibodies define antigens shared among monocytes and other blood cells. For example, monoclonal antibodies designated OKM1, Mo1, and MY4 are expressed on monocytes and granulocytes, while TA-1 and Mo4 are found on T-cells and platelets, re-

Table 7–5. Immunologic Function of Human T-Cell Subsets Recognized by Monoclonal Antibodies

Function	T-Helper T-Inducer (T 4$^+$)	T-Cytotoxic T-Suppressor (T 5/8$^+$)
Proliferation induced by		
Soluble antigen	+	−
I-region (D/DR) products	+	+
Concanavalin-A	+	+
Phytohemagglutinin	+	−
Helper induction in		
T-Mφ interactions	+	−
T-T interactions	+	−
T-B interactions	+	−
Suppressor effector in		
Antibody production	−	+
Cell-mediated reactions	−	+
Cytotoxic effector cell	−	+

spectively. Anti-OKM1 and anti-Mo1 also have reactivity against null cells. Deletion of OKM1-positive cells abrogates antibody-dependent cellular cytotoxicity (ADCC) and natural killer (NK) activity by human mononuclear cells. There are several rat anti-mouse monoclonal antibodies that define antigens expressed on macrophages alone as well as a number of reagents that detect antigens that are shared among myeloid cells. For example, anti–Mac-1 reacts with mouse macrophages, granulocytes, and some mouse cell lines as well as with human peripheral blood monocytes, granulocytes, and null cells. Of clinical significance is the observation that many of the mouse anti-human monoclonal antibodies are reactive with myeloid leukemia cells but not with malignant lymphoid cells. These reagents may prove useful not only for the diagnosis of myeloid leukemia when conventional methods are questionable, but also as specific immunotherapeutic agents for treatment of disorders of the reticuloendothelial system. Very recently, a series of monoclonal antibodies that are reactive with distinct stages of monocyte/macrophage differentiation have been developed. Similarly, monoclonal antibodies that are capable of defining functional macrophage subsets are now beginning to appear.

In addition to the above-described surface markers, nonlymphoid cells as well as B-cells, T-cells, and macrophages express on their surface, to varying degrees, antigens representing the gene products of the *major histocompatibility complex* (MHC) of the species. A detailed description of these alloantigens is found in Chapter 3, while their role in cellular interactions is discussed later in this chapter.

SURFACE RECEPTORS

Specific *receptors* with binding affinity for a variety of ligands are found on the surface of cells that participate in the immune response. Methods that have been developed for the detection of these receptors can also serve as a means of evaluating the quantity or quality of a particular cell type. One such method involves the formation of *rosettes* consisting of either a lymphocyte or a macrophage surrounded by an appropriate indicator cell. In humans, three types of rosettes can be distinguished that correspond to different cell surface receptors (Fig. 7–5). T-lymphocytes from normal humans, when

mixed with sheep erythrocytes (E), form spontaneous rosettes (Fig. 7–5A). While there is no specific immunologic basis for the formation of these *E-rosettes* (also called T-rosettes), the presence of E-receptors on the surface of mature T-cells has proved to be extremely useful for quantitating these cells in peripheral blood. A second type of receptor that is involved in rosette formation binds antigen-antibody complexes or aggregated immunoglobulin through the Fc portion of the IgG molecule (Fig. 7–5B). These *Fc receptors* are normally readily detectable on the surface of B-cells and macrophages and form *EA-rosettes* with sheep erythrocytes that have been coated with specific anti-sheep erythrocyte antibody (A). In addition to finding receptors for the Fc portion of IgG on B-cells and macrophages, the subset of human T-cells (called T_γ cells) that function as *cytotoxic and suppressor cells* (analogous to the $T1^+$, $T3^+$, $T5^+/T8^+$ cells) also possess Fc receptors, which can be detected using an IgG antibody prepared against ox erythrocytes. Receptors for the Fc portion of monomeric IgM are differentially expressed on macrophages and the subset of human T-cells (called T_μ cells) that function as *helper and inducer cells* (analogous to the $T1^+$, $T3^+$, $T4^+$ cell). Recently, lymphocytes and macrophages expressing Fc receptors for IgE and IgA have been described. These cells appear to have class-specific regulatory function on IgE and IgA antibody production. Finally, Fc receptors have been demonstrated on natural killer and K-cells (Chapter 9) involved in antibody-dependent cellular cytotoxicity (ADCC). The third type of receptor, found on some B-cells, some macrophages, and a limited number of other cell types, recognizes the third component of complement (C3b). These *EAC-rosettes* are formed with sheep erythrocytes coated with specific antibody and complement. The complement receptor does not appear to be a single molecular species. Recent studies indicate that there are unique membrane-binding sites for at least C3b, C3d, and C4. Lymphocytes bearing this receptor are referred to as *complement receptor (CR⁺) lymphocytes*. This receptor is useful in distinguishing immature B-cells (CR⁻) from mature B-cells (CR⁺) by rosette analysis.

ANTIGEN-BINDING RECEPTORS

The initiation of the immune response is dependent upon recognition of a foreign

PARTICIPATING CELL	SHEEP RED BLOOD CELL INDICATOR	ROSETTE

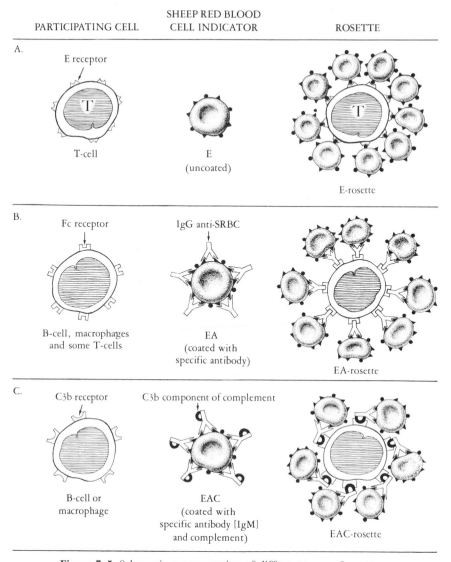

Figure 7–5. Schematic representation of different types of rosettes.

configuration (antigen) by specific receptors on B- and T-cells.

Receptors for Antigen on B-Cells. Immunoglobulin (Ig) can be readily detected on the surface of B-cells from human and most mammalian species through the use of fluorescent-labeled antisera prepared against various immunoglobulin classes. These surface Ig's are capable of binding specific antigens and function as antigen receptors that are likely to be involved in the differentiation events culminating in antibody synthesis. B-cells contain about 100,000 randomly distributed Ig molecules per cell. While it was originally thought that the Ig receptor on the B-cell was identical to the antibody product ultimately synthesized by the antigen-stimulated cell, current evidence indicates that surface-bound and secreted Ig differ somewhat in their C_H domains.

Specific Ig classes can be associated with B-cells. In humans and mice, IgM-bearing cells are more common than those bearing IgG. The relative proportion of κ and λ light chains on the surface of B-cells corresponds to that expressed on serum immunoglobulins. However, whereas the major serum Ig expresses the γ heavy chain, the major Ig expressed on B-cells bears the μ heavy chain. The cell surface IgM appears to exist predominantly in the monomeric form as IgM_S (8S), containing more carboxy-terminal hydrophobic amino acids and fewer carbohydrate moieties than are found in the pentameric serum IgM. In addition to expressing surface IgM, many B-cells also simultaneously express IgD on their surface. The immunoglobulin molecules on cells that· simultaneously express IgM and IgD appear to be limited to the same type of light chain and idiotype. There is also evidence that the surface and secreted Ig have the same specificity and affinity for their specific antigen, which suggests that they .possess the same V_L and V_H domains and the same idiotype.

The surface immunoglobulins are neither rigidly held in fixed position nor loosely bound; in fact, there is fluidity and movement of these molecules. For example, when a radiolabeled or fluorescein-labeled anti-immunoglobulin serum is reacted with living B-cells, changes can be observed at the cell surface (Fig. 7–6). If the reaction is carried out at low temperature (4°C), the labeled material can be seen in a *diffuse* arrangement over the entire cell surface, indicating that the surface immunoglobulin is randomly distributed. As the temperature is raised, the labeled material assumes a distribution of spots or patches over the surface. *Patch for-*

mation is independent of cell metabolism but is dependent upon the bivalence of antibody (e.g., F(ab')$_2$. This reaction is thought to depend upon cross-linking of the receptors. After a short time the label coalesces into a cap over one pole of the cell. *Cap formation* is an energy-dependent process. Following this the cap is either released or internalized within the cell, where the material is seen in vesicles. The cell surface remains devoid of immunoglobulin for a period of time before newly synthesized receptors can be detected. The same phenomenon can be demonstrated when B-cells expressing specific receptors bind a multivalent antigen. It has been suggested by some that these events are crucial to the triggering of cell differentiation and proliferation required for the initiation of the immune response. Others suggest that the above events function solely to remove excess antigen from the cell surface.

Receptors for Antigen on T-Cells. Based upon our understanding of the specificity of the antigen-antibody reaction, it would be

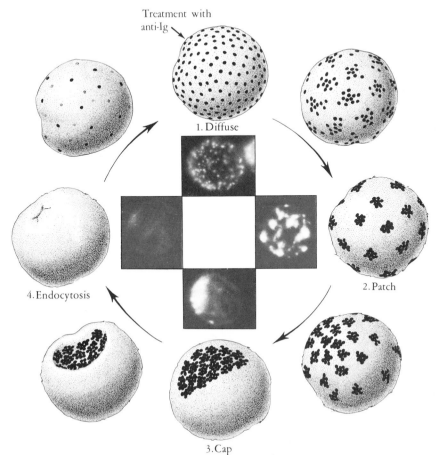

Figure 7–6. Redistribution of surface immunoglobulin as a consequence of treatment with anti-Ig. Inserts show cells treated with fluorescein-labeled anti-immunoglobulin. (Photomicrographs courtesy of Dr. Joseph Davie.)

logical to conclude that the T-cell receptor must also be represented by immunoglobulin. However, the nature of the T-cell receptor is controversial and, at present, uncertain. Immunoglobulin can be detected on the surface of T-cells, but only in trace amounts, and it is uncertain whether this is passively acquired from B-cells or made by the T-cell. The fact that anti-immunoglobulin antisera do not readily block the immunologic functions of these cells argues against the receptor's being an immunoglobulin. Those who favor the immunoglobulin nature of the T-cell receptor suggest that it is located deeper in the cell membrane than that of B-cells; that it is sterically hindered by other surface components; or that it belongs to a class of hitherto unidentified immunoglobulins that lack a conventional constant (C) region domain, since antisera to such domains react poorly, if at all, with T-cells. Studies on the genetic control of antibody formation have shown that antigen recognition by T-cells is regulated by genes closely associated with the major histocompatibility complex (MHC), called Ir genes (Chapter 3). It is currently believed that T-cell receptors for antigen are represented by variable (V) region domains, since their antigen-recognition units express idiotypes in response to activation by antigen, which are the same as those of antibody molecules stimulated by the same antigen. It is likely that these V-region domains on the T-cell are associated with MHC gene products rather than with conventional C-region domains.

In the human, an additional substance is associated with the cell surface. The material is a low molecular weight protein fragment found in association with the histocompatibility antigens (HLA). This β_2 *microglobulin* in many ways resembles the homology regions of immunoglobulins; its amino acid sequence is very similar to the homology regions in the constant portion of the light chain (C_L) and the heavy chain (CH_3) of IgG. It has been suggested, although this is no longer believed, that the β_2 microglobulin functions as the T-cell receptor by serving as the recognition site for B- and T-cell interactions or some regulatory substance. Its similarity in structure to immunoglobulin and its close association with HLA suggests an important evolutionary interaction between the products of the immune system and the histocompatibility system.

Blast Transformation. The recognition of an immunogen by specific receptors on B- and T-cells leads to the initiation of a series of events in which the cells increase in size, the nucleolus enlarges, rough endoplasmic reticulum and microtubules become prominent, the rate of DNA synthesis increases, and mitosis ensues. Figure 7–7 shows a typical blast cell. This process of *blast transformation* can also be induced by the addition of bivalent $F(ab')_2$, but not of monovalent Fab fragments of anti-immunoglobulin or anti-allotype antisera, to cultures of immunoglobulin-bearing lymphocytes. The addition of other agents, including certain plant proteins and endotoxin, called *mitogens,* to cultures of nonsensitized lymphocytes may also initiate blast transformation. These observations suggest that some membrane perturbation induced by the cross-linking of certain surface macromolecules stimulates the lymphocyte to divide.

Plant mitogens have the potential to activate large numbers of lymphocytes without regard to the antigenic reactivity of the responding cells. The different mitogens bind to and have specificity for diverse sugar moieties of glycoproteins on the lymphocyte membrane (e.g., concanavalin A [Con-A] binds to glycoproteins containing α-mannosyl moie-

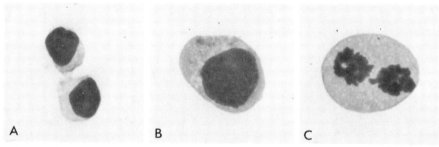

Figure 7–7. Photomicrographs of lymphocytes in the process of blast transformation. Giemsa stain, ×900. *A,* Unstimulated small lymphocytes; *B,* PHA-stimulated blast cell; *C,* PHA-stimuated lymphocyte in mitosis. (Courtesy of B. Zeligs.)

ties). Some of the mitogens have the ability to activate T-cells, others to activate B-cells, and some induce changes in both. It is important to note that a given mitogen will have diverse effects on lymphocytes obtained from different species. For example, whereas the lipopolysaccharide (LPS) of gram-negative bacteria is a potent mitogen for murine B-cells (but not for T-cells), it does not induce blast transformation in rabbit B-cells. Currently, there is question as to the mitogenic effect of LPS on human B-cells. Some believe that LPS induces a clonally restricted response in human B-cells (i.e., similar to that induced by any specific immunogen), but one report suggests that after an initial culture period in the absence of LPS, human B-cells will respond to the addition of LPS in a polyclonal manner. It is thought that the initial culture period is necessary to remove the influence of suppressor T-cells. Pokeweed mitogen (PWM) stimulates both B- and T-cell subpopulations of mouse and human lymphocytes. It has been suggested that stimulation of human B-cells by PWM depends on the presence of T-cells. Both phytohemagglutinin (PHA) and Con-A, in their soluble forms, selectively stimulate murine T-cells to synthesize DNA, divide, and produce a nonspecific factor that can replace the T-cell helper function in some immune responses. When rendered insoluble by attachment to large particles, Con-A and PHA induce blast transformation in both B- and T-cell subpopulations. In this case, B-cell stimulation could be indirect, since nonspecific products elaborated by PHA-stimulated T-cells initiate the activation of B-cells.

In addition to stimulating DNA synthesis in both T- and B-cells, certain mitogens, such as PWM, will initiate synthesis and secretion of IgM in cultures of B-cells, and others, such as PHA, will induce lymphokine production (Chapter 9) in cultures of T-cells and are called *polyclonal activators*. The reaction of lymphocyte populations to the various mitogens (Table 7–3) may, with caution, be used by the clinician to identify the type of cell (T- or B-cell) and to reveal developmental or functional deficiencies.

Macrophages

Although the involvement of macrophages in both *in vivo* and *in vitro* immune responses has been known for many years, their precise function still remains unclear. The basic functional property of a macrophage is its ability to engulf and remove foreign and effete materials. The endocytic processes of macrophages appear to be initiated by the interaction of the foreign material with the cell membrane. Phagocytosis can be facilitated by the presence of antigen coated with antibody, a process called *opsonization*. In addition, antibodies of a variety of specificities can be attached to the macrophage surface through its Fc receptor. This *cytophilic* antibody endows macrophages with enhanced abilities to recognize, engulf, and destroy antigenic substances. The receptors for complement components, which are independent of Fc receptors, also aid the macrophages in removing antigens from their environment.

Evidence for the role of the macrophage in humoral responses has been provided by numerous *in vivo* studies using irradiated animals, reticuloendothelial blockade, and anti-macrophage serum. The essentiality of macrophage participation in the *in vitro* immune response has been shown by experiments in which mouse spleen populations were separated into adherent (macrophage-rich) and nonadherent (lymphocyte-rich) populations. Neither of these populations by themselves can respond to antigen; however, when they are combined, an antibody response equivalent to that of the unseparated spleen cell population is obtained.

Numerous functional roles have been ascribed to macrophages participating in the immune response. In early experiments, it was thought that macrophages "*processed*" antigens into an immunogenic form that was recognized by a particular lymphocyte subclass. Processing appears to be an important event associated with the initial steps of the immune response to particulate materials; it is thought that this event may expose determinants otherwise unavailable to react with lymphocytes or may change pre-existing determinants into a recognizable form. In support of this concept, it has been shown that aggregation of soluble antigens leads to more efficient phagocytosis, which also results in enhanced immunogenicity.

It has also been suggested by some that processing of antigen by macrophages results in the production of a new class of macrophage-derived RNA that carries genetic information. Two fractions of macrophage-derived RNA have been described; however, one of these contains a portion of the original antigen. This antigen-RNA complex is more efficient in stimulating an immune response than the original antigen and has been referred to as a *superantigen*. In this case, the enhanced immunogenicity has been attributed to the adjuvant properties of the component nucleic acid.

The second class of RNA has been shown to be free of antigen fragments and is thought to have messenger RNA activity. It is referred to as *informational* RNA (i-RNA). This RNA has a molecular weight between 400,000 and 750,000 and selectively induces the formation of IgM antibody. Support for an informational role of macrophage-derived RNA was obtained from the following type of experiment. If, after incubation with antigen, macrophage RNA is prepared from cells of a strain of animal that produces antibody with a unique allotype marker (b^4b^4) and is added to lymphoid cells obtained from another animal that produces antibody of a different allotype (b^5b^5), the antibody molecules formed will be of the allotype of the macrophage donor animal (b^4b^4). Recent evidence has also shown that this i-RNA can direct the synthesis of 19S protein of a particular allotype in cell-free extracts, suggesting that the i-RNA functions as messenger RNA.

A second function attributed to the macrophage is *antigen presentation*. It has been amply demonstrated that after incubation of antigen with macrophages, a portion of the antigen remains associated with the macrophage surface. This macrophage-bound antigen is more immunogenic than an equivalent amount of free antigen. It is not clear whether the surface-bound antigen is derived from material taken up by the macrophage, processed, and subsequently exocytosed or whether it is a result of direct interaction of the material with components (e.g., antibody affixed to Fc receptors) on the macrophage membrane. This surface-associated antigen appears to be tightly bound and can be recovered in macromolecular form after limited treatment of the cell surface with proteolytic enzymes.

It is now clear that antigen presentation is mediated by a subset of macrophages bearing surface Ia molecules that are encoded by genes of the major histocompatibility complex (Chapter 3). Since anti-Ia antibody interferes with the presenting function of macrophages possessing membrane-bound antigen, it has been suggested that Ia and

specific antigen molecules "interact" on the macrophage surface. It is thought that it is the "Ia–antigen complex" on the *antigen-presenting cell* that is recognized by the responding lymphocyte subset. In spite of the current belief in this hypothesis, it must be considered with caution, since it has been difficult to demonstrate that antibody against the specific antigen can interfere with antigen presentation as has been shown to be the case with anti-Ia antibody.

An additional function attributed to macrophages is the production and secretion of a wide variety of biologically active factors that influence the activity of lymphocytes. Macrophage extracts or supernatant fluids from macrophage cultures can substitute for the function of intact macrophages in *in vitro* systems measuring antibody formation. However, it has also been shown that macrophage function can be replaced by 2-mercaptoethanol (2-ME) during the induction of the *in vitro* immune response to sheep red blood cells (SRBC) by mouse spleen cells. It has been suggested that in this system, 2-ME substitutes for macrophage function by acting in combination with a serum component of the tissue culture medium, leading to the activation of T-cells. An additional factor produced by macrophages that has a positive effect on lymphocyte function is *interleukin-1* (IL-1), formerly called lymphocyte activating factor. This material, which has been purified to homogeneity, stimulates maturation and proliferation in T-cells. In addition, IL-1 appears to stimulate the production of a second interleukin, IL-2, by T-cells, which acts together with the signals initiated by antigen and Ia such that T-cell activation is achieved. The production of IL-2 by helper T-cells has also been reported to be important for the stimulation of B-cells to proliferate and differentiate into immunoglobulin-secreting cells. Alternatively, macrophages may also suppress the activities of lymphocytes nonspecifically through the elaboration of other biologically active substances. These include: arginase, thymidine, complement-cleavage products, prostaglandins, interferon, and oxygen intermediates.

Although all of the above postulated functions of macrophages are worthy of further consideration, attention has been directed toward the surface membrane of the macrophage. Macrophage-bound antigen is highly immunogenic for T-cells. The fact that maximal stimulation is achieved when the macrophage and lymphocyte possess common histocompatibility molecules (Ia determinants) suggests that something more than antigen is required. Indeed, in several systems direct contact between macrophages and lymphocytes has been observed and suggests the necessity of cell surface interaction or the transfer of information from one cell to the other (Fig. 7–8) via soluble factors.

Null Cells

A relatively small proportion of lymphocytes can be detected that bear neither the Thy-l antigen nor the surface immunoglobulin that are characteristic of T- and B-cells,

respectively. These *null cells*, originally recognized for their ability to lyse tumor cells either spontaneously or through an ADCC mechanism (Chapter 9), have characteristics distinct from other types of lymphoid cells. This population, representing 5 to 15 per cent of the cells in peripheral blood, consists of hemopoietic stem cells, which are thought to include precursors of T- and B-cells, myeloid, erythroid, and thrombocytic series. Two types of cells are considered in this category.

KILLER CELLS (K CELLS)

This is a heterogeneous group of cells that, when taken from normal individuals, can lyse diverse target cells *in vitro* if incubated in the

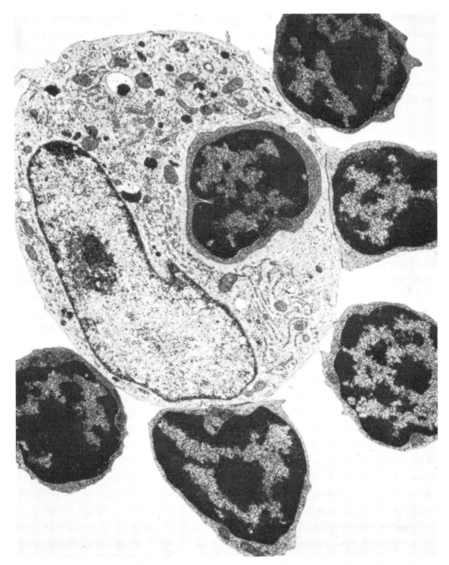

Figure 7–8. Photomicrograph of macrophage-lymphocyte interaction. (Reproduced from Lipsky, P. E., and Rosenthal, A. S.: Macrophage-lymphocyte interaction. I. Characteristics of the antigen-independent-binding of guinea pig thymocytes and lymphocytes to syngeneic macrophages. J. Exp. Med., *138*:900, 1973.)

presence of specific antibodies against surface antigens on the latter. Fc receptors for IgG on these cells can bind monomeric IgG, aggregated IgG, or IgG that has already reacted with antigen, e.g., on the surface of target cells. About 40 per cent of K cells possess receptors for SRBC, a typical T-cell marker, in addition to the Fc receptor for IgG. Another 40 per cent lack the T-cell marker as well as surface-bound immunoglobulin, a marker of B-cells, but possess receptors for complement components. The remaining 20 per cent of K cells do not possess any of the above-mentioned markers.

NATURAL KILLER CELLS (NK CELLS)

NK cells are nonphagocytic and nonadherent cells found in normal individuals of most mammalian species. They resemble large granular lymphocytes and compose about 5 per cent of peripheral blood and splenic leukocytes. They express surface receptors for the Fc portion of IgG and can function as K cells that mediate ADCC. Although these cells do not appear to be thymus-dependent, with significant levels of NK activity detected in athymic nude or neonatally thymectomized mice, these cells share T-cell–associated markers. About 50 per cent of human NK cells have receptors for SRBC, and the majority react with monoclonal antibodies against T-cell markers (e.g., T10$^+$) as well as monocyte/macrophage markers (e.g., OKM1). NK cells can react against a wide variety of target cells. Not only are tumor cells susceptible to lysis by NK cells but also fetal cells, virus-infected cells, and some subsets of thymus cells, bone marrow cells, and macrophages. Unlike the case with antigen recognition by T-cells, recognition by NK cells does not appear to require the sharing of histocompatibility antigens. The activity of NK cells can be augmented by interferon as well as other stimuli (e.g., retinoic acid). There is increasing evidence that these cells may play an important role in immune surveillance.

CELL INTERACTIONS IN THE INITIATION OF ANTIBODY FORMATION

The clonal selection theory of antibody formation proposed by Burnet states that an immunologically responsive cell (small lymphocyte) contains within its genome the genetic information to respond to a single immunogen (or a few related ones) even before the cell encounters the foreign configuration. Thus, the lymphocyte population of an individual is preprogrammed to contain a diverse library of cells, some of which respond to one antigen, others to a second, and so forth. The encounter between the immunogen and the precommitted cell results in the proliferation of the latter and the generation of a clone of differentiated antibody-forming cells (Fig. 7–9). This hypothesis implies that an antiserum prepared against a complex immunogen (e.g., bacterium) consists of a population of different antibodies, each produced by separate clones preprogrammed to respond to a particular antigenic determinant on the complex microorganism. In order to provide experimental evidence to support this hypothesis, attempts were made to determine the number of antibodies produced by single cells. It was found that a single plasma cell produces antibodies with a single antigen-binding specificity. The uniformity in primary structure of a given class of antibody produced by a single cell is similar to that of the myeloma protein produced in multiple myeloma and suggests that the immunoglobulin molecule is subject to *allelic exclusion;* that is, the cell expresses only one of its several alleles for the different polypeptide chains of the immunoglobulin molecule at any one time. However, in view of the fact that a single cell can be shown to produce more than one class of immunoglobulin (e.g., IgM and IgD) at one time, what was once referred to as the *one cell—one antibody* rule has now been modified to the *one cell—one idiotype* rule. Since the early immune response is characterized by the predominance of IgM antibody followed later by IgG, it has been suggested that cells can undergo an *IgM→IgG switch* during the course of the response. Immunologic evidence to support such a switch mechanism is based on the observation of patients with biclonal myelomas. One such patient produced both homogeneous IgM and IgG paraproteins. Analysis of these proteins revealed identity in primary amino acid sequence in all regions of the immunoglobulins except for the C_H region, which was μ in one protein and γ in the other. This switch can be explained on a genetic basis, whereby in making IgM the cell expresses genes for V_L, C_L, V_H, and Cμ regions (Fig. 7–10). The

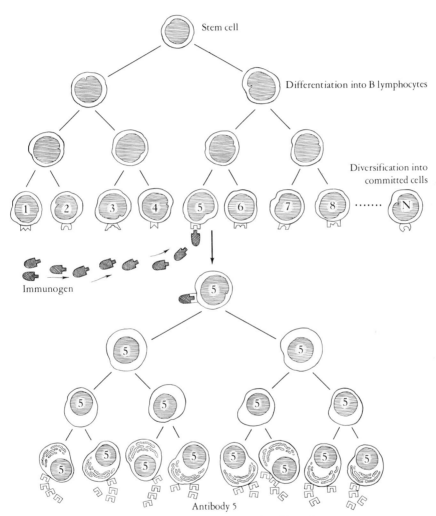

Figure 7–9. Schematic representation of clonal expansion of committed lymphocytes as a consequence of subsequent encounter with immunogen.

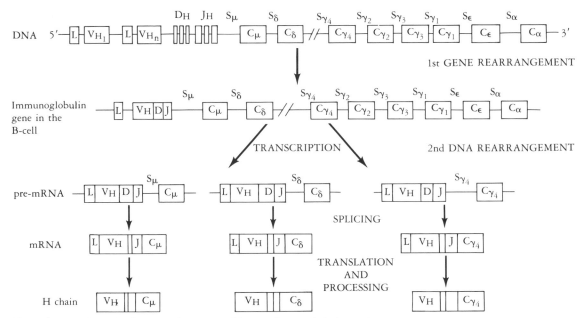

Figure 7–10. Schematic diagram of a proposed human heavy-chain locus demonstrating possible gene rearrangement involved in the dual expression of IgM and IgD as well as the IgM → IgG shift. L, leader sequences; V_H, variable region; J_H, joining segments; D_H, diversity segments; C, family of constant regions; and S, family of switch sites that precede each of the C-region genes. (After Rabbits, R. H., et al., 1981.)

switch to IgG synthesis preserves the expression of V_L, C_L, and V_H but involves a DNA rearrangement event in which Cγ gene can now be expressed. As indicated in Figure 7–10, the coding sequences for all C_H classes are found on the same chromosome separated at various lengths by intervening DNA segments containing specific switch sites (S). The Cμ gene is closest to the joining segment (J), and the Cα is farthest. A change in immunoglobulin class could occur when a switching site in the J-Cμ intervening DNA segment becomes joined to a switching site (S) between Cμ and any other C_H gene (e.g., Cγ$_4$). As a consequence of looping out and excision of the Cμ gene, the V_HJ sequence previously adjacent to Cμ will now be adjacent to Cγ$_4$. In a similar manner, the expression of IgD or other immunoglobulin heavy chains can be understood.

Compartmentalization of the Immune Response

Studies concerning the number of cells required for antibody formation have generated a vast amount of literature in the past decade. It was found that removal of the bursa of Fabricius from neonatal chickens, by either surgical or hormonal methods, re-

sulted in an impairment of the ability of these animals to synthesize antibodies. Similarly, injection of neonatal mice with anti-μ chain antiserum resulted in animals with severe deficiencies of the humoral immune response, as manifested by their inability to produce not only IgM antibodies but also IgG and IgA antibodies later in life. The clinical diseases observed in such animals are virtually identical to those seen in children suffering from a congenital sex-linked disease called Bruton's agammaglobulinemia. In none of the above situations is there impairment of cell-mediated immunity. On the other hand, removal of the thymus gland from neonatal animals resulted in a severely impaired cell-mediated response concomitant with variable deficiencies in the humoral response. Congenitally athymic (nude) mice display similar immunologic deficiencies of the cell-mediated response, although they respond normally to some immunogens and poorly, if at all, to others. In humans, a congenital developmental anomaly called the DiGeorge syndrome results in the birth of children lacking a thymus and displaying severe defects in cell-mediated immunity, along with variable defects in humoral immunity. Integration of these laboratory and clinical findings, which showed both a division of the immune response into humoral and cell-mediated immunity and combined immunodeficiencies related to the absence of the thymus, suggested, even before the nature of B- and T-cells was known, that cooperation between the cells of the two *central lymphoid organs* (bursa and thymus) was required for full expression of humoral immunity.

The current information regarding the mechanisms of cell cooperation involving macrophages, B-cells, and T-cells has been obtained from both *in vivo* and *in vitro* experiments. In 1966, it was first shown that thymus-derived and bone marrow–derived cells act synergistically in the restoration of the immune response of immunodeficient animals, and that if either population was omitted, a response did not take place. Subsequently, it was shown that depletion of spleen cell populations of adherent cells (macrophages) resulted in marked suppression of the immune response to SRBC and that this response could be restored by the addition of macrophages. Elegantly designed experiments showed that B-cells are the specific precursors of the antibody-forming cells and that T-cells, even though they do not differentiate into antibody-producing cells, can be stimulated to divide in response to antigen, can be specifically *educated* (have the ability to be primed by antigen and recognize it at a later time), and can provide a specific *helper* function for the initiation of the humoral response. Further understanding of the functions of B- and T-cells was obtained from studies of the carrier effect, in which it was shown that two receptors were involved in the elicitation of a secondary anti-hapten response, one hapten-specific, the other carrier-specific, and that B-cells carried the former, while T-cells carried the latter.

Cell Cooperation

In discussing potential mechanisms of antibody formation, two points should be addressed: The first is the mechanism by which the antigen-sensitive cell recognizes the immunogen, and the second is the nature of the signal required to trigger the B-cell to produce antibody. Regarding the first point, evidence has been presented that B-cells express clonally restricted immunoglobulin on their surface capable of reacting with a specific immunogen, and that this reaction leads to changes in the surface membrane, possibly

initiating proliferation and differentiation into an antibody-forming cell. While the precise nature of the T-cell receptor has not been defined, there is evidence to indicate that T-cells also express clonally restricted receptors for antigen on their surface, possibly in the form of idiotypic determinants. It is believed that interaction of the immunogen with these receptors contributes, in part, to the activation process in T-cells.

Influence of the Thymus on Immunogenicity

There is a growing body of evidence to suggest that the triggering of B-cells requires either one complex signal or two separate signals. Bacterial lipopolysaccharide, which has been shown to be mitogenic for murine B-cells, has the ability to activate B-cells nonspecifically. Such activation results in a *polyclonal* response, in which many clones of B-cells are activated in the absence of a specific antigen to make small amounts of their predetermined antibodies. Thus, a B-cell mitogen can provide a *nonspecific* signal to trigger B-cell activation. It is thought that the antigenic determinant carries a *specific second signal* that activates specific clones to produce large amounts of antibody. Thus, the triggering of B-cells appears to require two signals, a *specific signal* represented by the antigenic determinant that is recognized by the Ig receptor and influences the differentiation and proliferation of the clone. The specific signal is referred to as *immunogenicity* and the nonspecific signal as *mitogenicity* or *adjuvanticity*.

In recent years, by means of *in vitro* systems, some interesting observations have been made concerning the idea that the nature of the immunogen may influence the types of cells that interact in the immune response. A small number of immunogens appear to elicit B-cell responses in the absence of T-cell help. These so-called *T-independent antigens* have been characterized as polymeric substances having a large number of repeating identical determinants that are relatively resistant to degradation and include such substances as dextran, levan, ficoll, polyvinylpyrrolidone, lipopolysaccharide, polymerized flagellin, and pneumococcal polysaccharide (Fig. 7–11*A*). The immune response to these materials is characterized by the almost exclusive production of IgM

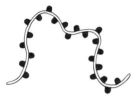

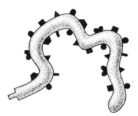

Figure 7–11. Schematic representation of T-independent and T-dependent antigens.

A. T-independent antigen -
contains many copies of identical
antigenic determinants (e.g., levan,
pneumococcal polysaccharide,
lipopolysaccharide)

B. T-dependent antigen -
few copies of many different
antigenic determinants (e.g.,
RBC, bacterium, protein)

with little or no IgG production and no production of immunologic memory. In addition to the lack of a requirement for T-cell help, the immune response to these materials was also thought to be independent of macrophage function. However, experiments using highly selective methods for the depletion of macrophages have suggested that these cells are required, albeit in small numbers, for responses to certain T-independent antigens. Interestingly, it has been found that T-cells may even play a suppressive role in the response to certain T-independent antigens (e.g., pneumococcal polysaccharide S-III), since removal of these cells by thymectomy or by treatment with anti-lymphocyte serum results in enhanced antibody production. Therefore, although these antigens appear to be independent of T-cell helper function, they may not be totally T-independent, in that T-cells may still play a regulatory role. To explain the triggering of B-cells it has been postulated, although not without controversy, that T-independent antigens carry both the specific and the nonspecific signal on the same molecule. The specific signal is represented by the ability of the multiple copies of the repeating antigenic determinant to cross link specific immunoglobulin receptors on the surface of B-cells. The nonspecific signal is represented by the ability of these substances, when introduced at high doses, to function as polyclonal B-cell activators, in that they stimulate multiple B-cell clones to proliferate and secrete immunoglobulin without regard to specific recognition by B-cell surface receptors. For example, LPS of *E. coli* is a polyclonal activator of mouse B-cells when given at high doses. However, while it also reacts with B-cells when given at low doses, it activates only those B-cells that are precommitted to make an anti-LPS antibody response. These results suggest that T-independent antigens possess separate antigenic and mitogenic sites and that these bind to separate receptors on B-cells (Fig. 7–12).

Almost all of the immunogens encountered in nature are not polymers of repeated similar antigenic determinants. Indeed, they are usually made up of a single copy or a few copies of diverse antigenic determinants (Fig. 7–11B). These substances induce immune responses, potentially involving all of the immunoglobulin classes and immunologic memory, and require T-cell help. Cells, proteins, glycoproteins, and hapten-carrier combinations are but a few examples of substances that make up the class of *T-dependent antigens.* It has been shown that the immune response to these antigens in T-cell–deficient animals is greatly suppressed and is limited, for the most part, to the IgM class of antibody, suggesting that T-cells are involved in the transition from IgM to IgG antibody synthesis.

T-Cell Subpopulations

It is now well accepted that there are three major subsets of murine T-cells that influence the activity of other T-cells as well as that of B-cells. These T-cell subpopulations, referred to as inducers, regulators, and effectors, have been defined through the use of antisera prepared against alloantigens described earlier in this chapter. Three T-cell subsets have been defined by cytotoxic antisera prepared against the murine Lyt alloantigens, which are coded for by two unlinked genetic loci (Lyt-1 on chromosome 19, and Lyt-2 and Lyt-3, which are closely linked on chromosome 6). These subsets have been designated as Lyt-1,2,3$^+$, Lyt-1$^+$, and Lyt-2,3$^+$. Of the T-cells found in peripheral lymphoid tissue, about 60 to 65 per cent are Lyt-1,2,3$^+$, 30 to 35 per cent are Lyt-1$^+$, and 5 to 10 per cent are Lyt-2,3$^+$.

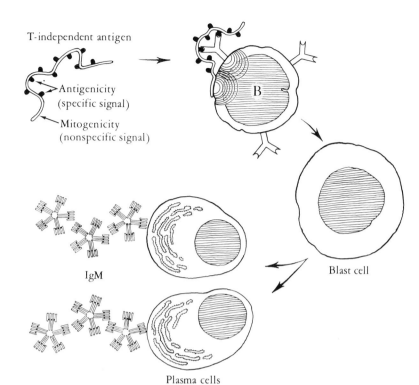

Figure 7–12. Schematic representation of a postulated mechanism for direct stimulation of B-cells by a T-independent antigen. Note that the molecule has the capacity to generate two signals.

The Lyt-1,2,3$^+$ cells are the earliest to appear in T-cell ontogeny and are greatly reduced in numbers in peripheral lymphoid tissue shortly after adult thymectomy. The Lyt-1$^+$ and Lyt-2,3$^+$ subsets appear in peripheral lymphoid tissue later, and their numbers are relatively unaffected by adult thymectomy. It is believed that the precursor of these T-cell subsets, designated as the TL$^+$ Lyt-1,2,3$^+$ cell, directly differentiates into the Lyt-1,2,3$^+$ cell with the loss of the TL antigen. It is also thought that the Lyt-1$^+$ and Lyt-2,3$^+$ cells arise from the Lyt-1,2,3$^+$ cell as two separate lines of differentiation rather than from sequential stages with one maturing into the other (Fig. 7–13).

Cytotoxic antisera have been used to selectively deplete lymphoid cell populations of specific Lyt-bearing cells in an attempt to define unique immunologic functions associated with these subpopulations. These studies revealed that the T-cell subsets were precommitted to serve a particular immunologic function during a process of thymus-dependent differentiation, which occurs before the cells encounter specific antigens. In other words, maturation of these cells is independent of antigen stimulation.

The Lyt-1$^+$ cell responds to immunogenic stimulation by proliferating and elaborating various factors (specific and nonspecific) that stimulate B-cells to differentiate into antibody-producing cells. Thus, the Lyt-1$^+$ cell is the carrier-specific T-cell in the hapten-carrier response and is the cell responsible for *T-cell helper function* (T$_H$). In addition, this T-cell subset also contains cells that help in the development of cytotoxic T-cells, which normally display the Lyt-2,3$^+$ phenotype as well as cells that function as effectors in delayed-type hypersensitivity responses. Thus, there is synergy between Lyt-1$^+$ and Lyt-2,3$^+$ T-cells in immune responses. The Lyt-2,3$^+$ population contains cells that manifest *T-cell suppressor function* (T$_S$) as well as cells that function as cytotoxic effectors involved in the destruction of tumor cells and transplanted allogeneic cells. Recent studies using the fluorescence-activated cell sorter have indicated that some Lyt-2,3$^+$ cells also bear the Lyt-1$^+$ marker, which could not be detected by conventional assays. The significance of this finding remains to be elucidated. The Lyt-1,2,3$^+$ cell appears to function as a precursor of

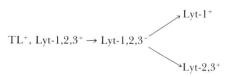

Figure 7–13. A proposed model of T-cell subset differentiation in the mouse.

both Lyt-1$^+$ and Lyt-2,3$^+$ cells as well as a cell that regulates the development of both T_H and T_S functional cell populations. This population functions as a precusor of killer cells that destroy virus-infected cells having altered self-antigens. In addition, these cells appear to interact with the Lyt-2,3$^+$ cells for other killer functions.

Further subdivision of the Lyt-1$^+$ and Lyt-2,3$^+$ subsets can be made on the basis of expression of MHC determinants. Some Lyt-1$^+$ cells also express markers coded by the Qa-1 region, while others lack these antigens. Similarly, some Lyt-2,3$^+$ T-cells also express I-J encoded markers, while others do not. The function of these cells will be discussed later in this chapter in the section on regulation of immune responses. Table 7–6 summarizes the properties of these murine T-cell subsets. As indicated previously, functional subpopulations of human T-cells have been defined by monoclonal antibodies. Table 7–7 outlines the similarities between human and mouse T-cell subsets with respect to their functional capabilities.

Genetic Control of Cell Cooperation

As indicated in Chapter 3, the immune response is subject to genetic influence at various levels, including that which encompasses cellular interactions. Such control can exist at the level of antigen presentation (macrophage), antigen recognition (T- and B-cells), and cell cooperation.

Advances in our understanding of the genetic control of cell cooperation were made possible by studies of the immune response of inbred animals, mainly mice and guinea pigs (Chapter 3). Specific responses to many antigens have been shown to be under the influence of autosomal dominant genes that are linked to the *major histocompatibility complex* (MHC), a multigenic system determining the structure and expression of a number of cell-surface glycoproteins. In the mouse, the H-2 is the major histocompatibility complex. Within the H-2 complex are two regions, *K and D,* which are approximately 0.5 centimorgan apart, a distance sufficient to include the genetic information for up to 2000 structural genes. The products of the K and D regions (called *Class I determinants*) are ubiquitously distributed cell-surface glycoproteins that appear to be in close association with β_2 microglobulin. These gene products are serologically defined antigens that elicit antibodies involved in graft rejection. The K and D gene products also appear to interact with cytopathogenic viruses, a process that has been shown to be necessary for recognition of virus-infected cells by cytotoxic T-cells. A new locus of undetermined function, called H-2L, has recently been described. This

Table 7–6. Characteristics of Lyt$^+$ Subsets of Mouse T-cells

Property	Lyt-1,2,3$^+$	Lyt-1$^+$	Lyt-2,3$^+$
Ontogeny	Early	Later	Later
Percent of T-cells in			
Periphery	60–65	30–35	5–10
Thymus	90	10	10
Helper activity for			
Antibody production	±	+	−
Generation of killer cells	±	+	−
DTH effector cell	±	+	−
Suppressor activity in			
Antibody production	±	−	+
Mixed-leukocyte reaction (MLC)	±	−	+
Regulator function			
Precursor	+	−	−
Amplifier	+	−	−
MHC reactivity			
I-region determinants	−	+	+
K/D region determinants	−	−	+
Killer potential	±	−	+
Cytotoxic effector	−	−	+

Table 7–7. T-Cell Subsets of Mice and Humans*

Human Marker	Mouse Marker	Function of Subsets
OKT 10,6,4,5† Leu-1	Lyt-1,2,3	$T_{regulator}$ $T_{precursor}$
OKT 4 Leu-3a,3b	Lyt-1	T_{helper} T_{DTH}
OKT 5/8 Leu-2a,2b	Lyt-2,3	$T_{suppressor}$ $T_{cytotoxic}$

*The Leu series of monoclonal antibodies is a trademark of Becton Dickinson Company, Sunnyvale, California. The OK series of monoclonal antibodies is the trademark of Ortho Pharmaceutical Corporation, Raritan, New Jersey.

†To date, no monoclonal antibody has been produced that is specific for this population of cells. However, the OKT 10,6,4,5 cell represents a cell that is found in the thymus but not in the peripheral lymphoid compartment, whereas the Leu-1 and Lyt-1,2,3 cells are found in the periphery as well as in the thymus.

locus lies close to, but is independent of, the H-2D locus. The murine K and D loci are equivalent to human B, C, and A loci (see Figs. 3–3 and 3–6).

Genetic markers have been identified between the K and D regions. The *S locus* contains structural genes coding for the synthesis of complement components (C3 and C4). An analogous region, coding for the second and fourth components of complement and the properdin factor B (BF) of the alternative pathway (Chapter 6) has been described in the human MHC.

Located between the K and S regions of the mouse MHC is the *I-region,* which controls immune responses to a large number of antigens and codes for cell surface glycoproteins (called *Class II determinants*) important in mediating cellular interactions. The I-region has been further divided into several subregions: I-A, I-B, I-J, I-E, and I-C. There are some questions about the existence of some of these regions. For example, it has been shown that some I-region functions can be explained by cooperation between I-A and I-E products on interacting cells. Whether I-B, I-C, and even I-J, which has been reported to be associated with certain T-cell subsets, actually exist is currently being evaluated. As with the K, D, and S regions, the human MHC possesses a region analogous to the murine I-region. This region is found close to the HLA-D locus and is referred to as the *D-related* (DR) locus. In addition to D and DR, several other yet incompletely defined loci have been detected in this region of the human MHC. These include DC, MB, and

SB. The products of the DR and SB loci appear to be analogous to the products of the murine I-E subregion, while the product of the human MB locus resembles that of the mouse I-A subregion.

The gene product of the I-region, referred to as *I-region–associated* or *Ia determinant (antigen),* plays an important role in antigen recognition by T-cells and in the interactions among macrophages, T-cells, and B-cells. These determinants have been defined by antibodies obtained by cross immunization between recombinant mice that differ in the I-region. Of the more than 20 Ia specificities currently recognized, the majority have been localized in the I-A subregion, with others having been identified in the I-E subregion. Some Ia specificities have also been described in the I-B and I-J subregions; the latter are thought to code for determinants present on suppressor T-cells. In contrast to K and D determinants, Ia determinants have a restricted distribution. They are found on B-cells, on some macrophages, and on certain T-cell subsets as well as on spermatozoa and epidermal Langerhans cells. It is now well documented that Ia determinants participate in the presentation of antigen by macrophages, since anti-Ia antibodies block the generation of T-helper cell activity. Ia determinants have been detected on both antigen-specific and nonspecific factors released by T-cells and macrophages. Ia determinants can be detected on killer T-cells, mitogen-responsive T-cells, MLR-stimulator T-cells, helper T-cells, and suppressor T-cells. It is likely that the Ia determinant represents the product of the postulated *cell interaction (CI) genes* located within the MHC that mediates cellular interactions.

The murine I-region also contains the so-called immune response genes (*Ir genes*) that appear to control the ability of an individual to respond to a specific antigen as well as the magnitude of the response to that antigen. These genes have been mapped primarily in the I-A subregion. A small number of Ir genes that appear to require complementation are found in both the I-A and the I-E subregions; their presence in the I-B subregion is not definitively established. Specific Ir genes have been delineated by measuring immune responses to structurally defined immunogens (Chapter 3). For example, the immune response to the synthetic branched copolymer of tyrosine, glutamic acid, alanine, and lysine, called (T,G)-A-L, has been shown to be under genetic control. Mice of the

C57Bl strain (responder) produce high titers of both IgM and IgG antibody to this T-dependent antigen. Mice of the CBA strain (nonresponder) produce a normal IgM primary response but do not produce IgG antibodies in the primary or secondary response. Thymectomized mice of responder strains react like nonresponders, suggesting that the product of the Ir gene is associated with the T-cell, since these cells appear to be needed for IgG production.

Additional information has been obtained from studies of the immune response of guinea pigs to poly-L-lysine (PLL). Inbred strain 2 guinea pigs (responder) respond well to DNP-PLL, giving high antibody titers to the haptenic (DNP) portion with cell-mediated hypersensitivity and helper activity to the PLL portion. Strain 13 animals (nonresponder) do not give the aforementioned responses. As with F_1 generations of responder × nonresponder mice, F_1 hybrids of strain 2 × strain 13 guinea pigs are all responders, as are about 50 per cent of the progeny of the backcross of hybrids to low-responder strains. Both nonresponder mouse and guinea pig strains will make anti-hapten responses like that of responder strains if the hapten is administered as a complex with an immunogenic carrier such as BSA (e.g., DNP-PLL-BSA or (T,G)-A-L-BSA). These findings suggest that the Ir gene product is concerned with the recognition of the carrier portion of the immunogen, a function normally ascribed to T-cells.

Although there are some studies that suggest that Ir gene control is also expressed at the level of the B-cell, the most convincing evidence points to the macrophage as the cell most intimately involved in I-region regulation of immune responsiveness. In an elegant series of experiments, Rosenthal and Shevach demonstrated that it was the I-region determinants on the macrophage, not the T-cell, that controlled the ability of lymphocytes to proliferate in response to *in vitro* stimulation by antigen. They immunized (2×13) F_1 guinea pigs simultaneously with DNP-GL (to which strain 2 responds, but strain 13 does not) and GT (to which strain 13 responds, but strain 2 does not). These antigens were then presented to lymphocytes from immunized guinea pigs either in their soluble form or in association with macrophages from strains 2,13 or (2×13) F_1 of normal animals (Table 7–8). Lymphocytes from (2×13) F_1 animals responded to both DNP-GL and GT when presented alone or by (2×13) F_1 macrophages. In a similar manner, strain 2 lymphocytes (responder to DNP-GL) or strain 13 lymphocytes (responder to GT) proliferated only when the antigen to which they normally respond was presented on strain 2 or strain 13 macrophages, respectively. No response was observed when DNP-GL was presented to (2×13) F_1 lymphocytes by strain 13 macrophages (nonresponder to DNP-GL) or when GT was presented by strain 2 macrophages (nonresponder to GT). On the other hand, proliferation of (2×13) F_1 lymphocytes occurred when DNP-GL was presented on strain 2 macrophages (responder for DNP-GL) and GT was presented on strain 13 macrophages (responder for GT). These results demonstrate that macrophages that present antigens to T-cells must share the same I-region determinants expressed by T-cells. In a manner similar to that described

Table 7–8. Regulation of T-Lymphocyte Proliferation by I-Region Determinants on Macrophages

Source of Sensitized T-Lymphocytes*	Antigen Used for In Vitro Challenge	Source of Macrophage for Antigen Presentation	Proliferative Response (DNA Synthesis)
Strain 2 (Responder)	DNP-GL	Strain 2 (Responder)	+ + +
		Strain 13 (Nonresponder)	−
Strain 13 (Responder)	GT	Strain 2 (Nonresponder)	−
		Strain 13 (Responder)	+ + +
(2×13) F_1	DNP-GL	(2×13) F_1	+ + +
		Strain 2	+ + +
		Strain 13	−
(2×13) F_1	GT	(2×13) F_1	+ + +
		Strain 2	−
		Strain 13	+ + +

*Animals were immunized simultaneously with DNP-GL and GT. (After Rosenthal and Shevach.)

for antigen-induced activation of helper T-cells described above, shared MHC determinants on macrophages are also required for the activation of killer T-cells involved in removal of virus-infected cells as well as allogeneic and tumor target cells and effector T-cells involved in delayed-type hypersensitivity responses. Whereas H-2K and H-2D determinants are involved in the activation of killer T-cells (Chapters 3 and 9), I-region determinants in the form of the Ia antigen participate in activation of helper T-cells and effector T-cells of DTH. Two models have been proposed in an attempt to explain the complex nature of the T-cell recognition unit (see Fig. 3–4). The *dual receptor* model suggests that T-cells either have two separate receptors or that the receptor consists of two distinct regions—one that recognizes antigen and the other that recognizes self-MHC determinants (either H2-K and H-2D or I-region). The second model, referred to as *altered-self*, suggests that the T-cell receptor is a single unit that recognizes a complex determinant generated by an interaction between antigen and MHC molecules. Both of these models indicate that T-cells cannot be activated by interacting with either antigen or self-MHC determinants alone. The ability of T-cells to recognize self-MHC determinants is acquired in the thymus during differentiation rather than being determined by the cell's own H-2 haplotype.

MODELS OF ANTIBODY FORMATION

The immune response to T-dependent antigens requires the activity of Ia-bearing accessory cells (represented by macrophages, dendritic cells, and epidermal Langerhans cells). Figure 7–14 depicts the postulated cellular events involved in T-cell activation. As indicated in the previous section, the initial stage of T-cell activation occurs as a consequence of the recognition of processed antigen in association with self-MHC (Ia) determinants. Possibly, as a result of surface changes due to ligand binding, the macrophages are stimulated to synthesize and secrete interleukin-1 (IL-1). This soluble mediator appears to provide a second signal that exerts its effect both by stimulating an increase in the number of receptors on the T-cell for a second distinct interleukin, called IL-2, and also by inducing the synthesis of

IL-2 by the T-cells. Whether the T-cells that synthesize IL-2 are the same as those that react with it is not clear at this time. As a consequence of IL-2 stimulation, full activation of T-cells is achieved. In addition to their ability to cooperate with other cell types for further expression of the immune response, activated T-cells release products that increase the reactivity of macrophages. Soluble materials released by activated T-cells appear to augment the density of Ia determinants expressed on the surface of macrophages, thereby augmenting the antigen-presenting capabilities of these cells.

In addition to the activation of T-cells resulting from direct cellular contact between histocompatible macrophages and T-cells, helper cells can be generated by soluble factors produced by macrophages. Two of these factors, designated genetically related factor (GRF) and nonspecific macrophage factor (NMF), have been described. GRF is released from macrophages only after they have been incubated with soluble antigen. The macrophages that release this factor share I-region determinants (I-A) with responding lymphocytes. GRF is a heat-labile protein with a molecular weight of 55,000 to 60,000 whose biologic activity cannot be absorbed with anti-immunoglobulin, but can be with anti-Ia antibody. This factor was shown to contain Ia determinants linked to a small antigenic fragment. The nonspecific factor, NMF, was shown to be released from normal macrophages. It activated T-helper cells only when the T-cells were obtained from animals immunized with particulate antigens. This factor is not I-region–restricted. Thus, T-cell activation has a twofold requirement: (1) the recognition of antigen in association with Ia determinants on the surface of accessory cells, and (2) the release of biologically active factors from accessory cells, which then act on T-cells.

Just as two signals seem to be needed for the activation of T-cells, two signals have been shown to be required for triggering of the B-cell differentiation process that leads to antibody synthesis. As indicated previously, one of these signals involves the recognition of antigen by immunoglobulin receptors on B-cells. The second signal, which is incompletely defined, appears to be mediated by helper T-cells, which induce proliferation in B-cells, probably through a soluble factor (e.g., B-cell activating factor). Several models have been proposed to explain the

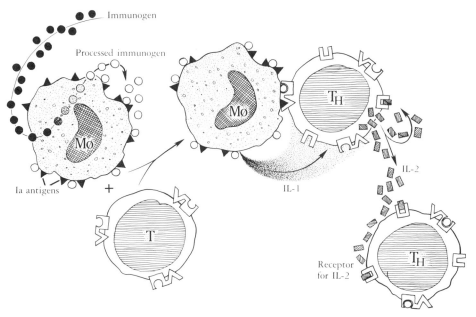

Figure 7–14. Schematic representation of the cellular events involved in T-cell activation.

interactions between helper T-cells and B-cells.

The *antigen-focusing hypothesis,* based on the carrier effect (see p. 123), suggests that there is simultaneous binding of complex antigens by T- and B-cells. In this model, the T-cell presents a polyvalent pattern of haptenic determinants whose critical function is the cross-linking of hapten-specific Ig receptors on the surface of B-cells. Evidence derived from *in vitro* experiments involving cellular interactions has cast doubt on the foregoing hypothesis, which relegates the T-cell to an essentially passive role. These experiments have demonstrated that cooperation between B- and T-cells can occur even when the two cell populations are separated by a membrane that is impermeable to the cells, and suggest that helper T-cells operate through soluble factors.

Two classes of soluble factors produced by T-cells have been shown to influence the activity of B-cells. The first of these factors is nonspecific (produced by T-cells in response to nonspecific stimuli) and can be generated in several ways. These factors have been used to replace the requirement for a carrier in anti-hapten secondary responses. One such factor has been produced by injection of allogeneic lymphoid cells into an animal primed with a hapten-carrier complex. For example, if animals primed with DNP-BSA are injected with allogeneic lymphoid cells from a donor whose cells will attack the host's

cells in a graft-versus-host reaction, and if at a later time they receive a second injection of DNP coupled to a non–cross-reacting carrier such as OA, then a secondary anti-DNP response can be elicited in the absence of OA-primed T-cells. The factor responsible for this so-called *allogeneic effect* is referred to as the *allogeneic effect factor* (AEF). The active factor appears to be a bimolecular complex consisting of 35,000 and 12,000 dalton subunits. The AEF contains determinants coded for by genes of the major histocompatibility complex of the mouse, since its activity can be removed by absorption with antisera prepared against the product of these genes, specifically anti-Ia. Similar nonspecific factors can be prepared from supernatant fluids of short-term cultures of histoincompatible mouse spleen cells that have participated in an *in vitro* mixed leukocyte reaction or from supernatant fluids of cells stimulated *in vitro* with T-cell mitogens such as Con-A or PHA. Together with the hapten-specific signal, these nonspecific factors are thought to function as a second signal in triggering the activation of B-cells.

T-cells have also been shown to elaborate antigen-specific factors, which cooperate with B-cells in immune responses. One such factor, produced by T-cells, was called "IgT" because it was initially thought to be a monomeric (8S) IgM molecule. This factor has the capacity to bind the specific antigen used to activate the T-cells and also has the ability to bind to the membrane of macrophages, probably through an Fc receptor. Using *in vitro* systems in which B- and T-cells were separated by a membrane permeable only by molecules, it was shown that upon stimulation with antigen, the T-cells release a factor that is complexed with antigen that can diffuse across the membrane and become associated with macrophages. The macrophage-bound antigen-"IgT" complex induces B-cells to respond specifically to the hapten determinants present on the molecule. Subsequent studies have shown that this factor, as well as other antigen-specific factors, are produced by Lyt-1^+ T-cells and that such factors carry Ia determinants coded for by the I-A subregion.

It has also been shown that (T,G)-A-L—activated spleen cells release an antigen-specific factor after *in vitro* challenge with the same material. This factor replaces the specific T-cell helper function and reacts with antisera prepared against molecules specified by genes located on the left side of the H-2 complex, specifically the I-A region. It has been demonstrated that both responder and nonresponder T-cells produce this "antigen recognition" factor. On the other hand, this factor, whether derived from responder or nonresponder animals, will cooperate effectively only with B-cells from responder animals. It has been suggested that B-cells carry an "acceptor" site for T-cell factors. Thus, a genetic defect that gives rise to a nonresponder animal may also be found at the level of the "acceptor" site (B-cell). In examining several strains for their ability to produce the "antigen-recognition" factor (T-cell) or the "acceptor" site (B-cell), investigators have found strains that are defective in T-cell factor, B-cell "acceptor," or both. These results suggest that two I-region genes are involved in the control of the response to (T,G)-A-L. One, expressed in T-cells, codes for an "antigen recognition" factor and is coupled to an "interaction" factor; the other, expressed in B-cells, codes for the "acceptor" site. It is the "interaction" factor that reacts with the B-cell "acceptor" site and thus facilitates cell cooperation.

Utilizing the foregoing information, it is possible to present a hypothetical model of antibody formation that illustrates potential interactions among T-cells, B-cells, and macrophages (Fig. 7–15). While it is clear that the immunogen plays an important role in selecting the specific receptor (idiotype)-bearing B- and T-cells that cooperate for antibody

production, it is also well accepted that these cellular interactions are under the control of genes coded for by the MHC. This model is based on *in vitro* events and may be subject to complete revision as new information arises and ideas and concepts change in this rapidly moving area of immunobiology.

In this model, the initial event most likely involves the interaction of the immunogen with an accessory cell (e.g., macrophage) in a nonspecific manner, leading to the processing of this material into an immunogenic form that is expressed on the macrophage surface. In the case of T-dependent antigens, the first specific recognition event involving carrier determinants occurs at the level of the T-cell and is mediated by the incompletely defined T-cell receptor, which recognizes the antigen in the context of self-MHC determinants on the macrophage surface. Full activation of T-cells in some systems involves the activity of a soluble factor produced by the accessory cell (interleukin-1), which stimulates the production and release of a second factor, interleukin-2 (also called T-cell growth factor [TCGF]), by the T-cell (Fig. 7–14). Additional antigen-specific factors that carry Ia determinants (e.g., GRF, described above) and are produced by macrophages have also been shown to be involved in T-cell activation. Alternatively, there is also some experimental evidence that helper T-cells can be activated as a consequence of the direct interaction of antigen with T-cell receptors. However, this appears to be unlikely, since current thinking suggests that those antigens that bypass the initial event of interacting with an accessory cell and react directly with the T-cell induce a population of suppressor T-cells rather than helper T-cells (see discussion on regulation later in this chapter).

Once activated, helper T-cells or their factors can cooperate with B-cells by one or more of several possible mechanisms. According to one mechanism, B-cell triggering involves the direct interaction of activated T-cells with B-cells possessing specific Ig receptors. In this case, there is some evidence to indicate that the cooperating cells must also share MHC-coded surface determinants in order for optimal interaction to occur. For reasons indicated earlier in this chapter, this does not appear to be the favored mechanism. The remainder of the mechanisms to be described involve soluble factors produced by activated helper T-cells. In the first of these, the activated T-cell has been reported

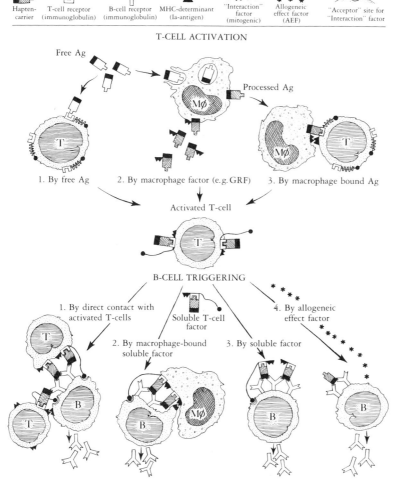

Figure 7–15. Schematic representation of cellular interactions involved in the generation of the humoral immune responses. Note that T-cells can be activated in three ways: (1) by free antigen (Ag); (2) by macrophage-processed antigen; or (3) by macrophage-associated antigen. In turn, B-cells may be triggered to produce antibody in four ways: (1) by direct contact with Ag-bearing activated T-cells; (2) by macrophage-bound factor; (3) by a soluble Ag-specific T-cell factor; or (4) by a nonspecific (allogeneic effect) factor produced by T-cells.

to release its receptor ("IgT")-containing antigen, which then becomes associated with the surface of a macrophage, possibly through Fc receptors. As a consequence of this binding, a lattice of repeating similar antigenic determinants, resembling that found on T-independent antigens, is thought to be created. Thus, both types of antigens can be visualized as being presented to B-cells in an analogous manner. While this hypothesis is attractive, it remains unproved.

An additional antigen-specific factor has been shown to contain MHC-coded determinants, specifically Ia. At present, it is not clear whether the B-cell and macrophage must share I-region determinants for efficient cooperation to occur. This mechanism of cell communication is also not favored in view of the fact that it requires a direct interaction between antigen and T-cell as the initial event, instead of the more widely held view that antigen first interacts with macro-

phages. An additional mechanism suggests that the activated helper T-cell can release an immunologically active substance containing an "interaction" factor that bears I-region determinants (Ia) and represents the mitogenic signal provided by the T-cell. This soluble material can react with a B-cell that carries both an antigen-specific Ig receptor and an "acceptor" site (which also may be coded for by an I-region gene) for the T-cell "interaction" factor. Since there is no direct contact between T- and B-cells, there may not be a requirement for the sharing of common MHC gene products. Indeed, efficient cooperation between soluble T-cell factors and B-cells has been achieved with various combinations of allogeneic cells. For example, the *allogeneic effect factor* described earlier is capable of providing the second signal to antigen-stimulated B-cells in certain experimental systems.

In each of the mechanisms described

above, the precommitted B-cell recognizes the appropriate antigenic determinants (hapten) through its surface Ig receptors, providing the antigen-specific signal. The non–antigenic-specific or mitogenic signal is provided by the activated helper T-cell or its product(s). The activated B-cell then goes through a series of events involving its differentiation into a plasma cell, accompanied by the proliferation of a clone of antibody-secreting cells. Our understanding of Ir genes, their control of complex cellular interactions in the immune response, and their relationship to the antigenic makeup of the individual is in a very early stage. This area of immunology is destined to have a strong impact on our understanding of disease processes.

REGULATION OF ANTIBODY FORMATION

It soon becomes apparent that there must be some regulatory mechanism(s) operating to control antibody formation. If this did not occur, antigen stimulation might lead to proliferation of antibody-forming cells comparable to that seen in neoplasia. Several potential mechanisms are described below.

Antigenic Competition

Simultaneous or close administration of two unrelated immunogens in some cases results in the transient and nonspecific suppression of the immune response to one of the antigens and a normal response to the other. This phenomenon, called *antigenic competition,* is defined as the inhibition of the immune response to one antigen or determinant as a consequence of the administration of another antigen or determinant. Competition between two separate antigens is called *intermolecular* antigenic competition, while that which occurs between antigenic determinants on the same molecule is called *intramolecular* antigenic competition. The maximum suppressive effect is observed when the second antigen is administered a few days after the first one. If the second antigen is given after a booster injection of the first one, competition is more apparent. The mechanism involved in antigenic competition is not known. Several possible explanations have been advanced, including (1)

activation of suppressor T-cells; (2) interference with the ability of macrophages to present antigen to lymphocytes owing to saturation of essential cooperating sites on the macrophage surface; (3) competition for nutrients; or (4) release of soluble suppressor factors.

Antigenic competition is of both theoretical and practical importance. For the immunologist, it is important to understand the mechanism by which two unrelated immunogens interfere with each other. This is difficult to understand if we accept the premise of the clonal selection theory, which states that antigen-sensitive cells are precommitted to produce antibody of one specificity. This phenomenon has been used as a major argument for multipotentiality of antigen-sensitive cells. For the clinician, antigenic competition has practical significance when vaccination programs are considered. For example, if appropriate dose adjustments of diphtheria and tetanus toxoids are not made in the DPT vaccine given to children, antigenic competition might occur. The clinician must also consider the immunosuppressive effects of this phenomenon in relation to disease processes. For example, in murine systems it has been shown that infection with leukemia viruses results in an immunosuppressed animal. Similarly, certain virus infections in humans (e.g., measles) can result in an immunosuppressed host.

Passive Antibody

It has been shown that the administration of preformed antibody can interfere with the host's ability to produce its own antibody in response to immunogenic stimulation. This suppressive effect can be achieved by injection of antibodies directed against different targets. For example, administration of anti-SRBC antibody (anti-immunogen) at the same time or soon after injection of SRBC results in suppression of anti-SRBC antibody formation in mice. This suppression is antigen-specific and most pronounced when the anti-immunogen antibody is given in relative excess. Antibodies of the IgG class are more effective at inducing suppression than are IgM antibodies, as are high-affinity antibodies compared with low-affinity antibodies. This phenomenon does not occur when passive antibody is given to previously immunized animals; thus, it does not appear to affect immunologic memory.

The clinician has made use of this phenomenon in the prevention of severe hemolytic disease of the newborn due to Rh incompatibility. Preformed antibody prepared against Rh^+ red blood cells is injected into Rh^- mothers at the time of delivery of Rh^+ babies. This antibody binds to and enhances the elimination of Rh^+ red blood cells that enter the maternal circulation as the placenta separates. This procedure prevents the immunization of the mother, who, if untreated, would produce a secondary IgG response to Rh^+ red blood cells in a subsequent Rh-incompatible pregnancy. These IgG antibodies are capable of crossing the placenta and could result in the destruction of fetal red blood cells. In addition to the desirable immunosuppressive effect of passive antibody described above, the clinician must be aware of undesirable effects that may occur naturally. For example, the placental transfer of maternal antibody against certain viruses (e.g., polio and measles) could interfere with the initiation of an active immune response against these agents in the young child. Therefore, the clinician must adjust the immunization timetable to allow for the disappearance of maternal antibody if successful active immunization is to be achieved. Although the mechanism of action of this feedback effect is not clear, it has been suggested that passive antibody acts by blocking antigenic determinants so that the appropriate antigen-sensitive cells cannot be stimulated.

As with passive administration of anti-immunogen antibody, injection of antibodies against the antigen-binding surface receptors on B- or T-cells also results in suppression of antibody formation. This type of suppression can be achieved using anti-receptor antibodies of various specificities. For example, injection of newborn animals with antibodies against the μ chain of IgM results in the loss of ability of the maturing animal to synthesize not only IgM but also IgG and IgA immunoglobulins. Passive transfer of anti-γ or anti-α antibodies interferes with the production of only IgG or IgA, respectively. This phenomenon, called *isotype suppression*, does not occur in adults and lends credence to the hypothesis that B-cells expressing IgM on their surface are precursors of cells that secrete other classes of immunoglobulin later in life.

Injection of newborn animals with antibody prepared against allotypic markers on paternal immunoglobulin molecules results in suppression of the appearance of Ig molecules bearing the paternal allotype. Normal Ig levels are maintained because of an overproduction of molecules bearing the maternal allotype. This phenomenon, called *allotype suppression*, usually lasts for several months even after the natural catabolic decay of the passively transferred Ig has occurred. This suggests that suppression is due to an active process. T-cells have been implicated in this phenomenon, since the cells responsible for suppression can be eliminated by treatment with anti-Thy-1 plus complement. Although the mechanism remains unclear, it has been suggested that suppressor T-cells exert their effect on helper T-cells rather than directly on the antibody-forming B-cell.

A third type of anti-receptor antibody can also suppress antibody formation. In this case, administration of antibodies against idiotypic determinants can suppress the production of immunoglobulins that bear that particular idiotype. This inhibition, referred to as *idiotype suppression*, can be of two types. One results from administration of high doses of anti-idiotypic antibody, causing immediate but transient suppression. A second type, resulting from low doses of anti-idiotypic antibody is characterized by delayed but chronic suppression. This type of suppression appears to play a major role in the regulation of antibody formation.

In 1974, Jerne proposed his *network hypothesis* in an attempt to explain the complex interactions that regulate antibody formation. He suggested that the immune system is self-regulating and is composed of a network of idiotypes and anti-idiotypic antibodies. According to this hypothesis, an antigen elicits the production of an antibody (Ab_1) that possesses a unique sequence of amino acids, called the idiotype (Id_1), in its antigen-binding region, which distinguishes it from other antibodies. The unique sequence displayed by Id_1 can also function as an immunogen in the same host (since this new array of amino acids is not recognized as self) and stimulates the production of another antibody (Ab_2) that has anti-idiotypic specificity for Ab_1 and at the same time displays its unique idiotype (Id_2). In a similar manner, Ab_2 will stimulate the production of Ab_3, which has its unique sequence (Id_3) and which displays anti–anti-idiotypic antibody activity against Ab_2, and so on, such that each idiotype that is expressed will stimulate the production of a corresponding anti-idiotypic antibody. From previous discussion it should be recalled that both B- and T-cells, as well as their soluble products (e.g., antibody, T-cell suppressor and helper factors) display idiotypic determinants. Further, inherent in the clonal selection theory is the fact that the idiotype of the Ig secreted by a B-cell is the same as its surface Ig receptor for antigen. In other words, each clone of B- or T-cells possesses a receptor capable of recognizing not only a specific antigenic determinant but also an idiotype expressed by the receptor on another clone of B- or T-cells. Figure 7–16 schematically presents the idiotype–anti-idi-

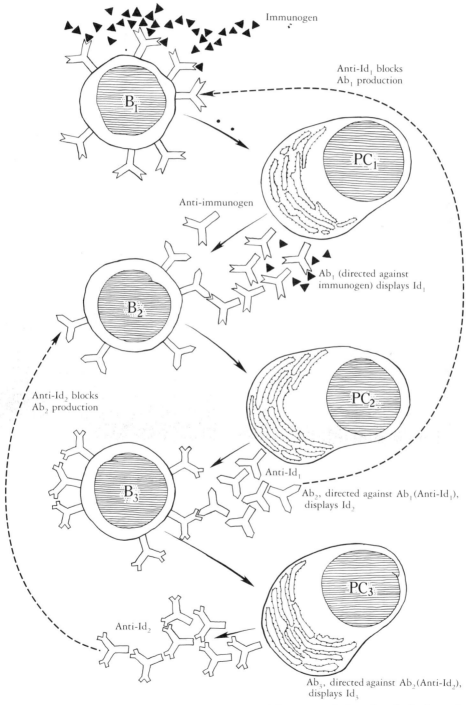

Figure 7–16. Schematic representation of idiotype–anti-idiotype regulation of antibody formation.

otype network operative in B-cells. In this scheme, the immunogen stimulates the first cell to produce its antibody (Ab_1). This antibody then stimulates another clone of B-cells, which has specific receptors for Id_1 of Ab_1, to make large amounts of Ab_2, which can suppress production of Ab_1 by a mechanism involving *idiotypic suppression*. The presence of Ab_2 can lead to the formation of Ab_3, which recognizes Id_2 and suppresses the formation of Ab_2, thereby terminating the suppression of Ab_2 on Ab_1 production. It should be noted that the network can also involve T-cells, whereby helper or suppressor T-cells can express idiotypes identical to those displayed on antibody molecules. Perturbation of this network, initiated by exposure to antigen, results in interaction between idiotypes, anti-idiotypes, and anti–anti-idiotypes that either turn on or turn off antibody formation through the activities of the various subsets of immunoregulatory T-cells.

Regulatory T-Cells

It has been amply demonstrated that in addition to the helper function provided by T-cells, the presence of this class of lymphocytes can also result in a reduction in the magnitude of the normal immune response or the level of immunoglobulin synthesis. The concept of a suppressor T-cell population was initially derived from studies involving the transfer of normal or immune cells to tolerant (Chapter 10) hosts and of tolerant cells to normal irradiated hosts. It was found that, as a result of the encounter of antigen with T-cells during the induction of tolerance, B-cells were "turned off" and could no longer cooperate with normal syngeneic T-cells to induce an immune response. This phenomenon is termed *infectious tolerance* and suggests a role for *suppressor T-cells* in the induction of tolerance.

Additional support for the presence of a population of suppressor T-cells can be summarized as follows: (1) In the immune response to T-independent antigens, removal of the thymus or treatment with anti-lymphocyte serum results in enhanced antibody formation; (2) T-cells from animals displaying chronic allotype suppression will cause allotype suppression by normal cells either *in vitro* or when passively transferred *in vivo*; (3) T-cells stimulated nonspecifically by mi-

togens (e.g., Con-A) suppress *in vitro* immune responses; (4) on the basis of studies of the hapten-specific IgE response, it appears that T-cells determine the class of immunoglobulin produced following antigenic stimulation; and (5) genetically defined nonresponder strains of animals appear to possess this characteristic owing to the presence of cells capable of suppressing immune responses to specific antigens.

It has been shown that suppression can be mediated by soluble factors that are either extracted from or released by T-cells. One such suppressor factor is involved in the regulation of the response to KLH in mice. This factor displays carrier-specific suppressor activity for IgG antibody production and appears to be under genetic control of the I-J subregion of the MHC. The target of this factor appears to be the carrier-primed helper T-cell rather than the hapten-primed B-cell. This observation indicates that interaction among T-cell subsets is responsible for the suppression of antibody formation. Further information regarding the nature of soluble regulatory factors produced by T-cells is expected in the near future in view of the development of techniques that enable T-cells to be immortalized as hybridomas in much the same way as B-cells have been for the production of monoclonal antibodies.

As indicated earlier in this chapter, it has been possible to further differentiate Lyt-bearing subsets of T-cells on the basis of their expression of MHC-associated determinants. For example, it has been shown that while interaction between both $Lyt\text{-}1^+$, $Qa\text{-}1^+$ and $Lyt\text{-}1^+$, $Qa\text{-}1^-$ T-cells is required for generation of helper activity for antibody production by B-cells, the $Lyt\text{-}1^+$, $Qa\text{-}1^+$ subset is also involved in a *feedback regulatory loop* that generates active suppression by the $Lyt\text{-}2,3^+$ subset of T-cells. Mobilization of the $Lyt\text{-}2,3^+$ suppressor subset occurs as a consequence of a signal transmitted by the $Lyt\text{-}1^+$, $Qa\text{-}1^+$ *inducer T-cell* to the $Lyt\text{-}1,2,3^+$ *regulator T-cell*, which, in turn, generates suppressor function in the $Lyt\text{-}2,3^+$ cells. Thus, two subsets of $Lyt\text{-}1^+$–bearing T-cells can be identified, one that is $Qa\text{-}1^-$ and is called a *helper-effector*, and a second that is $Qa\text{-}1^+$ and is called a *helper/suppressor-inducer*. Subpopulations of the $Lyt\text{-}2,3^+$ T-cell subset have also been delineated on the basis of their expression of I-J subregion products. While $Lyt\text{-}2,3^+$, $I\text{-}J^-$ cells function as *suppressor-effectors*, the $Lyt\text{-}2,3^+$, $I\text{-}J^+$ T-cells appear to transmit a signal, also through the Lyt-1,2,3$^+$ regulator T-cell, for a second feedback regulatory loop that turns off suppressor activity mediated by the Lyt-2,3$^+$, I-J$^-$ effector cells. This regulatory loop has been called *contrasuppression*, and the Lyt-2,3$^+$, I-J$^+$ T-cell that stimulates this loop is referred to as a *contrasuppressor-inducer*.

Figure 7–17 is a schematic representation of the proposed cellular interactions that might occur among the already recognized subsets of regulatory T-cells. Presentation of the immunogen on macrophages results in the activation of Lyt-1$^+$, Qa-1$^-$, I-J$^-$ (helper-effector T-cell) and Lyt-1$^+$, Qa-1$^+$, I-J$^+$ (inducer T-cell), which cooperate with B-cells to initiate antibody formation (Pathway 1). At the same time, the Lyt-1$^+$, Qa-1$^+$, I-J$^+$ (helper/suppressor-inducer T-cell) population is activated to stimulate Lyt-1,2,3$^+$, Qa-1$^+$, I-J$^+$ (regulator) T-cells, which influence the Lyt-2,3$^+$, Qa-1$^-$, I-J$^-$ (suppressor-effector) T-cells to exert their regulatory effect (Pathway 2). As mentioned previously, it is currently thought that the suppressive effects mediated by the Lyt-2,3$^+$, Qa-1$^-$, I-J$^-$ T-cells are manifest at the level of the helper-effector T-cells (Lyt-1$^+$, Qa-1$^-$, I-J$^-$), rather than by direct action on B-cells. In situations in which the immunogen appears to bypass interaction with macrophages (e.g., high anti-

gen dose), Lyt-2,3$^+$, Qa-1$^-$, I-J$^-$ (suppressor-effector T-cells) can be directly activated by antigen (Pathway 3). These cells also exert their suppressive effects at the level of the helper-effector T-cell. Finally, the contrasuppression circuit (Pathway 4), initiated by the activation of Lyt-2,3$^+$, Qa-1$^+$, I-J$^+$ T-cells, has a dual regulatory effect in that it appears to interfere with the suppressive activities of the Lyt-2,3$^+$, Qa-1$^-$, I-J$^-$ (suppressor-effectors) as well as to render the Lyt-1$^+$, Qa-1$^-$, I-J$^-$ (helper-effector) resistant to the activity of the suppressor-effector (Lyt-2,3$^+$, Qa-1$^-$, I-J$^-$) cells. This pathway also is thought to occur through the Lyt-1,2,3$^+$ regulator cell. Recently, it was demonstrated that similar T-T interactions are required for the generation of human suppressor-cell activity. In this system, cooperation between OKT4$^+$ and OKT5/8$^+$ T-cells was required for suppression to be exerted in an antigen-specific primary immune response.

The importance of regulatory T-cells is being recognized in clinical medicine. It has been shown that certain patients with common variable immunodeficiency (CVI) appear to have an increase in suppressor cell activity. This has been shown by the inhibition of immunoglobulin synthesis by normal cultured cells after the addition of lympho-

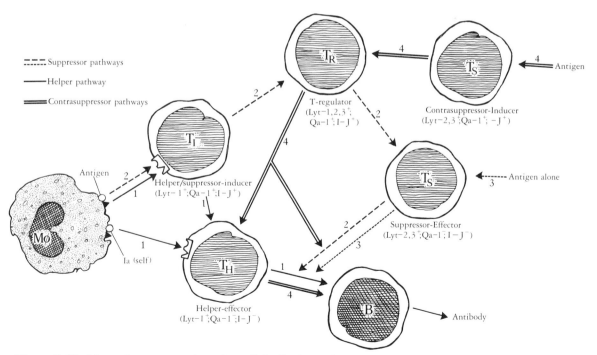

Figure 7–17. Schematic representation of T-cell feedback regulatory circuits involved in the control of antibody formation. (After Gershon and Cantor.)

cytes from CVI patients. Recently, a great deal of attention has been focused on gaining an understanding of the pathogenesis of acquired immunodeficiency syndrome (AIDS). Immunologic studies of several patients reveal a primary T-cell defect as indicated by a reduction in the absolute number of T-helper cells and depressed T-helper/T-suppressor cell ratios. Whether these immunologic aberrations are the cause or the effect of this newly described disease remains to be determined.

It has also been suggested that there is an enhancement of suppressor cell function in patients with multiple myeloma. The normal polyclonal response of the myeloma patient may be suppressed by these cells, resulting in an increased susceptibility to infection. Further, there is evidence to indicate that suppressor cells are closely involved in the control of autoimmune disease. It is thought that with advancing age there is a decrease in number or function of suppressor T-cells that allows for the expression of autoimmune disease. A similar argument has been advanced to explain the higher incidence of cancer in aging patients.

Thus, the reader can appreciate that a delicate balance exists between help and suppression, which serves to regulate the immune response.

THEORIES OF ANTIBODY FORMATION

The observation that an animal can produce antibody molecules not only against pathogenic microorganisms but also against foreign proteins and synthetic configurations has led to many speculations regarding the mechanism of antibody formation. The theories proposed fall into two categories that are based on the action of the immunogen, which can be either *selective* or *instructive* in the process of antibody formation.

In 1900, in what we would consider the Dark Ages of immunology, before the nature of the antibody molecule was known, before the nature of the reactions between antigen and antibody was known, before the nature of the cells that made antibody was known, Ehrlich proposed a theory of antibody formation that was remarkably similar to currently accepted ideas (see Fig. 1–11). He proposed that all cells of the body possess side chains on their surface, termed hapto-

phores (antibody), that function as receptors for metabolites, termed toxophores (antigens). As a result of the reaction between the metabolite and the receptor, the receptor is consumed and the cell compensates by synthesizing new side chains in excess, some of which are released into the circulation. Ehrlich's concept of selection of cells with pre-existing receptors for antigen was challenged in the 1930's by the work of Landsteiner, who showed that an animal could respond, by producing antibody, to a large number of synthetic haptens that it would never be expected to meet in nature.

At about the same time, *instructive,* or *template*, theories became popular. One of these theories proposed that antigen directs the formation of antibodies from its precursor molecules. Breinl and Haurowitz suggested that under the influence of antigen, the subunits of the antibody molecule (subunit structure was unknown at that time) combine with each other in an anomalous manner so that a specific antibody is formed. This modification was due to the presence of antigen within the antibody-forming cell, and thus the antigen served as a direct template. This view was expanded by Linus Pauling, who suggested that all antibody molecules have identical primary structure and differ from each other only in the conformation of their peptide chains. He proposed that antigen within the cell at the time of antibody synthesis serves as a template to stabilize a specific complementary conformation on the antibody molecule. These theories implied that antibody-forming cells are multipotent, that is, they can make all types of antibody specificities. They also predicted that antibody activity would be recovered from denatured antibody by renaturation only in the presence of specific antigen. When it was shown that antibody specificity resides in the primary sequence of amino acids in the antibody molecule, that antibody-forming cells have restricted potentiality, and that renaturation, in the absence of antigen, restores antibody activity, the direct template theory was modified.

An indirect template theory was put forth, in which it was suggested that antibody specificity is influenced directly though the action of antigen on DNA. This implies an alteration in the sequence of events in protein synthesis from the usual DNA $\rightarrow$ RNA $\rightarrow$ protein. It also implies that the antigen can function as a mutagen. These theories are untenable in view of our current knowledge of molecular biology.

In 1955, Jerne proposed a modern view of the selective theory, in which he suggested that the population of antibody-forming cells is endowed with a finite number of randomly distributed specific receptor molecules that arise spontaneously in the absence of antigens. These specific receptor molecules (natural antibodies) are released from individual cells, and antigen selects these specific receptors, thereby initiating antibody formation (natural selection). This hypothesis suggested that there are separate genes coding for each antibody molecule and that the entire library of genes required for all antibodies is present in each potential antibody-forming cell. This idea served as the basis of *germ-line* theories.

Burnet evolved the basic principles of the above-stated theory into the modern *clonal selection theory*. This theory suggested that there are a large number of previously programmed clones in the adult, each one carrying specific receptors on its surface capable of reacting with a specific immunogen. The outcome of the reaction between receptor and immunogen is either antibody formation or suppression (death of the clone if stimulated during fetal development or tolerance). Burnet suggested that the progenitor cells of the immune response are highly mutable omnipotent cells. He postulated that the diversity of specificities formed is the result of *somatic mutation*. Somatic development results in the differentiation of a population of individual antigen-sensitive cells, each of which has the capacity to respond to one or to a limited number of antigenic configurations. The antigen selects a specific precursor cell, which then proliferates into a clone of cells producing specific antibody. Although this theory, in its present form, leaves the explanation of certain immunologic phenomena unanswered, it is the most widely accepted among immunologists.

ANTIBODY FORMATION AT THE MOLECULAR LEVEL

The IgG molecule is a multichain protein that, upon partial reduction, yields two heavy chains and two light chains (Chapter 5). In addition, each chain is composed of a variable sequence of amino acids (V_H and V_L) associated with its antigen-binding activities, and a constant sequence of amino acids (C_H and C_L) reflective of that particular class of polypeptide chain. The observation that immunoglobulin polypeptide chains of the same type have identical sequences in the constant region but different sequences in the variable region seems difficult to reconcile with the dogma of molecular biology that states: "one gene, one polypeptide." Based on work done with the inheritance of allotypic markers, it was concluded that each constant region sequence is coded for by a single structural gene. In order to account for the great diversity of antibody specificities, it was postulated that there were multiple V region genes and that each V subgroup must be specified by at least one gene. It is now believed that one of many V region genes can become associated with a single C region gene for the synthesis of a single immunoglobulin chain (Chapter 5). Therefore, a departure from dogma exists and we now speak of *"two genes, one polypeptide."* The potential mechanism by which two genes recombine to direct the synthesis of a single polypeptide chain has been discussed (Fig. 7–10 and Chapter 5).

The early molecular events preparatory to the formation of antibody follow established patterns of protein synthesis. Following stimulation of the antigen-sensitive cell, there is a period of cellular proliferation accompanied by differentiation. The cells begin to synthesize DNA in as little as three hours after stimulation, and peak synthesis occurs three to four hours thereafter. Increases in RNA synthesis parallel those of DNA, with both mRNA and ribosomal RNA synthesis occurring. The use of inhibitors of nucleic acid synthesis during this time results in marked suppression of the immune response. Morphologic changes become apparent, with the cell displaying a well-developed endoplasmic reticulum and Golgi apparatus.

In the same manner that myeloma proteins have aided our understanding of the structure of immunoglobulins, studies of their synthesis have also aided our understanding of the molecular events of antibody formation. With the use of cell-free systems, it has been shown that only one mRNA molecule is involved in the synthesis of a single heavy or light polypeptide chain, rather than two mRNAs, where one codes for the variable and the other codes for the constant portion of the given chain. The base sequences and structure of several Ig mRNAs are now known. It has been shown that the precursor of mRNA, found in the nucleus, is of very high molecular weight and is processed into a smaller unit before it reaches the cytoplasm. Cytoplasmic mRNAs for both heavy and light chains contain a larger number of bases than can be accounted for in the translated polypeptide chains. The function of these extra bases is unclear at present.

After transcription and processing in the nucleus, the mRNA is transported into the cytoplasm, where it becomes associated with membrane-bound ribosomes to form the rought endoplasmic reticulum (Fig. 7–18). The individual polypeptide chains of the immunoglobulin molecule are made on separate polyribosome units. The immunoglobulin heavy chain is synthesized as a complete unit on heavy polysomes (16 to 18 ribosomes) having a sedimentation coefficient of 270S. Similarly, the light chains are synthesized as complete units on light polysomes (seven or eight ribosomes) having a sedimentation coefficient of 190S. It appears that both heavy and light chains are synthesized as larger precursors, containing an additional 20 N-terminal amino acid residues. This leader sequence of relatively hydrophobic amino acids, which appears to be involved in

membrane interactions with the Ig molecule, is cleaved as the chains enter the lumen of the endoplasmic reticulum. The newly formed L-chains are released from the polysomes and enter an intracellular pool of free L-chains. Although there is thought to be some assembly of L- to H-chain at the level of the heavy polysomes, most of it occurs postribosomally as the individual chains pass through the cisternae of the endoplasmic reticulum. Assembly into the full molecule containing two identical heavy chains and two identical light chains (H_2L_2) occurs by means of two major pathways with a variety of convalently linked intermediates. In the first pathway, two H-chains form an H_2 dimer followed by the addition of each of the L-chains to give H_2L, then the H_2L_2 molecule. In the second pathway, the H- and L-chains combine to form a half-molecule (HL), which then combines with another half-molecule (HL) through inter–H-chain disulfide bridges to give the complete molecule. While there is some preferential assembly by one of these pathways within a given species and Ig subclass, both have been shown to function.

Synthesis of H- and L-chains occurs at a

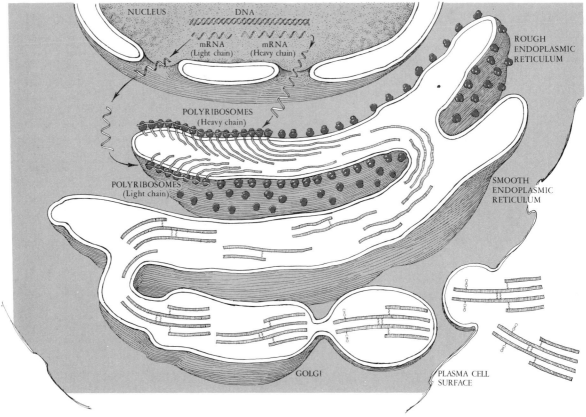

Figure 7–18. Schematic representation of immunoglobulin biosynthesis at the cellular level. (Adapted from Scharf.)

rapid rate, 60 seconds and 30 seconds, respectively. In spite of this, secretion of the newly synthesized molecule does not occur until after a lag of about 20 to 30 minutes. It is during this time that carbohydrate is added and the molecule is transported to the membrane. The H-chains, and in some cases the L-chains, are glycosylated in both the rough and the smooth endoplasmic reticulum. The assembled molecules traverse the Golgi apparatus and then move toward the cell surface. As they are transported to the cell surface in secretory vesicles, interchain disulfide bonds are formed and sugars are added successively to form oligosaccharide groups of the complete molecule. Most of the immunoglobulin molecules are secreted into the membrane and remain there for a period of time before being released.

In the case of IgM and IgA, polymerization occurs with the addition of the J-chain either shortly before or simultaneously with secretion of these molecules from the plasma cell. Finally, the mechanisms that control both the synthesis and the secretion of Ig molecules are not yet well understood, but should be of importance for the design of potential therapeutic modalities to be used in treatment of immunoproliferative diseases such as multiple myeloma.

Suggestions for Further Reading

The Fate of Immunogen

Ada, G. L., Nossal, G. J. V., and Pye, J.: Antigens in immunity. II. Distribution of iodinated antigens following injection into rats via the hind foot pads. Aust. J. Exp. Biol. Med. Sci., *42*:295, 1964.

Bellanti, J. A., and Herscowitz, H. B. (eds.): The Reticuloendothelial System—A Comprehensive Treatise, Vol. 6: Immunology. New York, Plenum Press, 1984.

Bierme, S. J., Blanc, M., Abbal, M., et al.: Oral Rh treatment for severely immunised mothers. Lancet, *1*:604, 1979.

Campbell, D. H., and Garvey, J. S.: Nature of retained antigen and its role in immune mechanisms. Adv. Immunol., *3*:261, 1963.

Dixon, F. J.: The metabolism of antigen and antibody. J. Allergy, *25*:487, 1954.

Mattingly, J. A., and Waksman, B. H.: Immunologic suppression after oral administration of antigen. I. Specific suppressor cells formed in rat Peyer's patches after oral administration of sheep erythrocytes and their systemic migration. J. Immunol., *121*:1878, 1978.

Antibody Formation in the Animal

Abramoff, P., and Brien, N. B.: Studies of the chicken immune response. I. Correlation of cellular and humoral immune response. J. Immunol., *100*:1204, 1968.

Eisen, H. N., and Siskind, G. W.: Variations in affinities of antibodies during the immune response. Biochemistry, *3*:996, 1964.

Fazekas de St. Groth, S., and Webster, R. G.: Disquisitions on original antigenic sin. I. Evidence in man. J. Exp. Med., *124*:331, 1966.

Mitchison, N. A.: The carrier effect in the secondary response to hapten-protein conjugates. II. Cellular cooperation. Eur. J. Immunol., *1*:18, 1971.

Uhr, J. W., and Finkelstein, M. S.: The kinetics of antibody formation. Prog. Allergy, *10*:37, 1967.

Cells of the Specific Immune Response

Bach, J. F.: Evaluation of T cells and thymic serum factors in man using the rosette technique. Transplant. Rev., *16*:196, 1973.

Binz, H., and Wigzell, H.: Antigen binding, idiotypic receptors from T lymphocytes: An analysis of their biochemistry, genetics, and use as immunogens to produce specific immune tolerance. Cold Spring Harbor Symp. Quant. Biol., *41*:275, 1976.

Cantor, H., and Boyce, E.: Regulation of the immune response by T-cell subclasses. Contemp. Top. Immunobiol., *7*:47, 1977.

Cooper, M. D., and Buckley, R. H.: Developmental immunology and the immunodeficiency diseases. JAMA, *248*:2658, 1982.

Cowing, C., Schwartz, B. D., and Dickler, H. B.: Macrophage Ia antigens. I. Macrophage populations differ in their expression of Ia antigens. J. Immunol., *120*:378, 1978.

Cramer, M., and Krawinkel, U.: Immunochemical properties of isolated hapten specific T-cell receptor molecules. *In* Pernis, B., and Vogel, H. J. (eds.): Regulatory T-Lymphocytes. New York, Academic Press, 1980.

Fishman, M., Adler, F. L., and Rice, S. G.: Macrophage RNA in the *in vitro* immune response to phage. Ann. N.Y. Acad. Sci., *207*:73, 1973.

Förster, O., and Landy, M. (eds.): Heterogeniety of Mononuclear Phagocytes. New York, Academic Press, 1981.

Greaves, M., and Janossy, G.: Elicitation of selective T and B lymphocyte responses by cell surface binding ligands. Transplant. Rev., *11*:87, 1973.

Herberman, R. B., and Ortaldo, J. R.: Natural killer cells: Their role in defenses against disease. Science, *214*:24, 1981.

Herscowitz, H. B., Holden, H. T., Bellanti, J. A., et al. (eds.): Manual of Macrophage Methodology: Collection, Characterization and Function. New York, Marcel Dekker, 1981.

Klinman, N., Mosier, D. E., Scher, I., et al. (eds.): B Lymphocytes in the Immune Response: Functional, Development and Interactive Properties. New York, Elsevier/North Holland, 1981.

Mishell, B. B., and Shiigi, S. M. (eds.): Selected Methods in Cellular Immunology. San Francisco, W. H. Freeman, 1980.

Moretta, L., Webb, S. R., Grossi, C. E., et al.: Functional analysis of two human T cell subpopulations: Help and suppression of B cell responses by T cells bearing receptors for IgM (T_M) and IgG (T_G). J. Exp. Med., *146*:184, 1977.

Nelson, D. S. (ed.): Immunobiology of the Macrophage. New York, Academic Press, 1976.

Pernis, B., and Vogel, H. J. (eds.): Regulatory T Lymphocytes. New York, Academic Press, 1980.

Pernis, B., Forni, L., and Amante, L.: Immunoglobulin

spots on the surface of rabbit lymphocytes. J. Exp. Med., *132*:1001, 1970.

Raff, M. C.: Surface antigenic markers for distinguishing T and B lymphocytes in mice. Transplant. Rev., *6*:52, 1971.

Reif, A. E., and Allen, M. J. V.: The AKR thymic antigen and its distribution in leukemias and nervous tissue. J. Exp. Med., *120*:413, 1964.

Reinharz, E. L., and Schlossman, S. F.: The differentiation and function of human T lymphocytes. Cell, *19*:821, 1980.

Taylor, R. B., Duffus, W. P. H., Raff, M. C., et al.: Redistribution and pinocytosis of lymphocyte surface Ig molecules by anti-Ig antibody. Nature [New Biol.], *233*:225, 1971.

Unanue, E. R., and Rosenthal, A. S. (eds.): Macrophage Regulation of Immunity. New York, Academic Press, 1980.

Vitetta, E. S., and Uhr, J. W.: Immunoglobulin-receptors revisited. Science, *189*:964, 1975.

Warner, N. L.: Membrane immunoglobulins and antigen receptors on B and T lymphocytes. Adv. Immunol., *19*:67, 1974.

Cellular Interactions in the Initiation of Antibody Formation

Bona, C. (ed.): Idiotypes and Lymphocytes. New York, Academic Press, 1981.

Claman, H. N., Chaperon, E. A., and Triplett, R. F.: Thymus-marrow combinations: Synergism in antibody production. Proc. Soc. Exp. Biol. Med., *122*:1167, 1966.

Early, P., Rogers, J., Davis, M., et al.: Two mRNAs can be produced from a single immunoglobulin μ gene by alternative RNA processing pathways. Cell, *20*:313, 1980.

Feldmann, M.: Cell interactions in the immune response *in vitro*. V. Specific collaboration via complexes of antigen and thymus-derived cell immunoglobulin. J. Exp. Med., *136*:737, 1972.

Feldmann, M., Rosenthal, A. S., and Erb, P.: Macrophage-lymphocyte interactions in immune induction. Int. Rev. Cytol., *60*:149, 1979.

Gillis, S., and Watson, J.: Biochemical and biological characterization of lymphocyte regulatory molecules. V. Identification of an interleukin-2–producing human leukemia T cell line. J. Exp. Med., *152*:1707, 1980.

Katz, D. H.: Adaptive differentiation of lymphocytes: Theoretical implications for mechanisms of cell-cell recognition and regulation of immune responses. Adv. Immunol., *29*:138, 1980.

Katz, D. H., Paul, W. E., Goidl, E. A., et al.: Carrier function in antihapten responses. III. Stimulation of antibody synthesis and facilitation of hapten-specific secondary antibody responses by graft-versus-host reactions. J. Exp. Med., *133*:169, 1971.

Lawton, A. R., III, and Cooper, M. D.: Modification of B lymphocyte differentiation by anti-immunoglobulins. Contemp. Top. Immunobiol., *3*:193, 1974.

Lee, K-C.: Regulation of T cell activation by macrophage subsets. Lymphokines, *6*:1, 1982.

McDevitt, H. O. (ed.): Ir Genes and Ia Antigens. New York, Academic Press, 1978.

Miller, J. F. A. P.: Influence of the major histocompatibility complex on T-cell activation. Adv. Cancer Res., *29*:1, 1979.

Miller, J. F. A. P., Basten, A., Sprent, J., et al.: Interac-

tions between lymphocytes in immune responses. Cell. Immunol., *2*:469, 1971.

Mishell, R. I., and Dutton, R. W.: Immunization of dissociated spleen cell cultures from normal mice. J. Exp. Med., *126*:423, 1967.

Mizel, S. B., and Mizel, D.: Purification to apparent homogeneity of murine interleukin-1. J. Immunol., *126*:834, 1981.

Moore, K. W., Rogers, J., Hunkapiller, T., et al.: Expression of IgD may use both DNA rearrangement and RNA splicing mechanisms. Proc. Natl. Acad. Sci. U.S.A., *78*:1800, 1981.

Mosier, D. E.: A requirement for two cell types for antibody formation *in vitro*. Science, *158*:1573, 1967.

Rabbits, T. H., Bentley, D. L., Dunnick, W., et al.: Immunoglobulin genes undergo multiple sequence rearrangements during differentiation. Cold Spring Harbor Symp. Quant. Biol., *45*:867, 1981.

Rajewsky, K. V., Schirrmacher, V., Nase, S., et al.: The requirement for more than one antigenic determinant for immunogenicity. J. Exp. Med., *129*:1131, 1969.

Rosenthal, A. S., and Shevach, E. M.: Function of macrophages in antigen recognition by guinea pig T-lymphocytes. I. Requirement of histocompatible macrophages and lymphocytes. J. Exp. Med., *138*:1194, 1974.

Shimpl, A., and Wecker, E.: Replacement of T cell function by a T cell product. Nature [New Biol.], *237*:15, 1972.

Smith, K. A., and Ruscetti, F. W.: T-cell growth factor and the culture of cloned functional T-cells. Adv. Immunol., *31*:137, 1981.

Tada, T., and Okumura, K.: The role of antigen-specific T-cell factors in the immune response. Adv. Immunol., *28*:1, 1979.

Waldmann, H., and Munro, A. J.: The interrelationships of antigenic structure, thymus independence and adjuvanticity. Immunology, *28*:509, 1975.

Watson, J., Frank, M. B., Mochizuki, D., et al.: The biochemistry and biology of interleukin-2. Lymphokines, *6*:95, 1982.

Zinkernagel, R. M., and Doherty, P. C.: MHC-restricted cytotoxic T-cells: Studies on the biological role of polymorphic major transplantation antigens during T-cell restriction-specificity, function and responsiveness. Adv. Immunol., *27*:52, 1979.

Regulation of Antibody Formation

Aune, T. A., and Pierce, C. W.: Preparation of a soluble immune response suppressor and macrophage-derived suppressor factor. J. Immunol. Methods, *53*:1, 1982.

Baker, P. J., Stashak, P. W., Amsbaugh, D. F., et al.: Evidence for the existence of two functionally distinct types of cells which regulate the antibody response to type III pneumococcal polysaccharide. J. Immunol., *105*:1581, 1970.

Beller, D. I., and Unanue, E. R.: Reciprocal regulation of macrophage and T-cell functions by way of soluble mediators. Lymphokines, *6*:25, 1982.

Benacerraf, B.: Genetic control of the specificity of T-lymphocytes and their regulatory products. *In* Fougereau, M., and Dausset, J. (eds.): Immunology 80. New York, Academic Press, 1980.

Bona, C., and Paul, W. E.: Cellular basis of regulation of expression of idiotype. I. T-suppressor cells specific for MOPC 460 idiotype regulate the expression of cells secreting anti-TNP antibodies bearing 460 idiotype. J. Exp. Med., *149*:592, 1979.

Cantor, H.: Control of the immune system by inhibitor and inducer T lymphocytes. Ann. Rev. Med., *30*:269, 1979.

Eichmann, K.: Expression and function of idiotypes on lymphocytes. Adv. Immunol., *26*:195, 1978.

Gershon, R. K.: T cell control of antibody production. Contemp. Top. Immunobiol., *3*:1, 1974.

Gershon, R. K.: Suppressor T-cells: miniposition paper celebrating a new decade. *In* Fougereau, M., and Dausset, J. (eds.): Immunology 80. New York, Academic Press, 1980.

Gershon, R. K., Eardley, D. D., Durum, S., et al.: Contrasuppression: a novel immunoregulatory activity. J. Exp. Med., *153*:1533, 1981.

Herzenberg, L. A., and Herzenberg, L. A.: Short-term and chronic allotype suppression in mice. Contemp. Top. Immunobiol., *3*:41, 1974.

Jerne, N. K.: Towards a network theory of the immune system. Ann. Immunol., *125C*:373, 1974.

Kohler, H.: Idiotypic network interactions. Immunol. Today, *1*:18, 1980.

Liacopoulous, P., and Ben-Efriam, S.: Antigenic competition. Prog. Allergy, *18*:97, 1974.

McDevitt, H. O.: The evolution of genes in the major histocompatibility complex. Fed. Proc., *33*:2168, 1976.

Moller, G., and Wigzell, H.: Antibody synthesis at the cellular level. Antibody-induced suppression of 19S and 7S antibody responses. J. Exp. Med., *121*:969, 1965.

Pross, H. F., and Eidinger, D.: Antigenic competition. A review of nonspecific antigen-induced suppression. Adv. Immunol., *18*:133, 1974.

Taussig, M. J., Munro, A. J., Campbell, R., et al.: Antigen specific T-cell factor in cell cooperation. J. Exp. Med., *142*:694, 1975.

Uhr, J. W., and Moller, G.: Regulatory effects of antibody on the immune response. Adv. Immunol., *8*:81, 1968.

Unanue, E. R.: The regulatory role of macrophages in antigen stimulation. Adv. Immunol., *31*:1, 1981.

Yamauchi, K., Murphy, D., Cantor, H., et al.: Analysis of antigen-specific, H-2–restricted cell-free product(s) made by "I-J⁻" Ly-2 cells (Ly-2TsF) that suppress Ly-2 cell–depleted spleen cell activity. Eur. J. Immunol. *11*:913, 1981.

Theories of Antibody Formation

Burnet, F. M.: The Clonal Selection Theory of Acquired Immunity. Nashville, Vanderbilt University Press, 1959.

Ehrlich, P.: On immunity with special reference to cell life. Proc. R. Soc. Lond. (Biol)., *66*:424, 1900.

Haurowitz, F.: The problem of antibody diversity. Immunodifferentiation versus somatic mutation. Immunochemistry, *10*:775, 1973.

Jerne, N. K.: The somatic generation of immune recognition. Eur. J. Immunol., *1*:1, 1971.

Pauling, L.: A theory of the structure and process of formation of antibodies. J. Am. Chem. Soc., *62*:2643, 1940.

Antibody Formation at the Molecular Level

Buxbaum, J. N.: The biosynthesis, assembly and secretion of immunoglobulins. Semin. Hematol., *10*:33, 1973.

Parkhouse, R. M. E.: Biosynthesis of polymeric immunoglobulins. Prog. Immunol. II, *1*:119, 1974.

Scharff, M. D., and Laskov, P.: Synthesis and assembly of immunoglobulin polypeptide chains. Prog. Allergy, *14*:37, 1970.

Scharff, M. D., Birshtein, B., Dharmgrongartama, B., et al.: The use of mutant myeloma cells to explore the production of immunoglobulins. *In* Smith, E. E., and Ribbons, D. W. (eds.): Molecular Approaches to Immunology. New York, Academic Press, 1975.

Sherr, C. J., Schenkein, I., and Uhr, J. W.: Synthesis and intracellular transport of immunoglobulin in secretory and nonsecretory cells. Ann. N.Y. Acad. Sci., *190*:250, 1971.

Stevens, R. H.: Distribution of immunoglobulin mRNA in mouse lymphocytes. Prog. Immunol. II, *1*:119,. 1974.

Williamson, A. R.: Biosynthesis of immunoglobulins. *In* Porter, R. R. (ed.): Defense and Recognition. London, Butterworth, 1973.

Chapter 8

Antigen-Antibody Interactions

Chester M. Zmijewski, Ph.D., and Joseph A. Bellanti, M.D.

The reactants of the specific immune response are either antibody, a product of the B-lymphocytes, or specifically sensitized T-lymphocytes. This chapter will deal with the reactions of antigen with antibody—the antigen-antibody interaction. Manifestations of the reaction of antigen with specifically sensitized T-lymphocytes and other cellular reactions, i.e., cell-mediated reactions, will be described in Chapter 9.

DEFINITIONS

Antigen-antibody interactions can be divided into three categories: (1) the *primary,* (2) the *secondary,* and (3) the *tertiary* (Fig. 8–1). The *primary* or initial interaction of antigen with antibody is the basic event and consists of the binding of antigen with an antibody molecule (Fig. 8–2). Since this interaction is rarely visible, its detection is usually accomplished by *secondary* reactions, which provide auxilliary means to visualize the reaction, e.g., precipitation. Tertiary reactions are biologic expressions of the antigen-antibody interaction that may be either beneficial or deleterious.

The measurement of *primary* antigen-antibody interactions can be accomplished by several techniques, including the ammonium sulfate precipitation method (Farr technique), equilibrium dialysis or visualization by immunofluorescence, ferritin labeling, or by a series of immunoassays, including radioimmunoassay (RIA), enzyme immunoassay (EIA), and fluoroimmunoassay (FIA) (Fig. 8–1). These methods are assuming clinical value in the measurement of antibodies important in disease processes, e.g., anti-

DNA antibody in lupus erythematosus determined by fluorescent technique, and hepatitis virus B antigen (HB$_s$Ag) or HB$_s$Ag antibody by radioimmunoassay.

The *secondary* manifestations of the antigen-antibody reaction include *precipitation, agglutination, complement-dependent reactions, neutralization,* and *cytotropic effects.* These reactions are of practical importance to the physician, since they form the basis of a number of laboratory tests used in the detection and identification of antigens, antibodies, or antigen-antibody complexes involved in disease processes.

The antigen-antibody interactions are sometimes expressed as *tertiary* manifestations (Fig. 8–1). Such reactions are by definition biologic expressions of the antigen-antibody interaction and at times may be helpful to the patient but at other times may lead to disease through immunologic injury. This chapter will be concerned only with the *in vitro* manifestations of the interaction of antigen with antibody. An interesting trend has been observed in recent years in which the earlier first-order immunoassays, e.g., RIA, are being replaced by second-order immunoassays, e.g., EIA (ELISA). It is likely that these too, in time, will be supplanted by third-order immunoassays, e.g., FIA (immunofluorescent techniques).

PRIMARY MANIFESTATIONS OF THE ANTIGEN-ANTIBODY INTERACTION

The primary interaction of antigen with antibody consists of the initial binding of

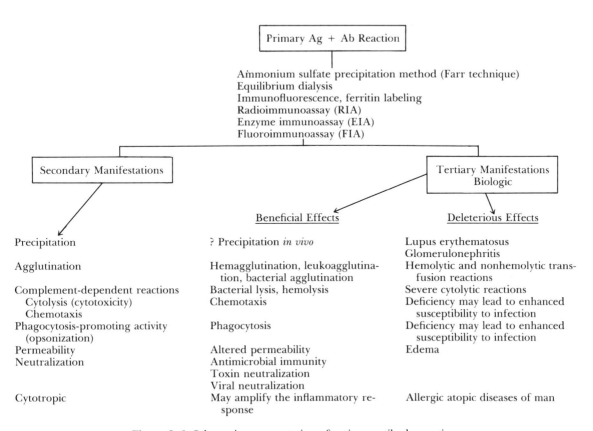

Figure 8–1. Schematic representation of antigen-antibody reactions.

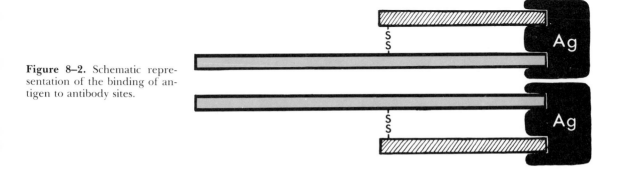

Figure 8–2. Schematic representation of the binding of antigen to antibody sites.

Table 8–1. Clinical Applications of Primary Antigen-Antibody Interactions

Label	Type of Assay	
	Quantitative Methods	Immunohistochemical Methods
Fluorescent	Fluoroimmunoassay (FIA)	Fluorescent antibody method
Radioactive	Radioimmunoassay (RIA)	Autoradiography
Electron-dense		Ferritin labeling
Enzyme	Enzyme immunoassay (EIA), e.g., enzyme-linked immunosorbent (ELISA)	Immunoperoxidase labeling

antigen with the two or more available antigen-binding sites on any given antibody molecule. This is shown schematically in Figure 8–2. The primary interaction of antigen with antibody is rarely directly visible, and visualization is usually accomplished by labeling antibody or antigen with fluorescent, radioactive, electron-dense, or enzymatic markers. These methods include both *quantitative* assays performed on sera and *immunohistochemical* techniques performed on tissues (Table 8–1).

Quantitative Methods for the Measurement of Antigen or Antibody Based on Primary Manifestations of the Antigen-Antibody Interaction

At present, the classic quantitative assay for the measurement of antigen-antibody reactions is the *radioimmunoassay* (RIA), in which a radioactively labeled substance (radioligand) is employed either directly or indirectly for the quantitative measurement of the unlabeled substance by a binding reaction to a specific antibody or other receptor system. Even substances that are not immunogenic by themselves (e.g., haptens) can be measured in these assays if they are coupled to larger carrier substances capable of inducing antibody to the low molecular weight material. Originally introduced as a method for the measurement of plasma insulin concentrations by Berson and Yalow, the technique has had an explosive impact upon all areas of medicine and has made possible the accurate measurement of small concentrations of a wide range of biologic substances, some of which could not be accurately measured previously, e.g., digoxin (Table 8–2). Although the vast majority of these assays employ an antigen-antibody reaction, some substances, e.g., hormones, may be assayed

by virtue of their binding to hormone receptors on cells or receptor proteins in the serum, e.g., thyroxin-binding protein (radioreceptor assay). These latter assays differ only in that receptors rather than antibody are used to bind the radioactive ligand. Radioimmunoassays are carried out either in solution, e.g., *liquid- or soluble-phase radioimmunoassays*, or on a supporting matrix to which the antigen (ligand) or antibody is adsorbed or covalently linked, e.g., *solid-phase radioimmunoassay* (Table 8–3). In contrast to the liquid-phase RIA, which depends upon a competitive binding principle and in which reactants are added together, the solid-phase RIA involves a two-step reaction, the first being the antigen-antibody binding and the second, the detection step.

LIQUID-PHASE RIA

The basic principle of the liquid-phase RIA is that the ligand to be measured (Ag) is assayed indirectly through its competition with a labeled derivative (Ag*) for binding a

Table 8–2. Examples of Substances Measurable by Radioimmunoassay

Serum proteins	Angiotensin
IgE (PRIST)	Bradykinin
IgE antibody (RAST)	Calcitonin
Anti-DNA	Glucagon
Carcinoembryonic antigen (CEA)	Kinins
	Drugs
Microbial agents and antibodies	Digoxin
HB_sAg or HB_sAb	Morphine
Hormones	*Metabolites*
Insulin	Cyclic AMP
ACTH	Cyclic GMP
Growth hormone	Folic acid
Steroid	Vitamin B_{12}
Estrogen	Intrinsic factors
Testosterone	
Thyroid hormones	

Table 8–3. Quantitative Radioimmunoassay Procedures

Type	Principle	Example
Liquid or soluble phase	Radioimmunoprecipitation	Ammonium sulfate method (Farr technique)
	Double-antibody method	
Solid phase	Competitive binding	Radioimmunosorbent test (RIST)
	Noncompetitive binding (sandwich)	Radioallergosorbent test (RAST) Paper radioimmunosorbent test (PRIST) HB$_x$Ag, Clq, DNA
	Competitive inhibition of binding	RAST inhibition assay

limited amount of antibody (Ab). This is shown schematically in Figure 8–3.

The assay is performed by reacting a standard quantity of Ag* with Ab in the presence of varying concentrations of unlabeled Ag in order to establish a standard curve (Fig. 8–4). In a similar fashion, the Ag containing the unknown is reacted with a standard quantity of Ag* plus Ab in a separate reaction mixture. When the reaction comes to equilibrium it is necessary to remove the Ag*Ab from the free Ag* in order to estimate the amount of unlabeled Ag present in the unknown. In the soluble phase, radioimmunoassay can be accomplished by the selective precipitation of the Ag*Ab complex from the solution by physicochemical techniques, e.g., ammonium sulfate method (Farr technique), or by the specific-antibody (double-antibody) method in which a second antibody is directed at the first. The amount of Ag in the unknown is then determined indirectly by the degree of binding of Ag* in the Ag*Ab complex from the standard curve.

SOLID-PHASE RIA

In addition to being performed in solution, the RIA assays have been modified so that the Ag or Ab can be immobilized or attached to a supporting medium (solid-phase RIA) (Table 8–3). The main advantage of this technique over the liquid phase is the simplicity of performance and the ease with which the Ag*Ab can be separated from the unreacted Ag*, either by washing or by centrifugation. One example of the competitive binding technique is the radioimmunosorbent test (RIST) for the quantitative measurement of IgE, which is represented schematically in Figure 8–5.

Other types of solid-phase RIA are the noncompetitive binding techniques for the measurement of Ag or Ab (Table 8–3). In this technique, represented schematically in Figure 8–6, either antigen or antibody is attached to a supporting matrix, and then the unknown specimen is added. When antibody is being analyzed, the antibody-containing specimen is added to the antigen-coated matrix, following which a second radiolabeled anti–gamma globulin reagent is added. When antigen is to be determined, antibody is immobilized on the matrix, the antigen-containing specimen is added, and a radiolabeled antibody to the antigen is added (Fig. 8–6). By means of this sandwich technique, which is a noncompetitive direct binding technique, specific antibody or antigen can be detected in a patient's serum. Examples of this technique include the radioallergosorbent test (RAST) for the measurement of specific IgE antibody to a variety of allergens, the PRIST test for the direct measure-

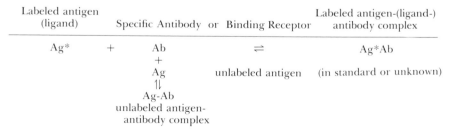

Figure 8–3. Schematic representation of the competitive binding radioimmunoassay.

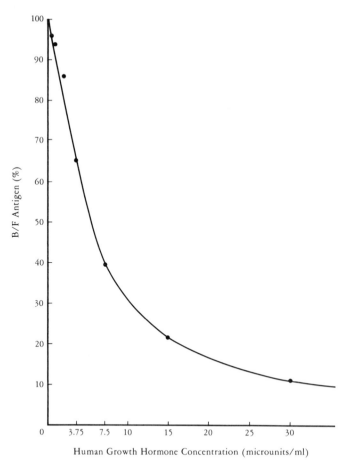

Figure 8–4. Standard curve for use in the radioimmunoassay of human growth hormone. (Courtesy of Dr. Malcolm M. Martin.)

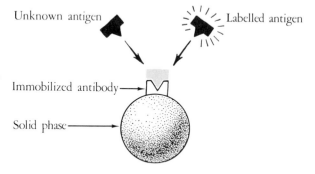

Figure 8–5. Schematic representation of the competitive binding RIA technique, e.g., RIST.

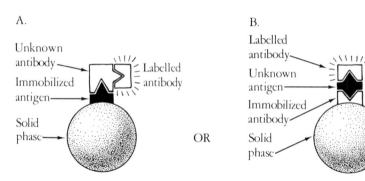

OR

Figure 8–6. Schematic representation of the noncompetitive (direct) RIA·binding technique illustrating the use of the test (*A*) in detecting unknown antibody, e.g., RAST and HB$_s$Ab, in which case antigen is immobilized, or (*B*) in detecting unknown antigen, e.g., PRIST and HB$_s$Ag, in which case antibody is immobilized onto the solid phase.

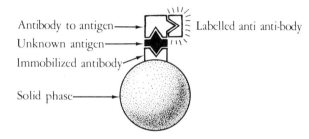

Figure 8–7. Schematic representation of the noncompetitive (indirect) RIA binding ("sandwich") technique.

ment of IgE globulin, and the measurement of hepatitis B antigen (HB_sAg) or specific HB_sAg antibody in the sera of patients with hepatitis. In some cases, the sandwich may be expanded to include an additional layer(s) (noncompetitive indirect binding technique) to increase the sensitivity of the assay or to allow the detection of antibody to antigens that cannot be readily attached to solid surfaces, e.g., penicillin RAST (Fig. 8–7).

Another modification of the solid RIA has been developed for the standardization of biologically active substances. This technique is illustrated in Figure 8–8 and consists of a two-step reaction: A solid-phase antigen is reacted with a known amount of Ab and radiolabeled anti-human gamma globulin, as in the direct sandwich technique described above; and (2) the unlabeled antigen to be assayed is added in a separate reaction mixture. The degree of inhibition of the reaction is used to quantitate the substance. The RAST inhibition assay is an example of this technique, which is currently being utilized for the standardization of allergenic extracts for use in immunotherapy of allergic disease in the human.

Another radioimmunoassay technique, the immunoradiometric assay, has been devel-

oped, in which purified antibody is radiolabeled and employed either in a liquid- or in a solid-phase radioimmunoassay. The primary advantage of this technique is its improved sensitivity and specificity; its main disadvantage is the complexity of the sophisticated technique required for antibody purification.

ENZYME IMMUNOASSAYS (EIA) AND FLUOROIMMUNOASSAYS (FIA)

Following the widespread use of radioimmunoassays during the past two decades, other markers have been introduced for the quantitative measurement of primary antigen-antibody interactions (see Table 8–1). One of these methods utilizes an enzyme as a label and is referred to as enzyme immunoassay (EIA) or enzyme-linked immunosorbent assay (ELISA). These assays have gained increasing popularity in recent years not only for their simplicity but also for a variety of factors both technical and regulatory (e.g., availability, elimination of the problem of disposal of radioactive wastes). The method utilizes an enzyme-linked antibody, e.g., alkaline phosphatase, and the end point of

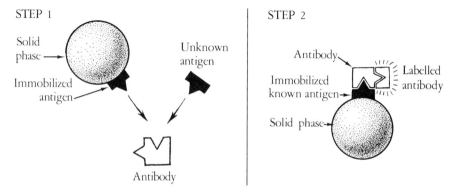

Figure 8–8. Schematic representation of competitive inhibition of binding, e.g., RAST inhibition assay. The assay is performed in two steps: (1) A known quantity of antibody is allowed to react in a competitive reaction between antigen immobilized on a solid phase and the unknown antigen to be measured, and (2) the bound antibody is measured, in a standard noncompetitive (direct) RIA assay, allowing the quantitation of the unknown antigen.

measurement is the enzymatic generation of a product from its substrate that can be measured colorimetrically or by the naked eye. This method has wide clinical application in the serodiagnosis of many diseases, including infectious diseases and particularly viral infections, for the detection of either antigen, e.g., hepatitis B antigen or antibody, e.g., rubella.

Another method for the detection of antigen and antibody is the fluoroimmunoassay (FIA), which utilizes a fluorescent label as a marker, e.g., fluorescein. Although the method can detect either antigen or antibody, thus far it has been used predominantly for the detection of antibody only.

Immunohistochemical Techniques

In addition to quantitative methods for the detection of antigen-antibody reactions, the manifestations of primary antigen-antibody interactions also form the basis of a wide variety of immunohistochemical techniques (see Table 8–1). These include the use of fluorescent-labeled antibody (e.g., immunofluorescence), enzymes (e.g., immunoperoxidase), electron-dense markers (e.g., immunoferritin labels), and radioactive markers (e.g., autoradiography).

Detection of Immune Complexes

Recent evidence indicates that antigen-antibody complexes play a major role in the pathogenesis of certain autoimmune diseases, in the modulation of graft and tumor rejection, and in several chronic infectious diseases, including the slow virus infections of man. Several techniques are now available for the detection of these immune complexes and are listed in Table 8–4. The clinical usefulness of these techniques has been

Table 8–4. Techniques for the Detection of Immune Complexes

Physicochemical methods (ultracentrifugation; gel filtration)
Precipitin reaction with Clq or monoclonal anti-IgG
Platelet aggregation
Binding to surface receptors of cultured RAJI cells
Clq binding test
Radioimmunoassays with monoclonal RF (MRF) or polyclonal RF (PRF)

rather limited, since several of them are research tools and are not readily demonstrated. However, newer techniques, e.g., the measurement of Clq, or monoclonal 19S anti-IgG, or the binding of immune complexes to surface receptors on cultured lymphoblasts (RAJI cells), have been developed that may allow new approaches to the elucidation of obscure diseases, which heretofore have been diagnostic and therapeutic orphans.

USE OF MONOCLONAL ANTIBODIES IN IMMUNOASSAYS

The principles of monoclonal antibody production from hybridomas has been described in Chapter 5. These monoclonal antibodies are finding application in a variety of immunoassays because they offer a number of distinct advantages over reagents prepared by more classic immunization techniques. These include a high degree of specificity, relative ease of *in vitro* production, great sensitivity, and almost limitless supply. The high degree of specificity may present potential pitfalls, however, because if monoclonal antibody is directed at the wrong antigenic specificity, an assay based on this reagent could give misleading results.

SECONDARY OR *IN VITRO* MANIFESTATIONS OF THE ANTIGEN-ANTIBODY INTERACTION

The humoral immune response to an immunogenic stimulus results in the production of circulating antibody belonging to one or more of the five major immunoglobulin classes: IgM, IgG, IgA, IgD, and IgE. Evidence for the presence of this type of response may be obtained from any of several serologic assay systems, listed in Figure 8–1, that are based upon secondary manifestations of the antigen-antibody interaction.

Precipitation, Agglutination, Phagocytosis, Cytotoxicity, and Toxin Neutralization

The type of assay system used to detect antibody depends not so much on the antibody produced as on the physical and chemical form of the antigen in question. Soluble antigens, when combined with their specific antibody, will lead to precipitation, in which the antigen-antibody complexes form large isoluble aggregates. The same antigens, if naturally or artifically attached to particulate matter, e.g., bacterial cells, red cells, latex particles, or bentonite particles, will form agglutinates or clumps. This process is referred to as agglutination. If living phagocytic cells, such as polymorphonuclear leukocytes, are added to the assay system, engulfment or phagocytosis of the antigen-sensitized particles may occur. Complement may or may not participate in this reaction; however, should antibody interact with cell-bound antigen to initiate the entire complement cascade, then cytotoxicity (cell death with lysis) may take place.

Toxin neutralization, the ability of specific antibody to neutralize toxin, forms one of the oldest of serologic reactions. It may be demonstrated *in vitro* or *in vivo*. The serum to be tested is first added to a potent toxin *in vitro* and then injected into a living animal or tissue culture system. The survival of the animal or the tissue culture is used as an index of toxin neutralization (LD_{50}) and will occur when antibody (antitoxin) is present in the test serum. On certain occasions, when a toxin is mixed *in vitro* with its specific antiserum, visible precipitation or flocculation will occur because of toxin-antitoxin forma-

tion. The Schick test for the detection of antibody to diphtheria toxin and the Dick test for the detection of antibody to scarlatinal toxin are examples of *in vivo* toxin neutralization.

To some degree, precipitation and agglutination may be considered as manifestations of the same antigen-antibody interaction, the only difference being the physical form of the test antigen. In both, a two-stage reversible chemical union takes place. In the first stage, antibodies present in the immune serum react with specific antigenic determinants present on the ligand. The ease of combination depends on several factors, notably pH, ionic strength, and temperature. For this reason, *in vitro* antigen-antibody reactions are carried out at specific temperatures in buffered media containing electrolytes. The union between antigen and antibody is accomplished by means of noncovalent binding, e.g., van der Waals forces. When the primary coupling reaction has reached equilibrium, the second stage, or *lattice formation*, takes place. During this phase, the unbound receptor sites on the antibody molecules attache to suitable receptors or additional antigen molecules, forming a lattice. This is represented schematically in Figure 8–9.

As in the first stage of the reaction, the

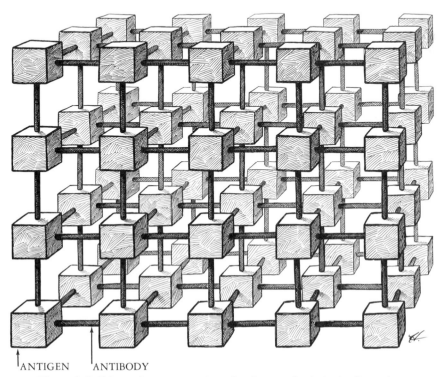

ANTIGEN   ANTIBODY

Figure 8–9. Schematic representation of antigen-antibody lattice formation.

second stage is also specific. Since two antigenic receptor sites of divalent antibody molecules are identical, an antibody with one specificity can link only identical antigens or antigenic determinants on the same molecule, never dissimilar ones. An illustration of this specificity can be noted in the following example:

When red blood cells from individuals belonging to blood groups A and B are mixed and then exposed to an immune serum containing only anti-A, the aggregates will be composed only of A cells. The B cells remain free in suspension.

In precipitation, the antigen is a soluble molecule. Therefore, a fairly large lattice must be formed before a visible aggregate is seen. In order to build a lattice of sufficient magnitude, a larger number of antibody molecules are required and the reactants must be present in optimal proportion. In agglutination, on the other hand, the antigen is part of a large insoluble particle, such as a red cell or a bacterial cell, and relatively fewer molecules are required for visible aggregation. Consequently, agglutination is a more sensitive serologic assay for antibody detection than is precipitation. This is an important consideration when choosing and interpreting serologic assay systems such as hemagglutination and bacterial agglutination. Sometimes it may become necessary to convert an ordinary precipitating system to an agglutinating system in order to increase the sensitivity of the assay. Shown in Table 8–5 are relative sensitivities of various antigen-antibody tests. In addition to the physical

Table 8–5. Sensitivity of Quantitative Tests Measuring Antibody Nitrogen of High-Avidity Antibody

Test	mg Ab N/ml or Test
Precipitin reactions	3–20
Immunoelectrophoresis	3–20
Double diffusion in agar gel	0.2–1.0
Complement fixation	0.01–0.1
Radial immunodiffusion	0.008–0.025
Bacterial agglutination	0.01
Hemolysis	0.001–0.03
Passive hemagglutination	0.005
Passive cutaneous anaphylaxis	0.003
Antitoxin neutralization	0.003
Antigen-combining globulin technique (Farr)	0.0001–0.001
Radioimmunoassay	0.0001–0.001
Enzyme-linked assays	0.0001–0.001
Virus neutralization	0.00001–0.0001
Bactericidal test	0.00001–0.0001

properties of the antigen, the nature of the antibody is important. On a molar basis, the IgM antibodies are more efficient agglutinators than are the IgG antibodies because of the greater number of antibody-combining sites on the IgM molecule; the IgG, on the other hand, are better precipitins than are the IgM.

Quantitative Precipitin Reaction

If increasing amounts of soluble antigen are mixed with a constant amount of antibody and the resultant precipitate is measured quantitatively, a dose-response relationship will be seen similar to that shown in Figure 8–10.

Initially, no precipitate will be formed. As the amount of antigen increases, small amounts of precipitate will result and gradually increase until the amount of precipitate is maximal. With continued addition of antigen, the amount of precipitate slowly diminishes until none is observed. This curve can be divided into the three zones shown in Figure 8–10.

In the first zone of the reaction, there is relative *antibody excess* (Fig. 8–10). Each of the two antigen-combining sites of an antibody molecule can react with a molecule of antigen, resulting in the formation of complexes composed of one antibody holding two antigens. No antigen is available for further union with the excess antibody, and therefore continued lattice formation with subsequent precipitation ceases. If the supernatant fluids are examined, it becomes evident that no free antigen exists. The composition of the supernatant fluids is shown in the accompanying inset of Figure 8–10.

In the middle, or equivalence, zone the concentrations of antigen reach optimal proportions (Fig. 8–10). Here the relative concentrations of antigen and antibody are such that maximal precipitation can occur. If, after removing the precipitates, the supernatant fluids are examined, it becomes evident that neither free antibody nor free antigen remains (Fig. 8–10). The multivalent antigen molecules are tightly held in a three-dimensional lattice by divalent antibody molecules.

The area to the right is known as the *region of antigen excess* (Fig. 8–10). Here, little precipitate is formed, although free antigen can be found in the supernatant. At this point, there is too little antibody to combine with

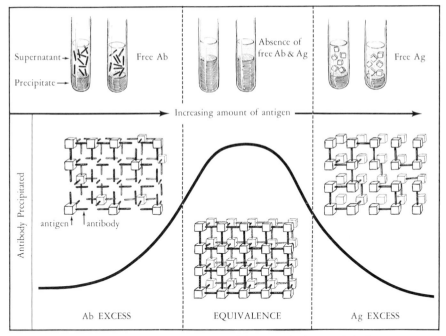

Figure 8–10. Schematic representation of the quantitative precipitation curve.

all the antigenic receptor sites. Examination of the supernatant fluid will reveal that free antigen is present in excess.

These relationships of antigen and antibody in precipitin reactions are most relevant to clinical medicine. Phagocytosis is efficient in the removal of aggregates that are formed in the region of optimal proportions. Antigen-antibody complexes formed in relative antigen excess, however, have the capability of initiating a sequence of destructive inflammatory damage, characteristic of the serum sickness type of disease. These complexes are small enough to remain soluble in the circulation but large enough to produce immunologic injury of tissues through complement activation.

Precipitation assays, apart from being performed in liquid media, are also carried out in semisolid media, e.g., agar, in which one or both constituents are allowed to diffuse into or toward the other. A solution of agar

is placed in a Petri dish; wells are cut into the gel; and antigen and antibody are placed in them. During incubation, both antigen and antibody diffuse toward each other from the wells and interact to form precipitates in the agar. A schematic representation of this reaction is shown in Figure 8–11. It can be seen that as diffusion progresses, concentration gradients of both antigen and antibody are established. When optimal concentrations are attained, a precipitate will form that is visible through the agar as a distinct band or line (Fig. 8–11). If the reaction is allowed to continue, the precipitin line may decrease in intensity or actually disappear owing to an excess of antigen or antibody.

The precipitin reaction is a useful analytic tool for the identification of unknown antibodies or antigens. If two different antigens, A and B, are each allowed to diffuse in agar from adjacent wells toward their specific antibody (anti-A or anti-B) in different plates,

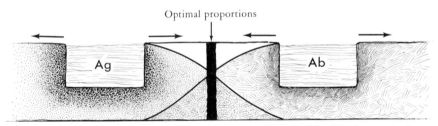

Figure 8–11. Schematic representation of Ouchterlony double diffusion method.

lines of precipitation will be obtained for each antigen-antibody system. The region of optimal proportion for the A–anti-A reaction may differ from that of the B–anti-B reaction. This may be due to differences in molecular weight or concentration, both of which can influence the rate of diffusion. With this technique, however, it is possible to determine whether two antigens are *identical, similar,* or *different* (Fig. 8–12) by juxtaposing the reactions between adjacent wells. For ex-

ample, an antiserum reactive with both antigens is placed in a central well surrounded by wells containing the two suspected antigens. Diffusion is allowed to take place and bands of precipitate are formed. If the two antigens are identical, they will diffuse at the same rate and the zone of optimal proportions will be reached in the same location. Therefore, the two bands will coalesce, as shown in Figure 8–12, in the *reaction of identity*. With further diffusion of antigen or

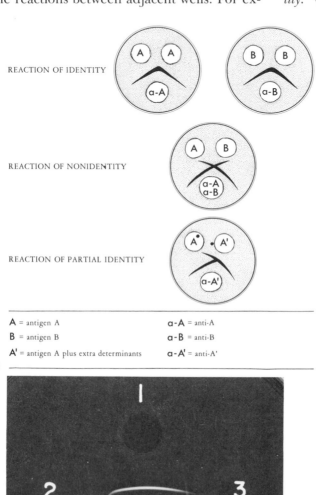

REACTION OF IDENTITY

REACTION OF NONIDENTITY

REACTION OF PARTIAL IDENTITY

A = antigen A

B = antigen B

A' = antigen A plus extra determinants

a-A = anti-A

a-B = anti-B

a-A' = anti-A'

A

B

RGG

Figure 8–12. *A,* Schematic representation of three types of Ouchterlony double diffusion reactions. *B,* Ouchterlony double diffusion plate showing the reaction of identity between fractions 1 and 2, the reaction of partial identity between whole rabbit gamma globulin (RGG) and fractions 2 and 3 and the reaction of nonidentity between fractions 1 and 3. (From Putnam, F. W., et al.: The cleavage of rabbit γ-globulin by papain. J. Biol. Chem., *237:*717, 1962; courtesy of Dr. Shunsuke Migita.)

antibody, the formation of soluble complexes will occur. Coalescence will be maintained, however, since the bands continue to form and dissolve at the same rate. If, on the other hand, the two antigens are completely different, the bands will cross in the *reaction of nonidentity*, as shown in Figure 8–12. In this case, the concentration of one antigen has little influence on the behavior of the other, and the two bands that form will cross over each other. Sometimes two antigens may be similar and share a common determinant; this results in spur formation—the reaction of partial identity (Fig. 8–12).

Precipitation in agar gels is widely used in diagnostic immunology. It is most useful in the quantification of immunoglobulin concentrations and in immunoelectrophoresis. In immunoquantification, the agar is impregnated by the antiserum and the material to be tested is placed in wells. The diameters of the concentric rings that form are directly proportional to the concentration of the antigen in question. In recent years, the method of detection of antigen-antibody precipitin reactions has been improved by nephelometric or light-scattering techniques, which have been used for the quantification of a wide variety of serum proteins and other body fluid proteins. These techniques are useful in the quantification of immunoglobulins in many disease states such as the immunoproliferative diseases and the immunologic deficiency states.

Agglutination Reactions

The same principles governing the antigen-antibody relationships seen in precipitin reactions also apply to agglutination reactions. The notable difference is that soluble complexes are not formed by the latter. Instead, in the region where antibody is in excess, visible agglutination may be inhibited. This is referred to as a *prozone phenomenon*. Owing to the particle size, electrostatic surface charge density, or immunochemical nature of the antibody, certain physicochemical conditions occur that affect agglutination reactions.

Any large particle, such as a red blood cell, suspended in solution contains a net surface electrostatic charge. This is due, in part, to cell surface chemical groupings that may be completely or partially ionized. Since red blood cell particles in any given reaction are similar, they carry an identical charge and therefore tend to repel each other. The strength of the effective electrostatic charge (zeta potential), as described below, tends to keep the particles at a given distance.

In agglutination, the first stage of the initial antigen-antibody union takes place as in precipitation and is dependent upon ionic strength, pH, and temperature. The second stage, lattice formation, is dependent upon overcoming the electrostatic repulsion forces of the particles. In the agglutination of red blood cells, for example, in which antigenic receptor sites may be located in deep valleys on the cell surface, antibody is firmly bound to receptor sites on one cell. Lattice formation cannot occur until its free receptor valence attaches to antigen between adjacent cells. If the cells are held apart by repulsive forces, the free end of the antibody molecule will not approach the antigen closely enough to make a firm bond. The repulsive forces may be overcome by physical methods that force the cells into closer proximity, e.g., centrifugation or sedimentation. With some antigen-antibody systems, however, such measures have no effect and agglutination cannot occur.

Those antibodies capable of reacting with antigen in saline solution have been termed *saline* or *complete* antibodies and, for the most part, consist of IgM antibody. Those incapable of reacting in saline have been termed *incomplete* or *blocking* antibodies and include the IgG antibodies. *It should be pointed out, however, that the terms "complete" and "incomplete" are misnomers, since all antibodies are functionally complete.* Certain types of 7S IgG antibodies cannot agglutinate red cells in saline suspension even though firmly attached to antigens. In these cases, the size of the antibody molecule and its wide spatial arrangement prevent agglutination. Even high centrifugal forces cannot overcome these electrostatic repulsion effects and allow lattice formation to occur. Nevertheless, if these same antibodies are mixed with red blood cells in a colloidal medium such as albumin, agglutination will occur. This principle becomes important in the interpretation of various types of antibody associated with alloimmunization, e.g., hemolytic disease of the newborn or transfusion reactions.

ZETA POTENTIAL

The distance between two particles in suspension is not solely dependent upon their net surface charge density. Ions in solution orient themselves around a particle so as to form a diffuse double layer or cloud. The difference in charge density between the inside and the outside of the ionic cloud creates an electrostatic potential known as the zeta potential. The zeta potential is the essential determining factor of the repulsion effects of two adjacent particles. By controlling this potential, it is possible to control the minimal distance two particles may achieve in suspension.

The zeta potential may be reduced by two methods: (1) pretreatment with enzymes, such as trypsin or neuraminidase, that alter chemical groupings on cell surfaces; and (2) the use of various colloidal diluents, e.g., serum albumin or Ficoll, that lower the zeta potential by changing the dielectric constant of the aqueous electrolyte solution. The net result is that the electrostatic repulsion effects are overcome and the cells or particles can approximate each other, permitting the firm coupling of antigen with antibody necessary for agglutination.

The Antiglobulin (Coombs) Reaction

In some cases, a short antibody molecule directed against a deeply located antigenic determinant cannot agglutinate, even when these various manipulations are employed. In such situations, a third type of serologic technique, such as the antiglobulin (Coombs) reaction, must be employed in order to demonstrate that antibody is present. The antiglobulin test consists of the addition of an antibody directed against gamma globulin, which provides a bridge between two antibody-coated cells (Fig. 8–13). Most commercially available Coombs reagents used in the clinical laboratory contain anti-human IgG in combination with some anti-human "nongamma" antibody to detect bound complement components. These are the so-called broad-spectrum Coombs sera and contain broadly reactive antiglobulin activity. Additional sera are available to detect class-specific antibody, e.g., IgG-, IgM-, IgA-associated antibody.

The Coombs test is performed in two ways: (1) the *direct* antiglobulin test, consisting of the detection of cell-bound antibody by the addition of the antiglobulin reagent directly to the cell suspension; and (2) the *indirect* antiglobulin test, detecting the presence of circulating antibody that is first adsorbed to the test red cells to which is added the antiglobulin reagent. For example, the direct Coombs test would be useful for the detection of IgG-sensitized red cells in an infant suspected of having hemolytic disease of the newborn; the indirect Coombs test would be useful for the detection of IgG-associated antibody in the serum of a mother suspected of being sensitized to the Rh antigen.

Passive Agglutination

Since agglutination tests are more sensitive indicators of antibody, it is sometimes desir-

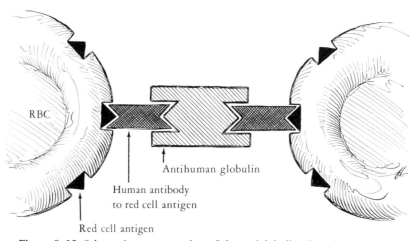

RBC

Antihuman globulin

Human antibody
to red cell antigen

Red cell antigen

Figure 8–13. Schematic representation of the antiglobulin (Coombs) reaction.

able to convert systems that precipitate to those that agglutinate. This is referred to as *passive agglutination* and can be accomplished by coating a small soluble antigen onto a larger insoluble particle, such as polystyrene, latex, bentonite, or red blood cells. Diagnostic tests employing this technique are in widespread use for the detection of a variety of antibodies, such as the rheumatoid factor (an IgM antibody directed against partially denatured IgG globulin).

Antigens may be coupled to erythrocytes by various techniques. Polysaccharide antigens readily adhere to the surface of unaltered red blood cells. Thus, specific polysaccharide antigens of certain bacteria adhere to erythrocytes and are used as test antigens for the detection of antibody. Protein substances may be attached to red cells that have been treated with tannic acid. The tanned-cell hemagglutination technique is valuable in detecting antibody to thyroglobulin in Hashimoto's disease. Finally, certain antigens may be attached to red cells by means of a chemical linkage such as the bis-diazotized benzidine (BDB) coupling reaction. Thus, both precipitation and agglutination provide very specific and sensitive tests in current use in diagnostic immunology.

COMPLEMENT-DEPENDENT REACTIONS

Complement has been described in detail in Chapter 6. Those complement-dependent effects useful in identifying antigen-antibody reactions include *lysis, phagocytosis, chemotaxis, opsonization, immune adherence, complement fixation,* and *altered permeability* (see Fig. 8–1).

Lysis

Lysis represents destruction of the cell membrane through the action of the late-acting complement components (C8, C9) that are activated by the reaction of specific antibody to a surface antigen and mediated through the activation of the complete complement sequence. These reactions usually result in the destruction of red blood cells (hemolysis), white blood cells (lymphocytotoxicity), or certain gram-negative bacteria (bacteriolysis).

Chemotaxis, Opsonization, Immune Adherence, Phagocytosis, and Altered Permeability

The interaction of antigen with antibody together with complement can also affect the inflammatory response through chemotaxis, opsonization, immune adherence, phagocytosis, and altered permeability. This involves a multiphasic act including the generation of chemotactic factor (C3a, C5a, C567), the activation of the phagocytosis-promoting factor (C3b), and the presence of complement receptors (C3b) and Fc receptors on the surface of phagocytic cells. The chemotactic and phagocytic factors can be initiated through the activation of either the classic or alternative complement pathway (Chapter 6). The antigen-antibody reaction usually leads to the activation of the classic pathway. Once initiated, these principles lead to the accumulation of phagocytic cells and to the enhancement of phagocytosis.

The activation of the complement cascade by the antigen-antibody interaction can also lead to the production of factors that alter the permeability of blood vessels. The action of these split products (C3a, C5a) is indirect and occurs through the release of vasoactive amines from mediator cells (Chapter 2).

Complement Fixation

The sera of all animal species contain varying quantities of complement. For many years, normal guinea pig serum was used as the primary source of complement in most serologic systems, since this species of animal contains high levels of complement having very efficient lytic properties. Different sources of complement are used in various *in vitro* tests; for example, in cytotoxicity tests used in transplantation, rabbit complement is the ideal source.

Lytic antibodies are rarely used directly in *in vitro* tests. The reasons for this are the low sensitivity of the method and the unavailability of antigen in proper form. For example, although it is possible to detect lytic antibodies against *Bordetella pertussis*, it takes at least one molecule of IgM antibody or two molecules of IgG antibody to initiate the complement sequence for the lysis of a single cell.

In order to produce a perceptible change by direct lysis, a huge number of bacterial cells would be required. The second limiting factor may be the type of antigen itself. There are certain organisms such as viruses, rickettsiae, fungi, and some spirochetes that are not susceptible to direct lysis.

For these reasons, the complement-fixation test capable of detecting the same antibody represents one of the most sensitive and frequently employed serologic tests in clinical medicine. The assay is based upon a two-stage reaction in which complement is consumed in the first stage of the antigen-antibody reaction. The binding of complement is assayed indirectly by a detection system consisting of antibody-coated erythrocytes that detect residual complement activity. In the first stage, the test antigen and the patient's heated serum (complement-inactivated) are incubated in the presence of a measured quantity of guinea pig complement. The amount of complement used is critical and represents a slight excess of that amount required to lyse a standard suspension of sheep red cells sensitized with rabbit anti–sheep red cell antibody (hemolysin or amboceptor). At the end of the primary incubation, the sensitized sheep red cells are added. If the patient's serum contains antibody directed against the test antigen, an antigen-antibody reaction occurs that consumes the complement. Therefore, little or no complement is available to lyse the sensitized sheep red cells. This is termed *complement fixation* and represents the presence of antibody. If, on the other hand, the patient's serum is devoid of antibody, no antigen-antibody reaction takes place in the first stage, and complement remains in the system and is available for the lysis of the added sensitized sheep cells. This represents the lack of complement-fixation and implies the absence of the complement-fixing antibody. This technique is much more sensitive than is the direct lysis of bacteria and provides a simple and quantitative method of antibody detection.

A special case of complement-dependent lysis is the *cytotoxicity test*. This assay employs a system in which the living cells are mixed with antibody and complement. When antibody to a cell-bound antigen is present, cell death will occur in the presence of complement. The end point or cell death can be ascertained by any of a number of methods, including supravital staining, gross appearance of cells, or enzymatic function. This assay has wide application in histocompatibility testing for organ transplantation and is also assuming importance in tests of cell-mediated immunity to viruses (Chapter 9) and tumor antigens. A specialized example of the use of lytic techniques *in vitro* is the Jerne plaque technique. In this method, a suspension of presensitized immunocompetent lymphoid cells is incubated in agar in which red cells, antigen, and complement are also present. The *in vitro* production of antibody by these cells is detected by clear areas of lysis surrounding each of the antibody-producing cells.

Cytotropic Effects

Cytotropic effects are a property of some classes of antibody that can bind to a limited number of mediator cells of the body, such as mast cells and basophils, and in most mammalian species, including man, appear to be primarily associated with the IgE class of immunoglobulin. When involved in antigen-antibody interactions, this class of immunoglobulin has the capacity to release from mediator cells a number of vasoactive amines important in localized and generalized forms of anaphylaxis. This class of antibody can be detected *in vitro* by means of the release of vasoactive amines from sensitized mediator cells (e.g., leukocyte histamine release) or by assays involving their effect on isolated target tissue (e.g., Schultz-Dale). In addition, these antibodies can be detected by radioimmunoassay tests (e.g., RAST).

SUMMARY

The manifestations of antigen-antibody interactions can be divided into three categories: the primary, the secondary, and the tertiary. The primary interaction of antigen with antibody is the basic event and may be demonstrated directly or through secondary manifestations, which include precipitation, agglutination, complement-dependent reactions, neutralization, and cytotropic effects. The secondary manifestations of antigen-antibody reactions encompass a number of physical and chemical interactions between antibody, antigen, complement, and the suspending medium in which the antigen-antibody reaction occurs. The tertiary manifestations of the antigen-antibody interaction are biologic expressions, which may be either beneficial or harmful to the host.

Suggestions for Further Reading

Haber, E., and Krause, R. M. (eds.): Antibodies in Human Diagnosis and Therapy. New York, Raven Press, 1977.

Henriksen, S. D. (ed.): Immunology. Baltimore, Williams & Wilkins Company, 1970.

Kabat, E. A. (ed.): Structural Concepts in Immunology and Immunochemistry. 2nd ed. New York, Holt, Rinehart and Winston, 1975.

Rose, N. R., and Friedman, H. (eds.): Manual of Clinical Immunology. 2nd ed. Washington, D. C., American Society for Microbiology, 1980.

Stites, D. P., Stobo, J. D., Fudenberg, H. H., et al.: Basic and Clinical Immunology. 4th ed. Los Altos, Lange Medical Publications, 1982.

Voller, A., Bidwell, D. E., and Bartlett, A.: Enzyme immunoassays in diagnostic medicine. Bull. WHO, 52:55, 1976.

Chapter 9

Cell-Mediated Immune Reactions

Joseph A. Bellanti, M.D., and Ross E. Rocklin, M.D.

The previous chapter describes those manifestations of the specific immune response concerned with the reactions of antibody with antigen—the *antigen-antibody interactions*. This chapter is concerned with those expressions of the immune response that involve the interaction of cells of the immune system with antigen and are termed *cell-mediated immune* (CMI) reactions. Until recently, these reactions were considered to be mediated only by T-lymphocytes independent of antibody; it is becoming increasingly clear, however, that they may also be carried out by a variety of cell types, humoral substances, or combinations of both.

Although the term "delayed hypersensitivity" has been used previously to include both normal and pathologic expressions of cell-mediated immunity, its use here will be restricted to include only those *in vivo* manifestations of the cellular immune response that lead to tissue injury. The more inclusive term "cell-mediated" or "cellular immunity" will be used to encompass both *normal* and *pathologic* events and will include both *in vitro* and *in vivo* expressions of specifically sensitized T-lymphocytes as well as those activities carried out by other cellular and humoral components of the immune response.

The series of reactions involved in this type of immunity seem to be characteristically associated with effector–target cell interactions involved in (1) acquired microbial resistance, particularly that associated with intracellular parasitism; (2) transplantation immunity; and (3) tumor rejection. In each of these situations, antigen is either intracellular or architecturally inaccessible, and antigen-antibody reactions appear to be relatively inefficient. Cellular reactions, on the other hand, appear to be more effective in the elimination of such sterically inaccessible antigens.

HISTORICAL ASPECTS

The phenomenon of delayed hypersensitivity was first discovered by Edward Jenner in 1798, during the course of his studies with cowpox virus immunization, when he observed that an inflammatory lesion occurred within 24 to 48 hours at the site of revaccination of a previously immunized individual. In the nineteenth century, during attempts at developing a vaccine for tuberculosis, Robert Koch observed a similar phenomenon. Following inoculation of culture broth of the tubercle bacillus into the skin of tuberculous guinea pigs, he observed a localized red lesion within 24 to 48 hours that occasionally became necrotic.

The following biologic characteristics of the delayed hypersensitivity reaction in skin are presented briefly to illustrate the basic immunobiologic principles underlying these effects.

Following the intradermal injection of antigen into a sensitized host, a reaction occurs at the localized skin site within 24 to 48 hours, reaching a maximum at 72 hours. The lesion consists of a firm indurated "red bump," whose intensity is directly related to the degree of sensitization of the host. For years, this *in vivo* method of testing for cell-mediated responses was the only procedure available and by its nature was difficult to quantify.

It was subsequently shown that this dermal reactivity could be passively transferred from a sensitized individual to a normal host by the use of living lymphoid cells, e.g., blood lymphocytes, but not by serum. Cell extracts of human leukocytes (transfer factor) were also shown to have the capacity to transfer this reactivity from sensitized donors to normal recipients.

The histology of the dermal skin site reveals the presence of mononuclear cells, basophils, and few neutrophils, in contrast to cellular reactions mediated by antibodies, in which neutrophilic infiltration and edema predominate. The early histologists were noncommital in their descriptions of these cells and used the term "round-cell infiltration." Recently, the predominant type of leukocyte in cell-mediated reactions has been shown to be the macrophage. In experimental studies in guinea pigs in which radioactively labeled macrophages were employed to determine the source of these cells, it was demonstrated that the macrophages present in the reaction site were those of the recipient and not the donor. Furthermore, most of the cells in the cell-mediated lesion appeared to be derived from rapidly dividing populations of macrophages originating in the bone marrow. These cells arrive at the test site via the motile form of the macrophage, the monocyte (Chapter 2).

CELL TYPES AND EFFECTOR MECHANISMS

There are a variety of cell types and cellular mechanisms involved in the expressions or regulation of cell-mediated reactions. Shown in Table 9–1 are the cell types with their sites of origin, surface characteristics, and mechanisms of action. These cell types include (1) T-lymphocytes, (2) macrophages, (3) killer or K-cells, and (4) natural killer or NK-cells.

T-Lymphocytes

The first cell type to be described is the T-lymphocyte (Table 9–1). In addition to its collaborative role with B-lymphocytes in either a "helper" or a "suppressor" function

(Chapters 7 and 10), it is now recognized that the T-lymphocyte, either alone or in concert with other subsets of T-lymphocytes, is important in the expressions of cell-mediated immunity. The clinically important reactions include the rejection of allografts, the rejection of tumors, and antimicrobial immunity.

The T-lymphocytes arise in the bone marrow and differentiate in the thymus; the mature forms contain characteristic markers (Table 9–1). Upon further differentiation these cells give rise to a population of cytotoxic T-cells that can destroy appropriate target cells either directly or through the elaboration of specific cell products, e.g., lymphokines. These cytotoxic lymphocytes can be generated *in vitro* in a mixed lymphocyte (MLC) reaction, *in vivo* during a graft-versus-host (GVH) reaction, or during the rejection of an allograft, tumor cell, or virally transformed or chemically modified target cell. Such cytotoxic cells can be demonstrated *in vitro* by the lysis of appropriate target cells.

Recently, cytotoxicity experiments in the murine system have suggested that certain genetic restrictions are involved in the recognition and destruction of virally infected or chemically modified target cells by T-lymphocytes. A requirement for identity at the H-2K or D locus has been demonstrated for both the sensitized T-lymphocyte and the target cell (Chapter 3). Although a similar relationship has not yet been demonstrated for the human, the biologic implications of these findings are very important with respect to antiviral immunity, autoimmunity, and malignancy. Furthermore, based upon these findings, the ability to differentiate between "self" and nonself" appears to be intimately related to histocompatibility and immune responsiveness. From an evolutionary standpoint, it has been suggested that minor alterations of these strong immuno-

Table 9–1. **Effector Cell Types Involved in Cell-Mediated Reactions**

| Cell Type | Precursor Cell or Site of Differentiation | Surface Markers or Receptors | | | | Mechanisms of Action |
		mIg	Fc	C3b	T Anti-gen	
T-lymphocytes	Thymus	−	−	−	+	Direct or elaboration of lymphokines
Macrophages	Monocyte precursor	±	+	+	−	Direct or armed with antibody; enhanced by MIF
K-cells	?	−	+	−	−	Armed with antibody (ADCC)
NK-cells	?	−	−	−	−	Direct

genic histocompatibility antigens by viruses or chemicals will immediately stimulate the immunologic system. Very recently, a genetic requirement for T-helper function in antibody synthesis by B-cells has also been demonstrated (Chapter 7).

Mononuclear Phagocytes

The mononuclear phagocytes make up a second set of cell types active in cellular immunity. These cells not only are important in the "processing" or "presentation" of antigen for the initiating events of T cell activation and antibody production by B-cells but also may perform an accessory function in the expressions of cell-mediated immunity by T-lymphocytes. Their actions are mediated in part through the elaboration of monokines such as interleukin-1, which is involved in the activation of T-cells, and colony-stimulating factor, neutral proteinases (plasminogen activator, elastase, and collagenase), and complement proteins, which are involved in various effector functions. Moreover, they may take part directly in the destruction of foreign substances by *phagocytosis* or by direct cytotoxic effect on target cells. In addition, some of the products of T-lymphocytes, e.g., migration inhibitory factor (MIF), may influence macrophage function by affecting cell movement or cellular metabolism. The enhancement of these macrophage functions by agents, e.g., immunopotentiators, is receiving widespread attention in cancer immunotherapy (Chapter 10).

The presence of an Fc receptor and a receptor for C3b may facilitate the uptake of complexes of antigen and antibody or antigen-antibody and complement, respectively. In addition, the presence of the Fc receptor may allow the cell type to participate in antibody-dependent cellular cytotoxic (ADCC) reactions, as described for the killer (K) cell.

Killer Cells

Another cellular type important in cell-mediated reactions is the killer or K-cells (see Table 9–1). Although their precise identity and site of origin are unknown, these cells are morphologically indistinguishable from small lymphocytes and Fc receptor–positive, surface immunoglobulin–negative (mIG—),

and C3b receptor–negative (i.e., null cells). These cells have been shown to have cytotoxic activity with target cells coated with specific IgG antibody in an antibody-dependent cellular cytotoxic (ADCC) reaction, in which an antibody molecule appears to form a bridge between the target cell and the effector cell. This presumably occurs through a binding of the Fab region of the immunoglobulin molecule with the antigenic determinants on the target cell and the Fc portion of the antibody with the Fc receptor on the surface of the lymphocyte. Complement does not appear to participate in these reactions, and unlike the situation with T-lymphocytes, these reactions can occur with nonsensitized K-cells.

Natural Killer Cells

A fourth cell type has very recently been described that appears to be a natural killer or NK-cell. The identity of these cells is also unknown; they contain no known T- or B-cell markers and do not require prior sensitization for their generation. These cells occur naturally and are found in increased quantity in mice lacking thymuses (nude mice). This finding may explain the apparent discrepancy in the immune surveillance theory, which would predict an increased incidence of tumors in such animals. The apparent increase in NK-cells may offer an explanation for the absence of increased tumorigenicity in these animals. These cells are thought to be involved in nonspecific killing of virally transformed target cells, allografts, resistance to some infections, and tumor rejection. Although their role in man is as yet undefined, these cells may be of profound biologic significance in immune surveillance of malignant diseases in the human.

Effect of Antibody on Cell-Mediated Reactions

In addition to its role in facilitating cell-mediated immunity through an ADCC mechanism, antibody may also exert a direct cytotoxic effect on a target cell through a complement-dependent reaction (Table 9–1) (Chapter 6). Alternatively, antibody directed against a target cell can "block" the cytotoxic effect of T-lymphocytes, macrophages, K-cells, or NK-cells, presumably by binding with antigenic determinants on the target cell surface. This interference by antibody or antigen-antibody complexes may have relevance for host immunologic reactions against certain tumors, and such "blocking antibody" may result in intensified tumor growth, a phenomenon referred to as *enhancement.* Other species of antibody formed in the tumor-bearing host can "unblock" this blocking antibody and lead to the destruction of the tumor. Whether this unblocking effect is related to direct complement-dependent effects of antibody or is favored by an ADCC effect is unknown.

COMPONENTS OF THE CELL-MEDIATED REACTION

Like the antigen-antibody reactions, the T-lymphocyte–antigen reactions may be divided into three stages: the *primary* stage, the *secondary* stage, and the *tertiary* stage (Fig. 9–1).

The Primary Stage: Combination of Antigen with Specifically Sensitized T-Lymphocytes

The cell-mediated reaction is initiated by the binding of antigen with an antigen receptor on the surface of a sensitized T-lymphocyte (Chapter 7). This may occur directly or, more likely, may be mediated by macrophage-bound antigen in association with "self" determinants. There are a number of other substances that can attach to the surface of the T-lymphocyte and either activate it, e.g., mitogens, or provide a basis for its identification, e.g., sheep erythrocyte binding in an E-rosette reaction (Chapter 7). Following the reaction of antigen with a sensitized T-lymphocyte, a sequence of morphologic and biochemical events occurs that forms the secondary stage.

The Secondary Stage: Morphologic and Biochemical Reactions

The second stage of the antigen–T-lymphocyte interaction is made up of the *in vitro* manifestations of cell-mediated immunity that presumably result from the membrane perturbations established following the primary interaction of the T-lymphocyte with antigen or mitogen, and are detected indirectly through morphologic or biochemical events. The morphologic changes of lymphocytes in tissue culture consist of blast cell transformation with subsequent mitosis. Many investigators suggest that the macrophage is essential for this reaction to proceed and that cell populations depleted of these cells may be deficient in lymphoproliferative activity. The biochemical events that occur during the secondary stage are revealed by *de novo* DNA, RNA, or protein synthesis, detected by use of radiolabeled precursors. Collectively, these morphologic and biochemical changes have proved to be of considerable clinical importance, since they are used in *in vitro* measurements to assess the functional reactivity of blood lymphocytes in patients suspected of having impaired thymic-dependent immunity.

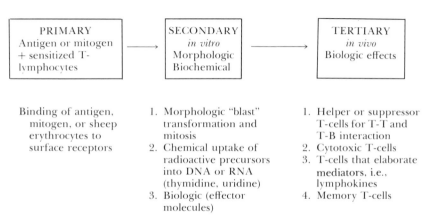

Figure 9–1. Schematic representation of cell-mediated events.

The Tertiary Stage: Biologic Expressions

The tertiary effects of cell-mediated immunity are the biologic expressions of these earlier events (Fig. 9–1). They consist of the following steps: (1) the generation of helper or suppressor T-cells for T-T and T-B interactions, including the role of macrophages; (2) the generation of cytotoxic T-cells; (3) the generation of T-cells that elaborate the effector molecules (mediators) of CMI; and (4) the generation of memory T-cells.

Thymocytes and thymus-derived lymphocytes (T-cells) are a heterogeneous population of cells. This heterogeneity is reflected in differences in organ localization, surface antigen properties, recirculation potential, and function.

T-lymphocyte development depends on the presence of a thymus. Immunocompetent cells migrate from the thymus to T-dependent areas in peripheral lymphoid tissue—the periarteriolar areas of the spleen and the deep cortical areas of the lymph nodes.

The genetic controls and immunoregulatory aspects of T-cell function in the mouse system have been described in Chapters 3 and 7, respectively. This section will focus primarily on the human T-cell–mediated immune responses.

Cell-mediated immune reactions are found to involve the sequential interactions of at least two types of thymus-derived lymphocytes (T-lymphocytes). T-lymphocytes in the mouse have been characterized by both Thy-1 (θ) antigen and a series of alloantigens termed Ly. One T-lymphocyte subpopulation bearing the Ly-1 marker responds to antigenic stimulation by proliferation and is responsible for T-lymphocyte proliferation in a mixed lymphocyte culture. A factor may then be elaborated (putatively Ia, see Chapter 3) that triggers a population of Ly-2,3-bearing T-lymphocytes. These cells mediate what has been termed cell-mediated lympholysis (CML) through a number of proposed mechanisms (lymphotoxin, for example). T-lymphocytes bearing Ly-1 markers may also produce factors such as MIF, which allows macrophages to provide additional help during an immune response against a tumor or tissue graft.

For ease of discussion, the cellular events that make up the tertiary stage of CMI in the human following interaction of antigen with T-lymphocytes are shown in Figure 9–2. T-helper/inducer (T_H) cells play a central role along with macrophages in providing positive signals for a number of cells that are involved in the expression of cell-mediated immune reactions. Initiation of cell-mediated immune reactions requires an antigen-presenting (processing) cell such as the macrophage. Other specialized cells, such as dendritic cells or cutaneous Langerhans cells, that are part of or related to the monocyte-macrophage lineage may also subserve this function. Initially, macrophages activate the small number of T-helper lymphocytes ($T4^+$) that possess receptors for the antigen in question by presenting the antigen to the T-cells in conjunction with "self-recognition" molecules (Ia). Activated T-helper cells elaborate lymphokines, some of which activate macrophages and also recruit other lymphocytes and monocytes-macrophages to participate in the reaction. Activated macrophages produce monokines, some of which are necessary for T-cell activation and induction of inflammation. Thus, a reaction that initially involves a small number of sensitized cells can be amplified and expanded to include a large number of cells that are not sensitized to the antigen that initiated the reaction.

Macrophages liberate interleukin-1, a monokine that seems identical to leukocyte pyrogen (the cause of febrile reactions) and is required for activation of T-helper lymphocytes. The later cells elaborate IL-2 and, together with IL-1, bring about the differentiation of the TDTH ($T4^+$) cells. The T_{DTA} cell activated by antigen and IL-1 then releases a series of molecules that can enhance the function of macrophages. One such factor(s) is macrophage activation factor (MAF); this may in fact be an activity due to multiple molecules, one of which seems to be γ interferon. When the macrophages are activated, they secreted not only interleukin-1 but also a series of enzymes (neutral proteases, e.g., colagenase and elastase) that can digest connective tissue, procoagulant molecules (tissue factor and factor VII) that can cause local coagulation via the extrinsic coagulation pathway, and a plasminogen activator. This last enzyme converts plasminogen to plasmin, and plasmin will digest fibrin and thereby slowly reverse clot formation. Fibrin is deposited at sites of DTH and an intermediate degradaton produce, "fibrinoid," is found in increased amounts in connective tissue diseases. Release of other lymphokines, such as

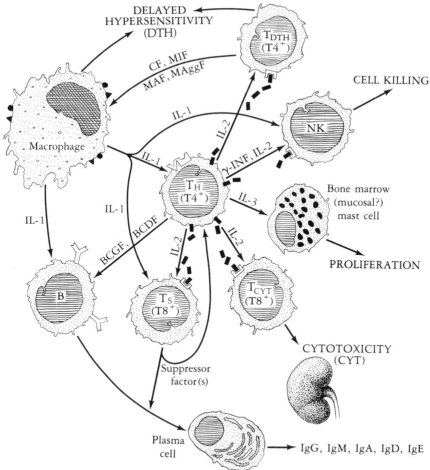

DELAYED
HYPERSENSITIVITY
(DTH)

CELL KILLING

CYTOTOXICITY
(CYT)

PROLIFERATION

Bone marrow
(mucosal?)
mast cell

Plasma
cell

IgG, IgM, IgA, IgD, IgE

Figure 9–2. Cellular events that make up the tertiary stage of CMI in the human, illustrating the central role of the T-cell in the immunoregulatory network.

macrophage chemotactic factor (CF), recruits the cells to the site of reaction, while migration inhibition factor (MIF) immobilizes macrophages and tends to localize them in the vicinity of the immune reaction. Release of another factor, a macrophage aggregation factor (MAggF), facilitates their adherence to each other. The latter factor appears to be fibronectin or fragments derived therefrom. Interleukin-2 (IL-2) is required for the proliferation of certain subpopulations of lymphocytes. IL-2 released by the T-helper cell interacts with an IL-2 receptor on T-suppressor cells (T8$^+$) and, in conjunction with IL-1, activates them. The T$_s$ cell regulates both T- and B-cells functions, usually by means of suppressor factors that block the activity of T-helper cells and the differentiation of B-cells into plasma cells. Also contained within the T8$^+$ subpopulation is a cytotoxic T-cell (T$_{CYT}$), whose function in cell-mediated immune reactions is that of transplant rejection and destruction of tumor cells.

The names "helper" and "suppressor" for these lymphocyte subpopulations refer in part to their role in the maturation and proliferation of B-cells to form antibody-secreting plasma cells (Chapter 7). The helper cell elaborates factors (B-cell growth factor [BCGF] and B-cell differentiation factor [BCDF], which facilitate differentiation of B-cells and secretion of antibody, while the suppressor cell produces factors that inhibit antibody formation. A proper balance between help and suppression appears necessary for regulation of all the immunoglobulin isotypes (IgG, IgM, IgA, IgD, and IgE). In some systems, IL-1 may also be required for B-cell activation. Once differentiation into a plasma cell has occurred, immunoglobulin synthesis proceeds.

Certain other lymphocyte functions have recently been shown to be mediated by lymphokines. For example, natural killer cells are lymphocytes that can kill target tissues, such as tumor cells, in the absence of antibody (killer function). Gamma interferon has been shown to promote the activity of these cells. There is also a third interleukin, IL-3, whose function in lymphocyte proliferation is as yet unclear. However, this molecule appears to stimulate the proliferation of bone marrow mast cells. The latter group of cells appears to populate mucosal lining tissue and represents a subpopulation of mast cells that differs from those usually identified within tissue.

EFFECTOR MOLECULES OF CELL-MEDIATED REACTIONS

Following the interaction of a sensitized lymphocyte with antigen, the lymphocyte is capable of elaborating an array of diverse substances. These factors have recently been shown to possess a variety of biologic activities that are thought to be the *in vitro* correlates of cell-mediated immunity. The physical and biologic activities of these effector molecules

Table 9–2. Products of Activated Lymphocytes

I. **Mediators Affecting Macrophages**
   (a) migration inhibitory factor (MIF)
   (b) macrophage activating factor
   (c) macrophage aggregation factor (? same as MIF)
   (d) factor causing disappearance of macrophage from perioneum (? same as MIF)
   (e) chemotactic factor for macrophages
   (f) antigen-dependent MIF
II. **Mediators Affecting Neutrophil Leukocytes**
   (a) chemotactic factor
   (b) leukocyte inhibitory factor (LIF)
III. **Mediators Affecting Lymphocytes**
   (a) mitogenic factors (Interleukin-2)
   (b) antibody enhancing factors
   (c) antibody suppressing factors
   (d) chemotactic factor
IV. **Mediators Affecting Eosinophils**
   (a) chemotactic factor*
   (b) migration stimulation factor
V. **Mediators Affecting Basophils (mast cells)**
   (a) chemotactic augmentation factor
   (b) histamine releasing factor
   (c) interleukin-3
VI. **Other Cells**
   (a) cytotoxic factors—lymphotoxin
   (b) growth inhibitory factors
      (1) clonal inhibitory factor
      (2) proliferation inhibitory factor
   (c) osteoclast activating factor (OAF)
VII. **Immunoglobulin Binding Factor**
VIII. **Procoagulant Activity**
IX. **Skin Reactive Factor**
X. **Interferon**
XI. **Immunoglobulin**

---

*Requires antigen-antibody complexes.

are shown in Tables 9–2 and 9–3. The knowledge of these effector molecules "has liberated immunologists from the firm, red bump" and allowed a better understanding of the dynamics of the *in vivo* reaction.

Transfer Factor

Following the *in vitro* interaction of the sensitized lymphocyte with its specific antigen, a substance is released that has the capacity to transfer delayed hypersensitivity to another nonreactive individual. This substance is referred to as transfer factor and has been described in the human and in primates. Lysates containing transfer factor are produced by freezing and thawing blood leukocytes. Both a dialyzable and a nondialyzable transfer factor have been identified. The dialyzable transfer factor has a molecular weight of less than 10,000, is stable at 37°C, and is resistant to treatment with DNase, RNase, and trypsin. The nondialyzable factor has not been well characterized. Transfer factor is immunologically specific; i.e., it will confer reactivity only toward the antigen that caused the factor to be generated initially. For example, transfer factor produced from the interaction of tuberculin with tuberculin-positive cells will confer the ability to react only with tuberculin, not with any other antigen. Transfer factor also has been shown to be capable of mediating homograft (skin) immunity.

Migration Inhibitory Factor

Migration inhibitory factor (MIF) inhibits the migration of normal macrophages *in vitro*. When cells from a peritoneal exudate of animals are put into a capillary tube, the macrophages migrate peripherally from the end of the tube. If one adds to the medium small quantities of antigen to which the animal exhibits CMI, the macrophages fail to migrate from the tube. This phenomenon, referred to as migration inhibition, is the *in vitro* assay for the substance migration inhibitory factor. This phenomenon has also been observed in humans; it is not species-specific and can be produced by antigen or mitogen stimulation of lymphocytes. The MIF generated by human lymphocytes, for example, can inhibit the migration of guinea pig macrophages (Fig. 9–3). MIF has a molecular

Table 9–3. Physical and Biologic Properties of Effector Molecules of Cell-Mediated Immunity*

	Molecular Weight	Physical Properties	Activities	
			In vitro	In vivo
Transfer factor(s)	<10,000 ?	Heat labile; (a) dialyzable polypeptide (b) nondialyzable	Mediator production Lymphocyte transformation	Transfer of reactivity to uncommitted lymphocytes
MIF (macrophage activating factor)	25,000–55,000	Heat stable; nondialyzable protein	Prevents random migration of macrophages; may activate macrophages	May lead to accumulation of macrophages; may increase phagocytosis and killing
Leukocyte inhibitory factor	68,000	Protein	Prevents migration of PMN's	Untested
Lymphotoxin(s)	25,000–150,000	Heat labile; nondialyzable protein	Target cell injury	May destroy target cells
Skin-reactive factor(s)	70,000			Localized cutaneous reaction
Chemotactic factors	12,000–60,000	Heat stable; nondialyzable protein	Attracts macrophages; attracts PMN's	Untested
Mitogenic factors	25,000	Heat stable; nondialyzable protein	Nonspecific lymphocyte transformation	Untested
Interferons	25,000–100,000	Heat stable; nondialyzable	Inhibits viral replication	Inhibits viral replication
Antibody	160,000	Heat stable; nondialyzable	Reactive with antigen	Varied

—— Involving thymic-dependent (T) lymphocytes,

– – – Involving thymic-independent (B) lymphocytes.

*Additional factors with undefined physical-chemical properties are listed in Table 9–2.

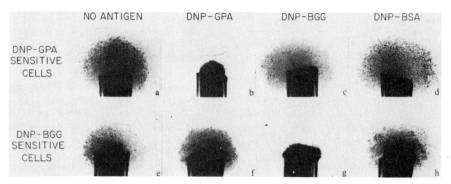

Figure 9–3. Inhibition of macrophage migration. *a–d*, Peritoneal exudate cells (macrophages and lymphocytes) from a guinea pig exhibiting delayed hypersensitivity to DNP coupled to guinea pig albumin (DNP-GPA). Migration of macrophages from the capillary tube has been inhibited (*b*) only by the immunizing antigen, not by DNP coupled to BSA (bovine serum albumin) or BGG (bovine gamma globulin). *e–h*, Cells from an animal exhibiting delayed hypersensitivity to DNP coupled to BGG. Again, this is the only antigen that inhibits migration. The experiment demonstrates the role of the carrier protein in determining the specificity of this *in vitro* correlate of delayed hypersensitivity. (From David, J. R., Lawrence, H. S., and Thomas, L.: J. Immunol., *93*:280, 1964.)

weight estimated to range from 25,000 to 55,000; is destroyed by trypsin and neuraminidase, but not by DNase or RNase; and is stable when heated to 56°C for 30 minutes. Guinea pig and human MIF have properties of an acidic glycoprotein.

MIF may be important *in vivo* as a substance that contains macrophages to the area of injury. It might also be involved in the formation of granulomatous lesions and those infectious diseases in which cell-mediated immunity and mononuclear infiltration are prominent features, e.g., the tuberculoma or tubercle granuloma. There is also evidence that MIF-rich fluids may alter morphology of macrophages, increase their ability to stick to glass surfaces, and augment their capacity to kill certain bacteria. Therefore, MIF, or some similar factor, may profoundly alter the functional capacity of macrophages, the net outcome of which has been termed "macrophage activation."

Lymphotoxin

Lymphotoxin (LT) is the term for a series of molecules (alpha, beta, gamma) liberated from specifically sensitized lymphocytes or nonspecific stimulants such as phytohemagglutinin (PHA). Lymphotoxin seems to be associated with target-cell injury and inhibits the capacity of cells to divide (Fig. 9–4). They have a molecular weight range between 25,000 and 150,000; are heat stable; and resist RNase, DNase, and trypsin but are destroyed by chymotrypsin. The biologic role of this mediator is unknown, but the obvious possibility exists that it destroys cells directly.

Skin-Reactive Factor

This material is also produced by the interaction of specifically sensitized lymphocytes with antigen and mitogens. When introduced into the skin of normal guinea pigs, skin-reactive factor or factors produce an indurated and erythematous lesion within three hours. The lesion reaches its peak at 10 hours and disappears by 30 hours. The histologic picture of the lesion is similar to that produced in the delayed-type cutaneous lesion. Its biologic activity may well be the sum of the factors described above.

Chemotactic Factors

Several chemotactic factors have been described that are released from the reaction of specific antigen with sensitized lymphocytes and can also be generated by nonspecific mitogens. One factor induces chemotactic migration of macrophages or monocytes; other factors are selectively chemotactic for neutrophils, eosinophils, and basophils. These substances have molecular weights ranging from 12,000 to 60,000.

Mitogenic Factor (Blastogenic Factor)

When sensitized lymphocytes are stimulated with specific antigen, a substance is released with the capacity to cause non-specific blast cell transformation and increase tritiated thymidine uptake. This factor has a molecular weight of 25,000 and, together with transfer factor, may be important in

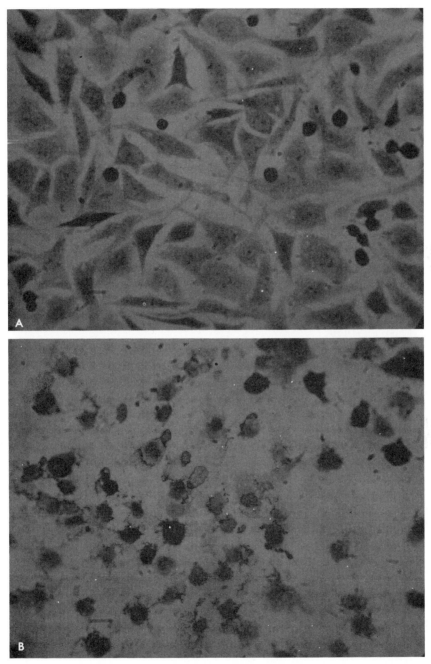

Figure 9–4. The effect of lymphotoxin on target cells. *A*, Control monolayer of L-strain fibroblasts. *B*, A similar monolayer after 24 hours of reaction with the supernatant from activated human lymphocytes that contained lymphotoxin. Extensive cell death is apparent. (Courtesy of Dr. G. A. Granger.)

augmenting or amplifying the cell-mediated response by recruiting uncommitted lymphocytes. This factor may be identical to the recently described interleukin-2, which causes proliferation of T-cells.

Interferons

The interferons are a group of substances whose approximate molecular weight ranges from 25,000 to 100,000. They are produced in cells following viral infection (nonimmune or α- and β-interferon). They are also released from sensitized lymphocytes (immune or γ-interferon) upon interaction with specific antigens and nonspecific stimulators such as PHA. These factors are known to be important effector molecules, significant not only in the recovery mechanisms of viral infections but also involved in immunoregulatory processes, including the activation of natural killer (NK) cells. The substances are particularly well suited to cell-mediated responses involving viral interactions *in vivo*.

Antibody

Antibody may also be released following interaction of antigen with specifically sensitized B-lymphocytes; however, it is not known whether antibody is produced by the same cells that elaborate MIF and other mediators. The role of antibody has been presented in previous chapters. Its function may be to augment the cell-mediated responses in a variety of ways, e.g., ADCC reactions.

Cell Types Elaborating Mediators

Studies in animals indicate that thymus-derived (T) lymphocytes are responsible for producing soluble mediators. The recent availability of methods to purify lymphocyte subpopulations with almost complete recovery of cells has permitted further investigation into the basis for antigen-induced lymphocyte activation. By use of purified populations, it has been shown that both T- and B-cells proliferate in response to mitogens such as PHA, Con-A, and pokeweed, but only T-cells proliferate directly in response to antigen. Both T- and B-cells produce MIF, chemotactic factor, and interferon in response to specific antigen or mitogens.

However, only T-cells produce lymphocyte mitogenic factor or interleukin-2.

Although the production of lymphocyte mediators may correlate with the presence of cell-mediated immunity, it is clear that these factors are not solely products of activated T-cells.

Lymphocyte-Macrophage Interactions

A surprising number of lymphocyte functions appear to be based upon low molecular weight substances. A small number of sensitized lymphocytes (effector cells) could amplify the total response by the recruitment of larger numbers of uncommitted cells (transfer factor, mitogenic factor). The elaboration of lymphotoxin could destroy unwanted foreign cells; the attraction of macrophages and polymorphonuclear leukocytes could be accomplished through the action of chemotactic factors; and interferon could be of particular value in inhibiting the replication of viruses. Finally, the role of antibody could participate in several of the antigen-antibody reactions or in ADCC reactions.

SUMMARY

Cell-mediated immunity includes those manifestations of the specific immune response expressed by a variety of cells and cell products. The hallmarks of these reactions, which differentiate them from humoral antigen-antibody reactions, are their delayed onset, the requirement for living lymphocytes or their products to elicit the response, and the recently discovered effector molecules with relatively low molecular weights, which appear to be the *in vitro* correlates of the *in vivo* response. This type of immunologic mechanism appears to be particularly well suited to antigens that are cell-bound or in other ways inaccessible to the antibody mechanism.

IN VIVO EXPRESSIONS

The *in vivo* manifestations of the immune response are a continuum consisting of the interactions of the host with all foreign macromolecular substances (immunogens) and include all the possible expressions of the immune response appropriate for the type of stimulus. The separation of these responses into "harmful" and "helpful" expressions of the immune response is artificial, since the total spectrum of the immune response is available for the disposal of a foreign substance. The types of *in vivo* expressions that are available are shown in Figure 9–5. They consist of phagocytosis, the inflammatory response, and those responses mediated by products of the specific immune response, antibody and cell-mediated immunity. The host response depends on whether the encounter is *initial* or a *repeat*.

The Body's First Encounter with Antigen

If a material is a particulate substance, such as a bacterium or a virus, the body will attempt to eliminate it by phagocytosis. Since this is the first encounter, there is no pre-existing antibody (opsonins) to facilitate engulfment. The fate of the disposal is decided by the efficiency of the unenhanced phago-

cytic process. If processing is successful, the material is eliminated and disease symptoms are not seen or are minimal. This is represented schematically in Figure 9–5. The specific immune response is induced to elaborate cells capable of antibody production or cell-mediated events (Fig. 9–5). Subsequent encounter with the same material will result in an enhanced efficiency of this process (see below). This is shown schematically in Figure 9–5 and represents the elimination of all exogenous antigens (bacterial organisms, viruses, and particulate matter) as well as altered or dead self components (effete red blood cells).

Phagocytosis may be unsuccessful because of the quantity or physical characteristics of the material or the general condition (health) of the host. For example, many encapsulated bacterial organisms (pneumococcus) escape engulfment because of the smoothness of the capsule. Other organisms may be engulfed but survive within the phagocyte (e.g., tubercle bacillus). In either event, active disease or death can occur (Fig. 9–5). The outcome of the disease is then determined by the effi-

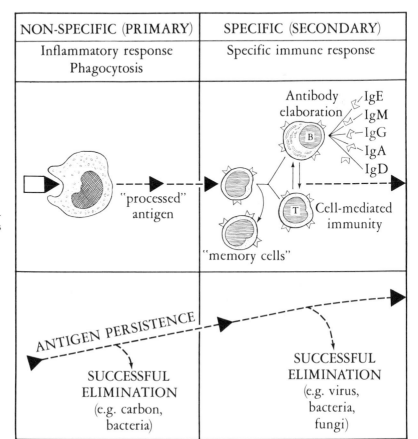

Figure 9–5. Schematic representation of the *in vivo* expressions of the immune responses.

ciency of the specific immune response, both antibody production and cell-mediated immunity. After the appearance of antibody, which with complement facilitates the uptake of an encapsulated organism, the phagocytes successfully destroy the disease-producing organism. Further, with the appearance of cell-mediated immunity and the elaboration of the effector molecules (MIF, mitogenic factor, and so on), phagocytosis by macrophages is enhanced, with elimination of organisms in this fashion.

Subsequent Encounters

All subsequent encounters of the host with a foreign substance lead to the same events described previously, except that the responses are greatly enhanced. Because of rapid recall, there is an increased number of cells involved in antibody production or in cell-mediated events resulting in products of the specific immune response. These processes, either alone or in concert with phagocytosis, expedite the elimination of the unwanted material (Fig. 9–5). However, even a subsequent encounter may be unsuccessful because of the general condition of the host, e.g., underlying disease, immunosuppressive therapy, or an overwhelming dose of challenge inoculum. The efficiency with which the immune response can dispose of foreign antigens determines whether the outcome will be beneficial or harmful. If antigen is successfully removed or eliminated by the more primitive responses of phagocytosis and inflammatory response, with or without enhancement by the specific immune response, then the outcome will be beneficial. If antigen cannot be eliminated, the more deleterious, devastating effects of the immune response (tertiary immune response) occur, manifested as the immunologically mediated diseases of man.

Summary

The *in vivo* manifestations of the immune response may be viewed as the total capacity of the host recognition system to dispose of foreign substances (antigens). These include the primitive responses of phagocytosis and inflammatory responses, which can dispose of most foreign substances. In the case of pathogens that have assumed virulent characteristics to evade these responses, a more sophisticated secondary system, the specific immune response, can lead to products that facilitate or enhance these primitive responses. The products include the elaboration of antibody or cell-mediated events that can effect disposal of the antigen, either alone or in concert with the more primitive responses. The outcome of this encounter of the host with a foreign configuration will be either beneficial or harmful, depending upon the efficiency with which the foreign substance can be eliminated.

Suggestions for Further Reading

Bloom, B. R., and Glade, P. R. (eds.): In Vitro Methods in Cell-Mediated Immunity. New York, Academic Press, 1971.

David, J. R., and David, R. R.: Cellular hypersensitivity and immunity: inhibition of macrophage migration and the lymphocyte mediators. Progr. Allergy, *16*:300, 1972.

Edelman, G. M. (ed.): Cellular Selection and Regulation in the Immune Response. New York, Raven Press, 1974.

Lawrence, H. S.: Transfer factor. Adv. Immunol., *11*:195, 1969.

Rocklin, R. E.: Clinical applications of in-vitro lymphocyte tests. Progr. Clin. Immunol., *2*:21, 1974.

Rose, N. R., and Friedman, H. (eds.): Manual of Clinical Immunology. Washington, D.C. American Society for Microbiology, 1980.

Williams, R. C., Jr., (ed.): Lymphocytes and Their Interactions. Kroc Foundation Series. Vol. 4. New York, Raven Press, 1975.

Chapter 10

Immunomodulation: Immunopotentiation, Tolerance, and Immunosuppression

Paul Katz, M.D.

The immune network in man involves a complex series of interrelated and mutually regulatory events. Under optimal conditions, that is, in the absence of certain diseases or pharmacologic agents, this scheme functions efficiently to rid the host of "foreign" configurations (e.g., microorganisms, tumors) while sparing native antigen-bearing tissues (i.e., "self"-antigens). In instances of disordered immunoregulation, the host may be unable to mount an immune response sufficient to eliminate detrimental antigens, resulting in widespread infection or malignancy, for example. Conversely, host responses may become aberrant and tissues bearing "self"-antigens may be incorrectly perceived as being foreign. Such circumstances would favor the development of the so-called autoimmune diseases.

Either intentionally or unintentionally, normal homeostatic responses may be modified by intrinsic alterations in the immune network or by exogenous influences. As noted previously, potentiation or suppression of immune responses may be either detrimental or beneficial. In some cases, immunomodulation is a desirable and often obtainable goal, while in other situations it must be combated in order to prevent undesirable and potentially life-threatening effects.

For ease of discussion, immunomodulation may be broadly defined as the overall regulation of immune responsiveness, which includes both *immunopotentiation* ("up-regulation") and *immunosuppression* ("down-regulation"). Further, we will examine tolerance, that is, the state of immunologic unresponsiveness.

IMMUNOPOTENTIATION

Immunopotentiation refers to the specific or nonspecific enhancement of immune responsiveness. This augmentation can be intrinsic, that is, arising from within the host, or extrinsic and secondary to exogenous influences. The overall potentiation of the immune response may occur by an alteration in any one of the many steps involved in the host's immunologic reactions. Thus, a given potentiator may increase an immunologic event by (1) shortening the "latent" time for the response to become manifest; (2) augmenting the overall "level" or "height" of a given response; (3) lengthening the duration of the response; (4) delaying the cessation of the response; or (5) developing a new response to a previously nonstimulatory antigen.

Immunopotentiation can occur in both the classic humoral and the cell-mediated immune systems. It is noteworthy, however, that a substance capable of enhancing a response in one system may be suppressive in the other system. Therefore, the overall biologic effects of a given response-modifying factor must be viewed as the sum total of potentially divergent reactions.

The concept of immunopotentiation has become increasingly important in recent years, particularly in regard to enhancing

Table 10–1. Nonspecific Immune Potentiators

Water and oil emulsions (e.g., Freund's adjuvant)
Microorganisms (e.g., BCG)
Microorganism components (e.g., lipopolysaccharides, endotoxin)
Synthetic polynucleotides (e.g., polyinosinic-polycytidylic acid)
Lymphokines (e.g., migration inhibitory factor, interferon)
Pharmacologic agent (e.g., levamisole)

responses against tumors and infectious agents above that which could be expected by exposure to the tumor or the infectious agent alone.

Compounds capable of augmenting immunologic reactivity may be divided into two classes: (1) *nonspecific* or *general* immune enhancers, which increase humoral and cell-mediated responses to a multitude of widely differing antigens; and (2) *specific* potentiators, which increase a restricted group of immune responses to an equally restricted group of antigens. Both of these classes will be examined.

Table 10–1 lists some of the nonspecific immune potentiators. These substances, often referred to as adjuvants, probably differ in their modes of action, yet their net responses are often comparable. Although the means by which these nonspecific stimulators exert their biologic effects remain elusive, one can postulate several potential mechanisms. The biologic half-life of a given antigen could be prolonged. Such is the case with the classic adjuvant, Freund's adjuvant, a mixture of oil and killed mycobacteria. Although prohibited for human use owing to the induction of granulomas, complete Freund's adjuvant, when administered with antigen, can markedly enhance the immune responses of animals to that antigen, in part secondary to a prolonged release of the antigen. Substances such as aluminum hydroxide and alum have shown comparable results, presumably related to the increased antigenic half-life.

These agents could also induce their biologic effects by attracting or activating immunocompetent cells at the site of the antigen. Such is probably the case for the lymphokines, the collective term applied to that group of antigen-induced, soluble, mononuclear cell–derived substances reviewed in Chapter 9. Likewise, complete Freund's adjuvant, as evidenced by its propensity to induce granulomas, can recruit immunoreactive cells.

Immune potentiators could induce the proliferation, differentiation, and activation of immunoregulatory cells. Such is clearly the case with nonspecific mitogenic substances such as lipopolysaccharide, endotoxin, and many of the lymphokines.

These substances could also exert a variety of effects on the metabolic pathways of cells involved in the immune response. Many of these agents, for example, are known to alter the intracellular concentrations of the cyclic nucleotides, cyclic adenosine monophosphate (cAMP) and cyclic guanosine monophosphate (cGMP). Considerable data have accrued indicating that cAMP or its intracellular inducers are capable of inactivating suppressor T-lymphocytes, with a resultant boost in antibody formation. Additionally, the increased intracellular cGMP:cAMP ratio noted after *in vitro* interferon treatment may account for the enhanced natural killer (NK) cell activity induced by this agent by increasing the release of lysosomal enzymes. These potential mechanisms of nonspecific induction and augmentation of immune responses are listed in Table 10–2.

Of the nonspecific immune potentiators, perhaps the best studied has been the attenuated strain of *Mycobacterium bovis*, bacille Calmette-Guérin (BCG). After the observation that tuberculous patients appeared to be relatively resistant to the development of certain other types of infections, a possible role as adjuvant was ascribed to the mycobacteria. Early animal studies suggested that BCG administration could induce the regression of transplanted tumors if the host were immunocompetent. Subsequent studies in man and continued studies in animal models have suggested numerous possible mechanisms by which immunopotentiation could occur. Included among these are: (1) activation of the reticuloendothelial system; (2) induction of lymphokine production by mononuclear cells, resulting in the attraction and activation of immunocompetent lymphoid cells; (3) stimulation of NK-cells; (4) cross-reactivity

Table 10–2. Potential Mechanisms of Action of Nonspecific Immunopotentiators

Prolongation of antigenic half-life
Attraction and/or activation of immunocompetent cells
Proliferation and/or differentiation of immunocompetent cells
Modulation of intrinsic metabolic pathways of immunocompetent cells

between tumor antigens and BCG, inducing an immune response against common antigenic determinants; and (5) increased susceptibility of tumor cells to destruction.

BCG has found some usefulness in the treatment of human malignancies, most notably malignant melanoma (Chapter 19). Although not without risk, BCG therapy may be valuable in certain clinical situations, particularly those in which other forms of therapy are also utilized.

Corynebacterium parvum is an anaerobic gram-positive bacillary organism that also has immunopotentiating capabilities. Used as a heat-killed suspension, *C. parvum* increases tumor resistance in animals, prevents the growth of established tumors, and diminishes the frequency of metastatic disease. As with BCG, the precise mechanism by which this organism augments immune responses is unclear; however, the ability of macrophages to phagocytose and kill is markedly enhanced. Paradoxically, some T-cell responses are depressed, including mitogen-induced proliferation and other blastogenesis-dependent processes, while B-cell activity is either normal or increased. Conceivably, *C. parvum* may act on various effector limbs of the immune response with an overall enhancement of immune reactivity favoring antitumor effects.

The synthetic polynucleotides, such as polyinosinic-polycytidylic acid (poly I:C) and polyadenylic-polyuridylic acid (poly A:U) have also demonstrated nonspecific immunoenhancing capabilities. Werner Braun very elegantly demonstrated that these agents could augment multiple aspects of the immune response. In particular, they increase antigen-specific antibody formation to a variety of antigens. Other effects have been demonstrated on helper T cell—mediated stimulation of B-cell responses and delayed-type hypersensitivity reactions. A direct B-cell effect has been reported, most likely mediated by changes in cyclic nucleotide concentrations. A considerable body of accumulated evidence has demonstrated that these agents can boost NK responses through their ability to induce interferon production by NK-cells.

As noted earlier, the lymphokines can potentiate immune reactivity. These compounds and their capabilities are reviewed in Chapter 9.

Of the pharmacologic agents with immunoenhancing capabilities, perhaps levamisole is the most exciting. This anthelmintic agent has been demonstrated to increase tumor resistance in certain animal models, perhaps through stimulatory action on macrophages and T-cells. Interestingly, this agent has shown promise in the treatment of diseases characterized by excessive immunologic activity, such as rheumatoid arthritis and systemic lupus erythematosus. It is quite possible that this agent eventually will be found to affect multiple limbs of the immune network.

Although agents that nonspecifically augment the immune response form the bulk of the immunopotentiators, there are some antigen-specific immunoenhancing compounds. Included in this group are the immunogenic RNAs and tranfer factor.

RNA obtained from murine or rabbit mononuclear cells has been shown to transfer specific antigenic responsiveness to an animal not exposed to that antigen. Subsequent studies have yielded considerable conflicting data, and it is not yet clear what the role of immune RNA is as an immune potentiator. RNA extracted from mononuclear cells of tumor-bearing animals reduced the tumor load in other tumor-bearing animals. Further work is clearly indicated in this area.

Transfer factor is a less than 10,000 molecular weight, dialyzable, cell-free extract of immune lymphocytes that can transfer cell-mediated immune responses from antigen-responsive to antigen-nonresponsive individuals. The activity transferred is antigen-specific, and a generalized immunoenhancement is usually reported. The original experiments using transfer factor demonstrated transfer of cutaneous reactivity to purified protein derivative (PPD) from a PPD-positive donor to a PPD-negative one.

Transfer factor is probably a heterogeneous group of compounds of T-cell origin that act on multiple different populations of T-cells. The factor is DNAase-resistant, dialyzable, and heat-sensitive. Although its mechanism(s) of action is unclear, transfer factor may induce lymphocyte proliferation, soluble mediator production and release, and the recruitment of immunocompetent cells. Conceivably, part of the effects of this agent could be secondary to adjuvant-like characteristics. Most clinical studies to date have employed transfer factor in the therapy of immunodeficient states, malignancies, and certain infectious diseases. These trials have met with varying degrees of success and failure, but, unfortunately, it is unlikely that transfer factor will be the hoped-for panacea to convey antigen-specific cell-mediated immunity.

SUPPRESSION OF IMMUNE RESPONSIVENESS

Just as it is necessary to potentiate the immune response in some instances, it becomes necessary at other times to benefit the host by manipulating the immunologic system in a negative way so that it cannot respond to the presence of a foreign configuration or, at best, will have a diminished response to it. As in the case of immunopotentiation, negative manipulation can affect both specific and nonspecific responses and collectively comes under the general heading of *unresponsiveness*. *Immunologic tolerance* is a form of specific unresponsiveness and may be defined as the inability to respond to a specific antigenic stimulation, based upon an immature or incompetent immunologic system, the genetic constitution of the host, or the properties of the antigen. *Immunosuppression* comes under the heading of nonspecific unresponsiveness, refers to the artificial prevention or diminution of expression of immune response, and involves a more generalized form of unresponsiveness.

Immunologic Tolerance: Historical Aspects

Implicit in all previous discussions of immunity is the fundamental ability of the immunologic system to differentiate "self" from "nonself." The idea that the body should never react with its own tissues was clearly enunciated by Ehrlich in his dogma "horror autotoxicus." One of the first challenges to this dogma came from the brilliant observations of Owen, who in 1945 demonstrated that each of nonidentical twin calves derived from two separate ova frequently shared two sets of red cells in their circulation, one set of its own, the other from its twin. This state is referred to as *mosaicism* or *chimerism*. Owen correctly assumed that this state of chimerism resulted from the well-known finding in such twin cattle of a common placental circulation that allowed the exchange of hematopoietic elements from one twin to the other early in fetal life. Paradoxically, if these same cells were introduced into the calf at a later time, they would lead to an immunologic response and their prompt rejection and destruction.

The second set of observations that challenged the classic dogmas of immunology were made in the late 1940s by Medawar, who used specifically inbred strains of mice. If, for example, one obtains two strains of mice, A and B (A with white skin, B with black), A will accept skin grafts from another A mouse but not from a mouse of the B strain; similarly, a B mouse will accept a graft from another B mouse but not from a mouse of the A strain (Fig. 10–1). However, when lymphoreticular cells of strain B were introduced into mice of strain A, the recipients treated were capable of accepting skin grafts from mice of strain B (Fig. 10–1). Medawar termed this effect "specific immune tolerance."

Once these observations were connected, further studies showed other ways to induce tolerance. The inoculation of embryos or young animals with antigens, for example, failed to elicit an immune response. Additional experiments showed that these animals actually became tolerant to the antigen with which the immature immune system had come in contact. In older animals, moreover, repeated high doses of certain antigens appeared to have a similar effect.

IMMUNOLOGIC TOLERANCE

Immunologic tolerance, a state of immunologic unresponsiveness, may, in many respects, be viewed as a form of immunosuppression. Strictly speaking, tolerance has been the term applied to that state in which exposure to an *immunogen* (an antigen capable of normally inducing immune reactivity) does not result in an immune response and appears to be secondary to a loss of immunoresponsive cell clones prior to their interaction with antigen. Under these circumstances, a "foreign" antigen is perceived in the same manner as a "self"-antigen and no response against that *specific* antigen is mounted. Tolerance should be viewed as antigen-specific, that is, tolerance to one antigen does not imply tolerance to all others.

Pseudotolerance or *immunologic paralysis* refers to that state in which antigen-responsive cells are present, but antigenic concentration is high enough that the binding to and neutralization of the antibodies formed occur. In this state, it seems reasonable to assume that persistent synthesis and elimination of antibody would also result in dissipation of the inciting antigen and a reduction in the pseudotolerant state. This situation is obviously quite distinct from true tolerance, in which the cells and their products needed to participate in the immunologic reaction are not available.

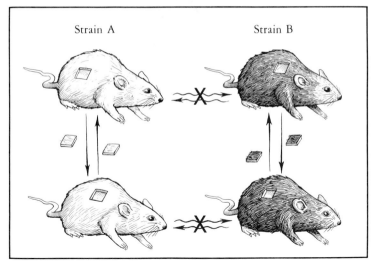

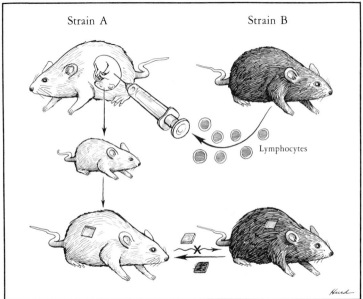

Figure 10–1. Representation of Medawar's experiment illustrating the fetal induction of tolerance in the mouse.

The induction of immunologic tolerance is dependent upon a variety of host and antigenic factors (Table 10–3). Immunologic immaturity greatly favors the development of tolerance, particularly in animal models, as described previously. Once an antigen-specific response has started, tolerance induction becomes progressively more difficult. In these circumstances, tolerance can be achieved by depleting the animal of antigen-reactive cells (e.g., with irradiation or anti-lymphocyte serum) and then reintroducing the antigen. Following the depletion of immunoreactive cells, the animal once again becomes immunologically naive and tolerance can be established. The ease of tolerance induction in the immature host may be, in fact, beneficial, as it enables the host to grad-ually accumulate self-antigens; the development of the tolerant state toward these antigens might then preclude autoimmune disease later in life.

Certain antigenic characteristics influence tolerance. For example, the physical state of gamma globulins in part determines their tolerogenicity. Aggregation of molecules favors immunogenicity, whereas monomers

Table 10–3. Factors Affecting the Development of Tolerance

Immunologic immaturity
Characteristics of antigen—physical state, complexity, persistence, distribution, etc.
Dose of antigen
Route of antigen administration
Genetic factors

more frequently evoke tolerance. Figure 10–2 shows how aggregated human gamma globulin (HGG) induces antibody formation by mouse spleen cells, whereas disaggregated HGG does not elicit an antibody response.

The complexity of antigenic structure also affects tolerogenicity. Substances of simple configuration equilibrate well between intra- and extravascular spaces and persist for some time. This is particularly true for simple antigens borne on replicating cells, where antigen persistence is readily achieved.

The dose of the antigen can likewise alter immunogenicity. As depicted in Figure 10–3, there is a certain dose of an antigen that will elicit a maximal antibody response. *Low-dose tolerance* is induced by antigens below the concentration for optimal responses. These low antigen concentrations may induce tolerance by an effect primarily on T-cells. Few antigens appear to be capable of producing low-zone tolerance. *High-dose tolerance* occurs when the dose of antigen is greater than optimal. This may be mediated by both a T- and a B-cell effect.

The route of administration also appears to be critical in determining immunogenicity and tolerogenicity. Soluble antigens administered intradermally with adjuvants induce antibody formation and cell-mediated immune responses. Conversely, intravenous inoculation favors tolerance, perhaps because of the high concentration of antigen achieved by this route.

Genetic factors may impair or enhance immune responsiveness. Studies in animal models have demonstrated that certain strains can be more easily tolerized than other strains.

It is apparent that T- and B-cell tolerance are separate and distinct. Induction of tolerance occurs more rapidly, persists longer, and requires less antigen in T-cells than in B-cells. It should be noted that apparent B-cell tolerance can be elicited by T-dependent antigens. Such antigens require T-cell help to provide the appropriate "signal" to B-cells to induce antibody formation. Tolerance to such antigens, then, may really be T-cell tolerance rather than B-cell tolerance, with a resultant net failure of antibody production. It is probably such T-cell tolerance that protects us from most self-antigens.

Tolerance does not necessarily imply an indefinite state of immunologic unresponsiveness. Elimination of the antigen by normal catabolism will reduce the concentration to a level at which the tolerant state can no longer be perpetuated. Tolerance can likewise end by the introduction of the inciting antigen in an altered form or by the use of a cross-reactive antigen. The precise mechanism by which tolerance is halted in these cases is not entirely clear.

IMMUNOSUPPRESSION

Suppression of naturally occurring immunologic responses can be either beneficial or detrimental to the host. Immunosuppression can occur in one of several ways: (1) secondary to normal immunoregulatory mechanisms; (2) secondary to an underlying disease or as a result of disordered immunoregulation; and/or (3) secondary to exogenous factors such as pharmacologic agents.

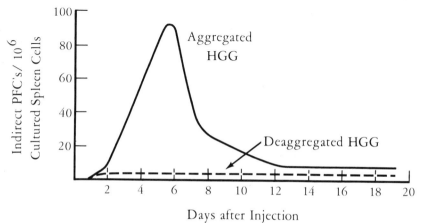

Figure 10–2. Antibody formation (plaque-forming cells, PFCs) by murine spleen cells after injection with either aggregated or deaggregated human gamma globulin (HGG). Aggregated HGG induces antibody formation, whereas deaggregated HGG is tolerogenic.

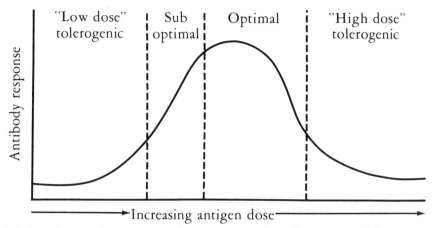

Figure 10–3. Relationship of antigen concentration to antibody formation. Low or high antigen concentrations prevent optimal antibody formation.

As discussed in the preceding sections, normal immunoregulatory mechanisms in combination with certain antigenic characteristics may induce specific immunologic unresponsiveness. This is quite obviously desirable in circumstances that prevent the immunogenicity of self-antigens. A breakdown in normal mechanisms of tolerogenicity could conceivably favor the development of autoimmune disease. It is also possible that immunosuppressive activities mediated by immunocompetent cells assist in the termination of a given immune reaction. This concept has been buoyed by the finding of naturally occurring suppressor cells in animals and man that may serve to down-regulate or modify ongoing immunologic activity. Such activities have been ascribed to various subpopulations of T-cells as well as cells of the monocyte-macrophage series, which are described more fully in Chapters 7 and 11.

It is not difficult to imagine how an overzealous suppressor network could result in or contribute to the pathogenesis of immunologic disease. In such circumstances, an overdampening of normal immune activities prevents the host from responding appropriately to specific or nonspecific signals. In 1974, Waldmann and coworkers reported a pioneering group of experiments involving the mitogen-induced B-cell responses of patients with common variable hypogammaglobulinemia (CVH). These investigators demonstrated that lymphocytes from these patients were unable to normally produce antibody *in vitro* in response to stimulation with the polyclonal B-cell activator pokeweed mitogen. Coculture of CVH lymphocytes with normal lymphocytes suppressed normal B-cell activity, indicative of excessive sup-

pressor cell function. It was determined that excessive suppressor T-cell activity was responsible for these abnormalities and that removal or inactivation of CVH suppressor T-cells abrogated these responses. Subsequently, numerous cases of excessive suppressor cell activity have been reported in a variety of immunologically mediated immunodeficiency states, infectious diseases, autoimmune disorders, and malignant states. One must be wary of extrapolating too much from the situation *in vitro* to the situation *in vivo*. Furthermore, it is often unclear whether the *in vitro* phenomenon antedates the development of the disease or merely reflects subsequent nonspecific immunologic aberrancies.

Excessive suppressor cell activity can be mediated by a specific subpopulation of T-cells. These cells have been phenotypically characterized in a number of systems as bearing Fc receptors for IgG (T-gamma cells), or as bearing antigens recognized by the OKT8 monoclonal antibody, or both. An alteration in the frequency of these cells does not necessarily imply a relative or absolute alteration in suppressive capabilities, however. Cells of the monocyte-macrophage series have also shown excessive suppressor function in such diverse diseases as multiple myeloma, sarcoidosis, Hodgkin's disease, and tuberculosis. It is quite likely that the mechanisms of T-cell suppression and monocyte suppression are distinct. Studies to better characterize these activities are currently in progress in a number of laboratories. In some instances, it has been possible to abrogate excessive immunosuppressive activity by pharmacologic agents. Such abrogation has been demonstrated with corticosteroids in sarcoidosis and with indomethacin in Hodgkin's disease. Whether the elimination of excessive suppressor influences alters immune reactivity is not defined at present.

Perhaps the greatest degree of immunosuppression that is clinically observed is that which occurs as a direct result of the treatment of an underlying condition, usually a malignant or autoimmune disorder. It should be noted that in many cases it may be difficult to distinguish between immunosuppression secondary to drug treatment and immunosuppression resulting from the primary disease.

The agents most commonly reponsible for immunosuppression today are the corticosteroids and the cytotoxic drugs.

Corticosteroids alter the immune response by their effects on leukocyte function or circulatory kinetics or both. A variety of *in vitro* studies have shown myriad effects on immunologic activity. Many of these studies, however, have employed drug concentrations that are unobtainable *in vivo*, and therefore these results are uninterpretable. Furthermore, corticosteroids can transiently induce changes in the composition of leukocytes in the intravascular space by redistributing certain cell types to extravascular compartments while limiting the egress of other cells. It should be noted that the degree of immunosuppression induced by these drugs will vary depending on the corticosteroid preparation, the dosage, and the dosage schedule.

Cytotoxic drugs have been increasingly utilized in the therapy not only of tumors but also of immunologically mediated diseases. Both by intent and by happenstance, these agents can powerfully dampen selected aspects of the immune response. In most cases, the suppression of aberrant immune responses cannot be separated from the suppression of desirable immune responses, rendering patients so treated susceptible to a variety of infectious complications.

The two agents most widely utilized to achieve immunosuppression are cyclophosphamide and azathioprine.

Other immunosuppressive agents that have been used clinically include antilymphocyte serum (ALS) and antithymocyte globulin (ATG). These antisera have been employed primarily in transplantation in the hope of preventing allograft rejection. Radiation therapy has long been used in tumor therapy and has recently been used experimentally in rheumatoid arthritis. It is probable that ionizing radiation destroys replicating cells nonspecifically and prevents the further propagation of an abnormal immune response. Cyclosporin A is a fungal metabolite recently employed in bone marrow transplantation. This agent somewhat selectively permits engraftment while preventing graft-versus-host reactions.

SUMMARY

The complicated array of interconnecting immunologic networks is obviously susceptible to augmentation and suppression. A variety of seemingly diverse innate factors, exogenous agents, and diseases can induce relative and absolute immunopotentiation or immunosuppression. This alteration in immune reactivity either may be harmful to the host or may, in fact, be a sought-after goal.

Suggestions for Further Reading

Immunopotentiation. Ciba Foundation Symposium 18. Amesterdam, Associated Scientific Publishers, 1973.

Katz, D. H., and Benacerraf, B.: The regulatory influence of activated T cells on B cell responses to antigen. Adv. Immunol., *15*:1, 1972.

Steinberg, A. D.: Immunoregulatory agents. *In* Kelley, W. N., Harris, E. D., Jr., Ruddy, S., et al. (eds.): Textbook of Rheumatology. Philadelphia, W. B. Saunders Company, 1981.

Waldmann, T. A., and Broder, S.: Suppressor cells in the regulation of the immune responses. Progr. Clin. Immunol., *3*:155, 1977.

Chapter 11

A Unifying Model for Immunologic Processes

Joseph A. Bellanti, M.D.

It may now be possible to construct a unifying model for immunologic processes based upon the various principles of the immunologic system described in Chapters 1 through 10. The model, which is an adaptation of one suggested by Talmage, will also serve as a framework for further study of immunologic mechanisms and the clinical applications of immunology. For ease of discussion, we may speak of five components of the host's encounter with foreignness: (1) *the environment,* (2) *the target cell,* (3) *the phagocytic cells,* (4) *the mediator cells* and mediator products, and (5) *the specific antigen-recognition cells* (B-lymphocytes and T-lymphocytes) and their products.

THE ENVIRONMENT

Since most substances that confront, and ultimately activate, the host's immunologic system arise from the exterior world, the place to begin in any discussion of the immunologic system is with the external environment (Fig. 11–1). Included within the external environment are the myriad foreign substances that range from the simplest of low molecular weight chemicals to the most complex microbial agents. It should also be emphasized that the immunologic system may be activated not only by foreign substances that arise from the external environment, but also by those that present from the internal environment, e.g., transplanted cells or altered self-components (virally or chemically altered or malignant cells). Those substances that have the capacity to evoke immunologic responses are referred to as *immunogens* or *antigens,* and all share the common characteristic of being recognized as *foreign* by the host (Chapter 4). Occasionally,

the encounter with a foreign configuration may lead to an inability to respond, a state that is referred to as *immunologic tolerance;* such configurations are referred to as *tolerogens* (Chapter 10). Allergens are a specialized class of immunogen and take part in hypersensitivity (allergic) reactions. Antigens may be complete and lead to an immune response *per se* (immunogens), or they may be incomplete (haptens) and require prior attachment to a carrier protein to become fully immunogenic (e.g., penicillin). As our environment becomes more complex, not only does the number of antigens increase but also the potential number of allergens to which we are exposed (Fig. 11–1). In addition to those diseases that are triggered by the effects of the immune response to an environmental agent, e.g., allergy, recent evidence suggests that a number of diseases may result from the direct toxic effects of environmental agents, e.g., heavy metals, on the immunologic system. Collectively, these adverse effects fall under the heading of *immunotoxicology* and are becoming increasingly important as our environment becomes more polluted and complex. Thus, the physician must be constantly aware of the many types and varied routes of exposure to immunogens and allergens and toxins that compose our complex environment, not only to prevent and treat certain diseases (e.g., vaccines), but also to be able to recognize the possibility of immunologically mediated diseases that may take unexpected forms or masquerade as other entities.

TARGET CELLS

The introduction of an environmental agent into a host may have an adverse effect

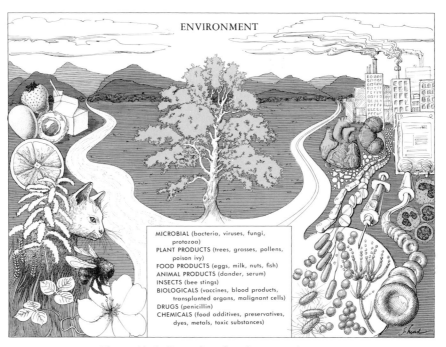

Figure 11–1. Examples of environmental agents.

on a target cell (Fig. 11–2, Table 11–1). There are a variety of target cells upon which an environmental agent may impact. They vary according to their type and location as well as the portal of entry of the foreign substance. It is important to emphasize that the target cells may be normal host cells that become the adventitious targets of injury by the environmental agents or immunologic processes, or they may represent altered host cells that have become modified through the interaction with the environmental substance (e.g., chemical), by infection (e.g., virus), or by malignant transformation (e.g., tumor cells); alternatively, the target cell may be a foreign cell introduced by transplantation. The target cell may thus sustain direct injury from the environmental agent or indirect injury through immunologic processes. The net effect leads to disruption of cell function or cell death. Some of the more common target cells are shown in Table 11–1. Included are cells of the skin, gastrointestinal tract, respiratory tract, and circulatory system. For example, disruption of epidermal cells following contact with an environmental agent, e.g., poison ivy, could lead to dermatitis; destruction of mucosal cells of the gastrointestinal tract secondary to ingestion of an environmental agent, e.g., an offending food substance, may result in gastrointestinal bleeding. If the target cells are smooth mus-

cle and glandular cells of the respiratory tract, the impact of the environmental agent may lead to increased contractility with bronchospasm and increased secretion of mucus characteristic of bronchial asthma. Alternatively, endothelial target cells of blood vessels

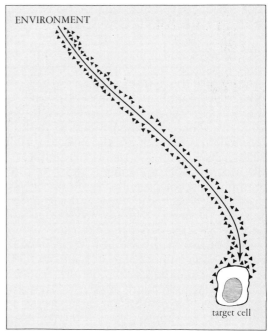

Figure 11–2. Effects of environmental agents on target cells.

Table 11–1. Effects of the Environment on Target Cells

Location of Target Cell	Example of Effect	Result
Skin	Disruption of epidermal cells	Dermatitis
Gastrointestinal tract		
Mucosal cell	Destruction	Gastrointestinal bleeding
Smooth muscle	Increased contractility	Diarrhea, vomiting
Glandular cell	Increased secretion	Increased mucus production
Respiratory tract		
Smooth muscle	Increased contraction	Bronchospasm
Glandular cell	Increased secretion	Increased mucus production
Circulatory system		
Endothelial cell	Increased intercellular pore size	Edema
Formed elements	Destruction of erythrocytes	Anemia

might respond by showing an increase in intercellular pore size with resultant loss of fluids and the production of edema. The impact of the foreign substance on the formed elements of the blood, such as red cells, might lead to their destruction and the development of anemia.

During the course of evolution, a number of *nonspecific* and *specific* immunologic mechanisms have appeared within the vertebrates (Chapters 1 and 2). This collection of cellular elements, referred to as the lymphoreticular system, is distributed strategically throughout the body and lines the lymphatic and vascular channels. Its function may be considered the protection of the target cell from injury. *Phagocytosis* and the *inflammatory response* are the body's first line of defense and represent the most primitive of the nonspecific immune responses (Chapter 2).

THE PHAGOCYTIC CELLS

The phagocytic cells are those elements that are involved in the process of engulfment and uptake of particles from the external environment; subsequent digestion of these substances may lead to their elimination (Chapter 2). The phagocyte may be considered, then, as a barrier between the environment and the target cell, protecting the target cell from subsequent injury (Fig. 11–3, Table 11–2). In the human, phagocytosis is carried out primarily by mononuclear phagocytes (macrophages), neutrophils, and eosinophils (Chapter 2). These phagocytic cells, together with the effector mechanisms triggered by or involved in their mobilization, are shown in Table 11–2. There are a variety of chemotactic factors—generated from the complement system (Chapter 6) or derived from specific lymphocytes, e.g., the lymphokines

(Chapter 9) or from the phagocytic cells themselves—that can lead to the accumulation of phagocytic cells in an area of inflammation. The net effect of these processes is the mobilization of phagocytic cells into areas in which their action is required for the protection of target cells from injury. However, on occasion the phagocytic cells themselves may contribute to tissue injury by the release of intracellular products, e.g., lysosomal enzymes, as seen in the autoimmune diseases.

MEDIATOR CELLS

Certain cells of the body contain macromolecular and low molecular weight sub-

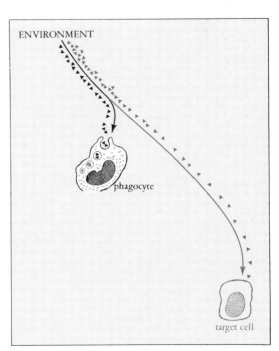

Figure 11–3. Phagocytic cells: mobilization factors and functions.

Table 11–2. Mobilization Factors and Functions of Phagocytic Cells

Phagocytic Cell	Agents Responsible for Mobilization of Cells	Cell Product or Function
Macrophages (monocytes)	Chemotactic factors, e.g., migration inhibitory factor (MIF), lymphokines	Processed immunogen, removal of environmental agent, prostaglandins
Neutrophils	Chemotactic factors (complement-associated and bacterial factors), lymphokines	Kallikreins (producing kinins), basic peptides, prostaglandins
Eosinophils	Identical with neutrophils, specific chemotactic factors, lymphokines	Ingestion of immune complexes, antagonize effects of mediators, e.g., leukotrienes (formerly SRS-A)

stances with biologic properties that can amplify the effects of the phagocytic cells or that may have a direct effect on the target cells. These cells are referred to as mediator cells. Following their interaction with the environmental agent, they perform their function by the release of chemical substances having a variety of biologic activities, e.g., the increase of vascular permeability or the enhancement of the inflammatory response (Fig. 11–4, Table 11–3). The mediator cells, like the target cells, represent a heterogeneous collection of morphologic types that includes mast cells, basophils, platelets, enterochromaffin cells, and neutrophils (Table 11–3). The best studied of these are the mast cells and basophils, which are important in certain immediate hypersensitivity diseases of man.

The term "mediators" encompasses a group of substances that are formed and released by mediator cells in response to an environmental agent (Fig. 11–5, Table 11–4). The best studied of these substances include histamine, serotonin, kinins, and, recently, the products of metabolism of arachidonic acid (eicosanoid system), including prostaglandins, thromboxanes, and leukotrienes, slow reactive substance of anaphylaxis (SRS-A) (which has now been identified as leukotrienes C_4, D_4, and E_4), eosinophilic chemotactic factors of anaphylaxis (ECF-A), and platelet-activating factor (PAF). Other macromolecular substances are derived from the phagocytic cells, e.g., lysosomal enzymes. Although most of these substances are synthesized in the mediator cells, some mediators, e.g., the complement and coagulation components, are synthesized in other cells and are found predominantly as serum components (Chapter 6).

Once they are released or generated, the

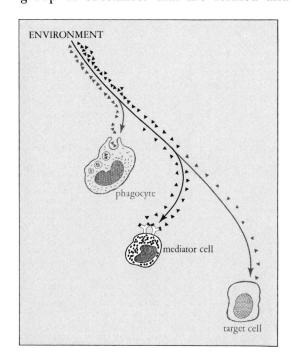

Figure 11–4. Mediator cells: products (mediators) and functions.

Table 11–3. Products and Functions of Mediator Cells

Mediator Cell	Product	Action
Mast cells	Histamine, leukotrienes C_4, D_4, E_4 (formerly SRS-A), prostaglandins, ECF-A	Increased vascular permeability, bronchoconstriction, eosinophilotaxis
Basophils, platelets	Vasoactive amines (histamine, serotonin)	Increased vascular permeability, smooth muscle constriction
Enterochromaffin cells	Serotonin	Vasodilation
Neutrophils	SRS, ECF	Contractility of smooth muscle, eosinophilotaxis

mediators have a twofold effect on the nonspecific immunologic responses and act with (1) the target cell, e.g., allergy, or (2) the phagocytic cells, e.g., promotion of chemotaxis (Fig. 11–5, Table 11–4).

CELLS OF THE SPECIFIC IMMUNOLOGIC SYSTEM: THE SPECIFIC ANTIGEN-RECOGNITION CELLS

These cells, in contrast to those of the nonspecific immunologic system, interact with the environmental agent in a highly specific way. The responses display *specificity*, *memory*, and *heterogeneity* and are basically carried out by two universes of lymphocytes: (1) the bone marrow or bursal-dependent B-lymphocytes, which provide humoral immunity; and (2) the thymus-dependent or T-lymphocytes, which participate in cell-mediated immunity (Chapter 2).

The B-lymphocytes are those cells that ultimately respond to the environmental agent, through either immunization or infection (Fig. 11–6). The exquisite specificity for the recognition of antigen by the B-cell is a function of immunoglobulin on the surface of these cells. As a consequence of the binding of antigen with the surface receptor, the cell differentiates into clones of antibody-secreting plasma cells, each of which secretes a single class of immunoglobulin that is specific for the antigen. There are five classes (isotypes) of immunoglobulins, IgG, IgM, IgA, IgD, and IgE, each differing in physical, chemical, and biologic properties (Chapter 5). The primary effect of antibody is its direct binding with the environmental agent (Fig. 11–6). In addition, antibody may interact with the phagocytic cells, the mediator cells, or the target cells. The effect of antibody on phagocytic cells is shown in Figure 11–7. Three types of interactions are seen: (1) the direct binding of antibody to the surface of the phagocytic cells (cytophilic antibody), (2) the uptake of antigen-antibody (Ag-Ab) complexes through the Fc receptor, and (3) the

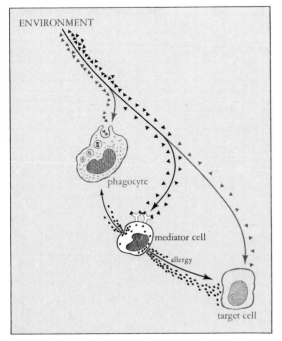

Figure 11–5. Mediator products and their effects on target cells (e.g., allergy) or phagocytic cells.

Table 11–4. Mediators Released in Response to Environmental Agents

Low molecular weight mediators (< 1000)
  Histamine
  Serotonin
  Kinins
  Slow reactive substance of anaphylaxis (SRS-A) (now leukotrienes C_4, D_4, E_4)
  Prostaglandins
  Eosinophilic chemotactic factors of anaphylaxis (ECF-A)
  Platelet-activating factor (PAF)
Macromolecular mediators (> 1000)
  Lysosomal enzymes
  Cationic proteins of polymorphonuclear leukocytes
  Complement and coagulation components

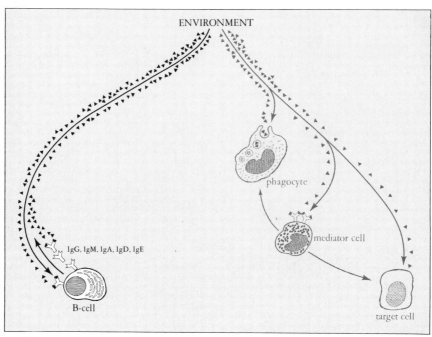

Figure 11–6. Reaction of B-lymphocyte to environmental agent through its surface receptor, with resultant antibody production.

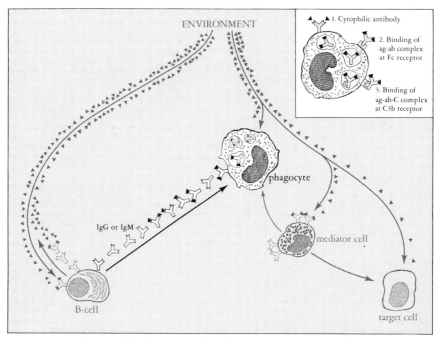

Figure 11–7. Responses of antibody with phagocytic cells.

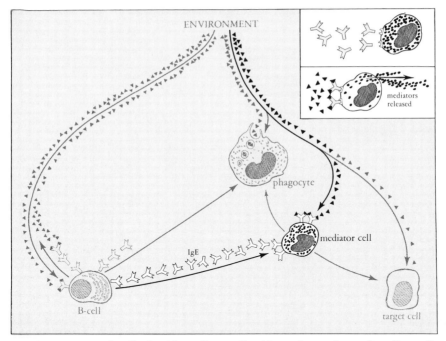

Figure 11–8. Responses of antibody with mediator cells with resultant release of mediators (insert).

uptake of antigen-antibody-complement (Ag-Ab-C) complexes through the C3b receptor (Fig. 11–7 inset). The coating of certain encapsulated bacterial organisms by immunoglobulins (IgG, IgM) or by certain complement components (e.g., C3b) facilitates their uptake by phaogcytic cells; collectively these substances are referred to as opsonins. The effect of antibody on mediator cells is shown in Figure 11–8. Certain classes of gamma globulin, e.g., IgE, can attach to the mediator cells by virtue of their Fc fragments. Following the interaction of at least two of these membrane-bound molecules with antigen, the release of mediators occurs (Fig. 11–8 inset). Occasionally, under abnormal circum-

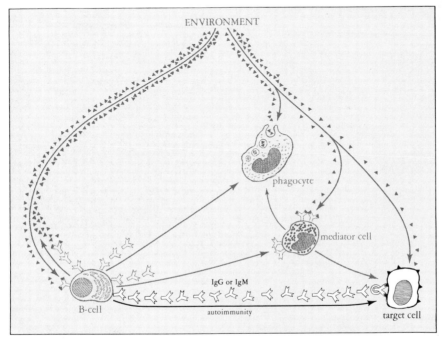

Figure 11–9. Effects of antibody on target cells with resultant autoimmunity.

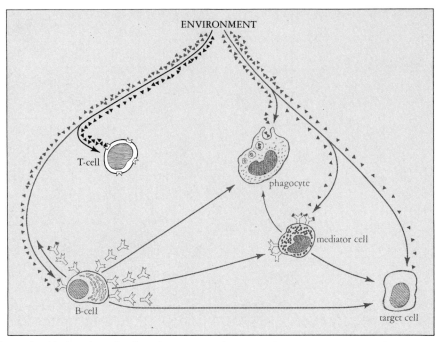

Figure 11–10. Reaction of T-lymphocyte to environmental agent through its surface receptor.

stances, antibody may be directed against the target cells (Fig. 11–9). This is a totally anomalous situation but is seen in some of the immunologically mediated diseases of man—the autoimmune diseases.

The T-lymphocytes are those cells responsible for cell-mediated immunity (Chapter 9).

These cells respond to the environmental agent through surface receptors (Fig. 11–10). Although not intact immunoglobulin, these receptors are analogous to the antigen-binding receptors (the V-region determinants) on the B-cells (Chapters 5 and 7).

Following the interaction of the environ-

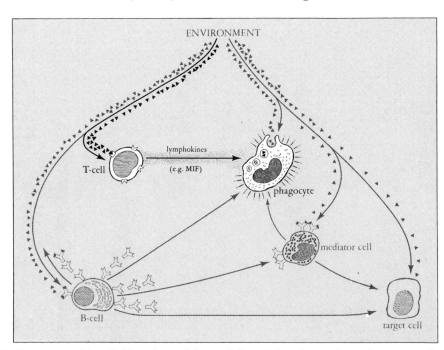

Figure 11–11. Responses of lymphokines (e.g., elaborated from T-lymphocytes) on phagocytic cells (e.g., macrophages).

mental agent with the T-cell, a series of morphologic, biologic, and biochemical events occur, in which the cell may function either directly or through the elaboration of certain products, the lymphokines (Chapter 9). The best studied of the lymphokines is migration inhibitory factor (MIF), which not only inhibits the migration of macrophages but also can activate the cell metabolically (Fig. 11–11). In addition, the T-lymphocyte can participate in the recognition of antigen on the surface of foreign target cells in any of three ways (Fig. 11–12). The cell may participate in direct lymphocyte-dependent cytotoxicity; or the elaboration of cytotoxin may lead to target-cell destruction; or certain subsets of lymphocytes, the killer or K cells, may lead to target-cell destruction through antibody-dependent cytotoxicity (ADCC) reactions (Fig. 11–12 inset).

An additional pathway of target cell destruction is mediated by a group of cells (natural killer or NK cells), which does not require prior sensitization by antigen, whose lineage is of uncertain origin (monocytic or T-cell), but which can directly destroy target cells. These cells appear to be enhanced by the action of interferon(s) and are importantly involved in transplant and tumor rejection.

The T-lymphocytes may also interact with the B-cells in two ways: (1) A subset of T-cells (the helper [T4] cells) can interact with B-cells to facilitate the production of antibody, and (2) another subset of T-cells (the suppressor/cytotoxic [T5/T8] cells) can inhibit the production of antibody by B-cells (Fig. 11–13).

The macrophage has been shown to be an essential cell that interacts with the T- and B-lymphocytes and is necessary for the induction of T-cell responses as well as T cell–dependent B-cell responses to antigen. Moreover, these cellular interactions of macrophages, T-cells, and B-cells appear to be genetically restricted by products (Class I and Class II molecules) of the major histocompatibility complex (MHC) locus, which are located on the surface of these cells (Figure 11–14) (Chapter 3). A number of cell prod-

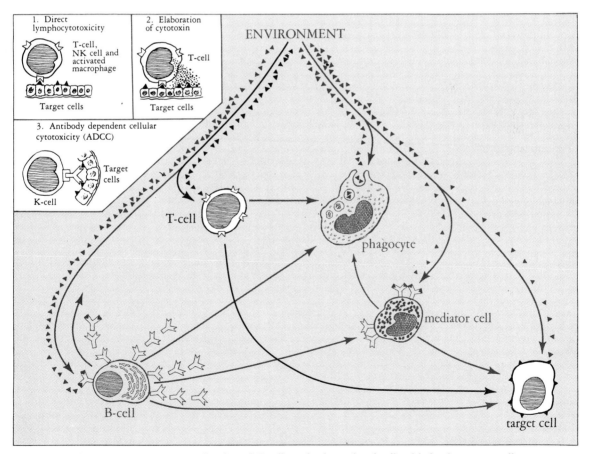

Figure 11–12. Responses of activated T-cells and other related cells with foreign target cells.

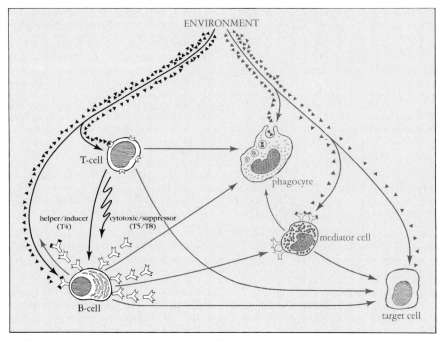

Figure 11–13. Helper and suppressor effects of T-lymphocytes on B-lymphocytes.

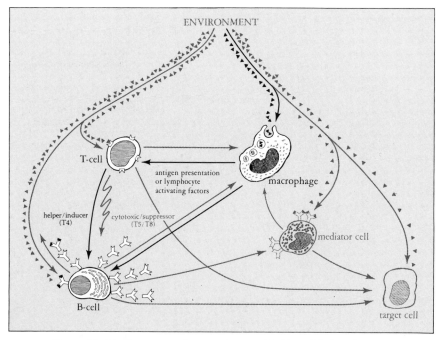

Figure 11–14. Responses of macrophages with T- and B-lymphocytes.

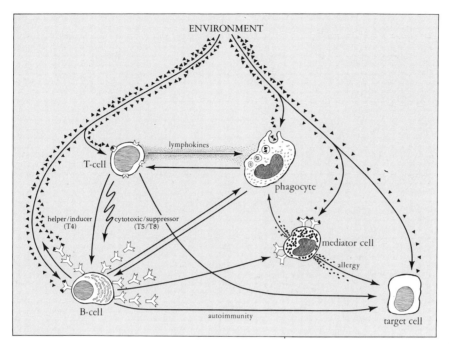

Figure 11–15. Total array of immunologic responses to the environment.

ucts (e.g., monokines and lymphokines), produced respectively by both macrophages (e.g., interleukin-1) and lymphocytes (e.g., interleukin-2), play an important role in the intercellular communication (Chapters 7 and 9).

Thus, the immunologic system may be viewed as a multicellular system involving the interaction of foreign substances with a wide variety of cell types (Fig. 11–15). The immunologic responses concerned with the recognition and disposal of foreignness are termed immunity when they lead to a beneficial response; when the interaction of the immunologic components and the environmental agent leads to injury of target cells, the responses are referred to as hypersensitivity or allergy; when the target cells of the host are injured directly by immunologic

mechanisms, these responses are referred to as autoimmunity. Occasionally, when the immunologic surveillance of a foreign target cell, e.g., tumor cell, is evaded, the manifestations of malignant disease may be manifested. The total array of these responses is shown in Figure 11–15.

Suggestions for Further Reading

Bellanti, J. A., Balter, N. J., and Gray, I.: A unifying model for immunotoxicology: A summation presentation. *In* Dean, J. H., and Podarthsingh, M. (eds.): Biologic Relevance of Immune Suppression as Induced by Genetic, Therapeutic and Environmental Factors. New York, Van Nostrand Reinhold Company, 1981.

Fauci, A. S., et al.: Activation and regulation of human immune responses: implications in normal and disease states. Ann. Intern. Med., *99*:61, 1983.

Index

Note: Page numbers in *italic* type indicate illustrations; page numbers followed by (t) refer to tables.